OTC
DRUGS

AN OVER-THE-COUNTER DRUG RESOURCE
FOR HEALTH PROFESSIONALS

REFERENCE BOOK
DO NOT REMOVE FROM
LIBRARY

Middlesex County College
Library, Edison NJ 08818

MOSBY'S OTC DRUGS

AN OVER-THE-COUNTER DRUG RESOURCE FOR HEALTH PROFESSIONALS

Richard P. Donjon, RPh
Director of Pharmacy Services,
St. Mary's–Good Samaritan, Inc.
Mount Vernon, Illinois,
Centralia, Illinois

Bryon J. Goeckner, PharmD
Formerly Clinical Manager of Pharmacy Services,
BJC North Region,
BJC Health Systems,
St. Louis, Missouri

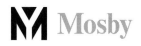

St. Louis   Baltimore   Boston   Carlsbad   Chicago   Minneapolis   New York   Philadelphia   Portland
London   Milan   Sydney   Tokyo   Toronto

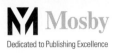

Mosby
Dedicated to Publishing Excellence

A Times Mirror
Company

Vice President and Publisher: Nancy L. Coon
Editor-in-Chief: N. Darlene Como
Senior Developmental Editor: Laurie Sparks
Project Manager: Carol Sullivan Weis
Production Editor: Karen M. Rehwinkel
Designer: Jen Marmarinos
Manufacturing Supervisor: Karen Boehme
Cover Art: Jill Christman

A NOTE TO THE READER

The authors and publisher have made every attempt to check
dosages and other content for accuracy. Because the science of
pharmacology is continually advancing, our knowledge base
continues to expand. Therefore we recommend that the reader
always check product information for changes in dosage or
administration before recommending or administering any
medication. This is particularly important with new or
infrequently used drugs.

Copyright © 1999 by Mosby, Inc.

All rights reserved. No part of this publication may be reproduced,
stored in a retrieval system, or transmitted, in any form or by any means,
electronic, mechanical, photocopying, recording, or otherwise, without
written permission of the publisher.

Permission to photocopy or reproduce solely for internal or personal use is
permitted for libraries or other users registered with the Copyright Clearance
Center, provided that the base fee of $4.00 per chapter plus $.10 per page is paid
directly to the Copyright Clearance Center, 222 Rosewood Drive, Danvers, MA,
01923. This consent does not extend to other kinds of copying, such as
copying for general distribution, for advertising or promotional purposes,
for creating new collected works, or for resale.

Composition by Graphic World, Inc.
Printing/binding by R. R. Donnelley & Sons Company

Mosby, Inc.
11830 Westline Industrial Drive
St. Louis, Missouri 63146

Library of Congress Cataloging-in-Publication Data

Mosby's OTC drugs : an over-the-counter drug resource for health professionals /
|edited by|
    Richard P. Donjon, Bryon J. Goeckner.
        p.   cm.
    Includes bibliographical references and index.
    ISBN 0-8151-8395-X
    1. Drugs, Nonprescription—Handbooks, manuals, etc.   I. Donjon,
Richard P.   II. Goeckner, Bryon J.
    |DNLM: 1. Drugs, Non-Prescription handbooks.   QV   735M894   1999|
RM671.A1M67   1999
615′.1—dc21
DNLM/DLC
for Library of Congress   98-39429
                                                                                  CIP

98   99   00   01   02   /   9   8   7   6   5   4   3   2   1

Contributors

Tricia Berry, PharmD
Assistant Professor of Pharmacy Practice,
St. Louis College of Pharmacy,
St. Louis, Missouri

Stefanie M. Davis, PharmD
Clinical Services Manager,
Managed Pharmacy Benefits,
St. Louis, Missouri

M. Patricia Fuhrman, RD, CNSD
Clinical Director, Nutrition Support Service,
St. Louis University Hospital,
St. Louis, Missouri

JaCinda Jones, PharmD
Manager, Pharmaceutical Care and Disease Management,
Medicine Shoppe International, Inc.,
St. Louis, Missouri

Melissa Matlock, PharmD
Clinical Pharmacy Coordinator,
St. Louis Children's Hospital,
St. Louis, Missouri

James E. Preston Jr., PharmD, BCPS
Clinical Pharmacist,
BJC Health Systems,
St. Louis, Missouri

Aaron Roberts, PharmD
Staff Pharmacist,
Walgreens, Inc.,
St. Louis, Missouri

Scot E. Walker, PharmD, BCPS
Director of Research,
Esse Health,
St. Louis, Missouri

Michael J. Willman, RPh
Pharmacist,
Gainesville, Florida

Consultants

Mindy K. Bingham, MSN, ARNP, C-S
Adult Nurse Practitioner,
Internists of North County,
St. Louis, Missouri

George DeMaagd, PharmD, BCPS
Assistant Professor of Pharmacy Practice;
Clinical Pharmacist, Michigan State University,
Kalamazoo Center for Medical Education;
Clinical Pharmacist, Bronson Methodist Hospital,
Kalamazoo, Michigan

Patricia A. Howard, PharmD, BCPS, FCCP
Clinical Associate Professor,
Department of Pharmacy Practice,
University of Kansas Medical Center,
Kansas City, Kansas

Joanne LaRocca, RN, MSN, FNP
Family Nurse Practitioner,
NE Iowa Family Practice Center,
Waterloo, Iowa

John Mitchell, PharmD
Editor,
Medical Education Systems, Inc.,
Canton, Michigan

Charlene Reeves, MSN, RN, CNS
Assistant Professor of Nursing,
Midwestern State University,
Wichita Falls, Texas

Roberta J. Secrest, PhD, PharmD, RPh
Scientist/Manager,
US Medical Research,
Hoechst Marion Roussel,
Kansas City, Missouri

Amy B. Sharron, MS, RN, CS, GNP
Geriatric Nurse Practitioner,
UMASS Community Physicians,
University Commons Nursing Care Center,
Worcester, Massachusetts

Preface

This book is not intended to be a compendium of all available information regarding nonprescription drugs and products. Rather, it is intended to be a convenient pocket guide. We recognize that excellent references exist but that their physical size limits their usefulness. The intent was to write a book that was portable and would fit into the pocket of a lab coat.

It is assumed that the user of this work will be a health care professional with at least a rudimentary knowledge of pharmacology, physiology, and pathology. As with any other reference, the guidelines and suggestions must be considered general in nature. Several reviewers suggested that cost information would be helpful to the user of this book. Although we agree that such information would be helpful, it would be virtually impossible to provide because prices vary widely among the different retailers of these products. We do recommend that generic or store-brand products be purchased when they are available. These products contain the same ingredients as the brand-name product but are less expensive. They are usually located next to the brand-name products on store shelves. It is hoped that the information contained in *Mosby's OTC Drugs: An Over-the-Counter Drug Resource for Health Professionals* will serve as a handy resource.

In the preparation of the manuscript, we frequently relied on several reference works. We wish to acknowledge this fact and to recommend the following references to persons seeking additional information:

Handbook of Nonprescription Drugs, ed 10, Washington, DC, 1993, American Pharmaceutical Association.

Drug Facts & Comparisons, St. Louis, Facts & Comparison, Inc.

Pediatric Dosage Handbook, ed 4, Hudson, Ohio, 1997, Lexi-Comp, Inc.

Geriatric Dosage Handbook, ed 3, Hudson, Ohio, 1997, Lexi-Comp, Inc.

Physician's Desk Reference for Nonprescription Drugs, ed 16, Montvale, NJ, 1995, Medical Economics Data Production Company.

Goodman & Gilman's The Pharmacological Basis of Therapeutics, ed 9, New York, 1996, McGraw-Hill.

The Effects of Drugs on the Fetus and Nursing Infant, Baltimore, 1996, The Johns Hopkins University Press.

We also wish to acknowledge the assistance of Michael Jobe and Heather Middendorf, pharmacy students at St. Louis College of Pharmacy, for their assistance in preparing the Product Information tables.

Richard P. Donjon
Bryon J. Goeckner

Guide to Using
Mosby's OTC Drugs

Information about nonprescription drugs is provided in a uniform format to make *Mosby's OTC Drugs* an easy-to-use reference. Each section is divided into the following topics:

- Pharmacology
- Side Effects
- Drug Interactions
- Lifespan Considerations
    Geriatric
    Pediatric
    Pregnancy
    Nursing Mothers
- Patient Education
- Product Selection
- Suggested Readings

Pharmacology

The emphasis of this section is the basic pharmacology and major mechanisms of action for the drugs being discussed. It is not intended to be an exhaustive review of the topic. Readers wishing in-depth pharmacologic information are referred to the appropriate textbooks, such as *Goodman & Gilman's The Pharmacological Basis of Therapeutics*.

Side Effects

An effort has been made to emphasize clinically significant side effects. We have attempted to differentiate theoretical and/or idiosyncratic side effects from those likely to be seen in clinical practice. When considering the possibility of side effects, one must remember that reported side effects such as nausea, vomiting, diarrhea, and headache frequently occur in patients receiving placebo in clinical trials. It is often difficult to separate true side effects from the "placebo effect."

Drug Interactions

There are hundreds of theoretical drug–drug interactions but relatively few drug interactions with true clinical significance. It is important to remember that the possibility of drug interactions does not necessarily preclude use of the interacting drugs. Rather, health professionals must be able to manage drug interactions and to take steps to minimize their occurrence. Additionally, most of what is known about drug interactions involves the combination of only two drugs at a time. As the number of drugs taken concurrently increases, the possibility of drug interactions increases. Given the number of possible permutations, it is virtually impossible to predict how large numbers of drugs might interact with each other to produce unwanted effects. For this reason, drugs should be prescribed and recommended only when necessary and only after obtaining a medication history.

Lifespan Considerations

Geriatric

Older patients tend to take more medications than younger patients. Much of the increase in usage is related to the increased prevalence of chronic disease in the elderly. Older patients tend to be more sensitive to the effects and side effects of drugs. Normal, age-related changes in physiologic function cause this increased drug sensitivity. Some of these changes in physiology include:

- **Age-related decline in renal function:** On average, glomerular filtration rate (GFR) decreases by approximately 50% between the ages of 20 and 70 years. Drugs eliminated by renal excretion can accumulate when renal function decreases.
- **Age-related changes in hepatic function:** Hepatic blood flow, hepatic size, and functional capacity of hepatic drug-metabolizing enzymes decrease with age. Drugs metabolized by the liver can accumulate when hepatic metabolism becomes less efficient.

The general rule of "go low and go slow" should be followed when recommending drug products to older patients. Therapy should be initiated with the lowest dose possible and titrated upward until the desired effect is achieved or side effects become evident. Polypharmacy must be avoided whenever possible to minimize the possibility of drug–drug interactions.

Pediatric

Many drugs are not approved for use in children, not because they are unsafe but rather because they have not been adequately studied in the pediatric population. Much of what we know about pediatric drug dosing is based on the experience of pediatricians treating sick children. The available pediatric dosing guides are a compilation of the published and unpublished work of these physicians.

Although diminished organ function is the major reason for altered drug effects in the elderly, immaturity of organ systems is a major reason for altered drug effects in neonates and young children. Some of the physiologic factors involved include the following:

- **Altered gastrointestinal function:** Neonates have very low gastric-acid secretion at birth and delayed gastric emptying. Low gastric pH can interfere with the absorption of acidic drugs, and delayed gastric emptying can lead to increased absorption of drugs that are absorbed in the stomach. Drugs absorbed in the intestine may have decreased or delayed absorption.
- **Altered drug distribution:** Neonates have low concentrations of plasma proteins, resulting in a larger unbound and active fraction of drug. This can lead to increased drug effects and toxicity.
- **Altered drug metabolism:** Drug-metabolizing hepatic enzyme systems mature at different rates. This can lead to higher plasma concentrations of some drugs and increased risk of toxicity.
- **Immature renal function:** Neonates have approximately 30% of the glomerular filtration rate and renal tubular secretion capacity of adults. At approximately 5 weeks of age, neonates can be given standard pediatric doses of drugs. At 9 to 12 months of age, an infant's renal capacity is equal to that of an adult.

Another reason that some drugs are not approved for use in children is the fact that neonates and young children may be unable to verbalize how they feel. An evaluation by an experienced health care professional familiar with the physical signs and symptoms of illness in children may be necessary to adequately diagnose and monitor treatment of children.

Pregnancy

With rare exceptions, any drug that exerts a systemic effect in the mother will cross the placenta and reach the embryo or fetus. If a drug is administered during pregnancy, the advantages of therapy must clearly outweigh the risks. The pregnancy risk of most drugs is unknown because drugs are not purposely tested in pregnant women. Available information is based on epidemiologic studies of patients who must receive certain drugs during pregnancy. Pregnancy-risk information is provided as a guide; however, no drug should be prescribed or recommended to a pregnant patient without consulting with the patient's obstetrician.

Nursing Mothers

Many drugs producing systemic effects in the mother find their way into the breast milk. The significance of maternal drug use depends on the degree to which the drug is distributed into the breast milk. When available, the recommendation of the World Health Organization (WHO) or the American Academy of Pediatrics is relayed in this section.

Patient Education

Key educational points important to successful therapy are presented in this section. Although it is not possible to anticipate all of the possible educational needs of the patient, this section serves as a reminder for the health care professional.

Product Selection

In this section, additional facts important to the decision-making process are provided. Specific recommendations are not routinely made because therapy must be individualized based on patient-specific factors.

Product Information Tables

The product information tables list the most commonly available products. The reader is cautioned that products are sometimes renamed, reformulated, or discontinued.

Suggested Readings

When appropriate, additional references are provided for those wishing additional information.

SUGGESTED READINGS

Ahronheim J: Practical pharmacology for older patients: avoiding adverse drug effects, Mt Sinai J Med 60(6):497-501, 1993.

Greenblatt DG, Sellers EM, Shader RI: Drug disposition in the elderly, New Engl J Med 306:1081-1088, 1982.

Radde IC: *Pediatric pharmacology and therapeutics*, St. Louis, 1993, Mosby.

Antepartum management of normal pregnancy. In Cunningham FG et al, editors: *Williams Obstetrics*, ed 20, Stamford, Conn, 1997, Appleton & Lange.

Contents

MOSBY'S
OTC
DRUGS

AN OVER-THE-COUNTER DRUG RESOURCE
FOR HEALTH PROFESSIONALS

PART I

Introduction

Approximately 30% of all drug expenditures in the United States are for over-the-counter (OTC) drug products. In 1995, OTC medications generated over $20 billion in sales (Snyder, 1997). It is estimated that by the year 2000, OTC sales could exceed $34 billion. Important factors fueling the growth of OTC sales include the following:

- The self-care movement
- Movement of prescription products to nonprescription status

SELF-CARE MOVEMENT

Over the past several decades, health care consumers have taken a strong interest in self-care. Approximately 70% of all consumers medicate themselves regularly (Box 1-1 lists common conditions that may benefit from self-medication). Some of the factors stimulating the self-care movement include the following:

- **Aging of the population.** Older patients are frequent users of OTC medications. This is due largely to the fact that chronic health problems tend to increase with age. Consumers believe OTC drugs can treat many of these chronic conditions.
- **Rising educational levels of the general population.** As the educational level of the population has risen, consumers have become more willing to accept greater responsibility for their own health and to attempt self-treatment.
- **Greater dissemination of health information.** In the past, information about medications and treatment of health conditions was available only to health professionals. However, in recent years there has been an explosion in the amount and quality of information available directly to the public. The Internet has made tremendous resources available to anyone with a computer and modem.
- **Lack of available medical services to some patients.** Although physicians may not be readily available to all consumers, OTC drugs are widely available. Nonprescription products can be purchased

---

Box 1-1   Common Conditions Possibly Benefited By Self-Medication

Aches and pains	Head lice
Acne	Headache
Allergic rhinitis	Heartburn
Anemia	Hemorrhoids
Athlete's foot	Insect bites/stings
Boils	Insomnia
Burns	Jock itch
Calluses	Motion sickness
Canker sores	Nasal congestion
Colds	Nausea/vomiting
Constipation	Pharyngitis
Contact dermatitis	Pinworm
Corns	Premenstrual syndrome
Cough	Prickly heat
Cuts (minor)	Scrapes
Dandruff	Sprains
Dental care	Strains
Diaper rash	Sunburn
Dry skin	Vaginal yeast infection
Dysmenorrhea	Vitamin/mineral deficiency
Feminine hygiene	Warts
Fever	Xerostomia
Flatulence	

---

easily at a wide variety of outlets, including grocery stores, mass merchandisers, discount stores, and pharmacies.

- **Growing dissatisfaction with conventional medicine and increased interest in "natural medicine."** The growth of managed-care medicine has resulted in a growing distrust of the traditional medical system. Manufacturers of natural products have positioned their products as alternatives to traditional medicine. In addition, best-selling books extoll the virtues of natural products and claim that the established medical system refuses to acknowledge the value of natural products. Fostering this conspiracy theory furthers the cause of those promoting natural products.
- **General increase in consumerism.** The modern consumer movement dates from the early 1960s when President John F. Kennedy announced a Consumer Bill of Rights. Since then, consumers have become increasingly vocal. They no longer passively wait for businesses to

Box 1-2 Recent Prescription to OTC Switches	
Product	**Indication**
Actron (ketoprofen)	Analgesic
Axid AR (nizatidine)	Acid reducer
Children's Advil (ibuprofen)	Antipyretic
Children's Motrin (ibuprofen)	Antipyretic
Femstat One (butoconazole)	Vaginal yeast infection
Monistat 3 (miconazole)	Vaginal yeast infection
Nasalcrom (cromolyn)	Allergy prevention and treatment
Nicoderm CQ (nicotine transdermal)	Smoking cessation
Nicorette (nicotine polacrilex)	Smoking cessation
Nicotrol (nicotine transdermal)	Smoking cessation
Orudis KT (ketoprofen)	Analgesic
Pepcid AC (famotidine)	Acid reducer
Rogaine (minoxidil)	Hair grower
Tagamet HB (cimetidine)	Acid reducer
Vagistat-1 (tioconazole)	Vaginal yeast infection
Zantac 75 (ranitidine)	Acid reducer

recognize their needs and wants. Instead, consumers make their demands known.

SWITCHING OF POPULAR PRESCRIPTION MEDICATIONS TO NONPRESCRIPTION STATUS

Since 1972, 51 active ingredients have been transferred from prescription status to OTC status by the United States Food and Drug Administration (FDA). Boxes 1-2 and 1-3 list recent switches from prescription to OTC drugs and future candidates for switching, respectively. Given the pharmaceutical industry's recent successes with transferring medications from prescription to OTC status, the "switch phenomenon" is expected to accelerate. Incentives for manufacturers to transfer their products from prescription to OTC status include the following:

- High profit margins for OTC products
- Tremendous success of recent prescription to OTC switches
- Access to a larger group of prospective purchasers
- Desire of consumers to self-medicate
- Aging of the population

Box 1-3	Future Candidates for Prescription to OTC Switch
Brand name	**Indication**
Carafate	Ulcers
Claritin	Allergic rhinitis
Clinoril	Analgesic
Colestid	Cholesterol reduction
Diflucan	Vaginal yeast infection
Dolobid	Analgesic
Feldene	Analgesic
Flexeril	Muscle relaxant
Habitrol	Smoking cessation
Hismanal	Allergic rhinitis
Intal	Asthma prevention
Mycostatin	Antifungal
Nizoral A-D shampoo	Dandruff
ProStep	Smoking cessation
Proventil	Asthma (bronchospasm)
Soma Compound	Muscle relaxant
Spectazole	Antifungal
Theo-Dur	Asthma
Ventolin	Asthma (bronchospasm)
Zithromax	Infections
Zovirax	Herpes

- Potential to extend the "patent life" of products, prohibiting generic competition

HOW IS OTC STATUS DETERMINED?

Determinants for changing a medication from prescription to OTC status include the following:

- **Safety.** An OTC drug is considered to be safe if it has a low incidence of adverse reactions or significant side effects under adequate directions for use, as well as low potential for harm, which may result from abuse under conditions of widespread availability. In other words, can the average consumer take the product safely without physician supervision?

- **Effectiveness.** An OTC drug is effective if there is a reasonable expectation that when used under adequate directions for use, with warnings against unsafe use, it provides clinically significant relief of the type claimed for a significant portion of the target population. In other words, will most patients experience improvement in symptoms?

- **Manufacturer's marketing strategy.** Given the high cost of drug development, testing, and marketing, most manufacturers apply for prescription status or new product. Each year, new prescription drugs are approved that could be sold without a prescription if the manufacturer chose to pursue it. Instead, the drug companies opt for the lucrative prescription market and attempt to switch to OTC status after the patent runs out and generics become available, or when prescription sales decline to a certain point.

LABELING OF OTC PRODUCTS

Whereas prescription drug labels carry minimal information for the patient, the FDA requires that OTC labels be much more detailed to enable consumers to properly use the products without the advice of a health professional. Figure 1-1 shows a sample label on an OTC product.

ABUSE POTENTIAL OF OTC DRUGS

OTC drugs do not cause physical addiction like some prescription drugs; however, OTC drugs are used incorrectly and inappropriately. Consumers often assume that because OTC drugs are sold without a prescription, they are free from side effects. Some may exceed the labeled dosage, assuming that the larger dose will increase efficacy. In most cases, the additional benefit is offset by the increased likelihood of side effects. Table 1-1 lists common examples of side effects caused by OTC drug abuse.

USE OF OTC DRUGS BY SPECIAL POPULATIONS

Pediatric Patients

Many OTC drug products are not recommended for children. It is not that they are unsafe, but rather that they have not been tested in children. Given the prohibitive cost for drug studies, it is unlikely that such testing will ever be completed for many OTC products. When children's dosing is given, it is usually the result of experience gained when the product was sold by prescription.

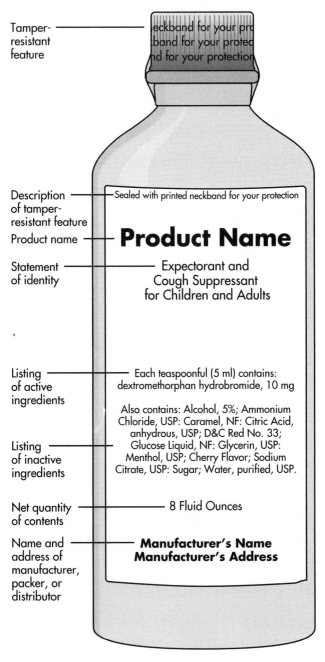

FRONT

Fig. 1-1 Required labeling information on OTC drug products.
Continued

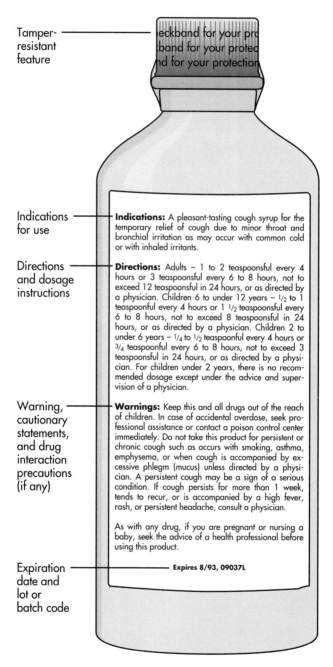

Tamper-resistant feature

eckband for your pro
band for your protec
nd for your protection

Indications for use

Indications: A pleasant-tasting cough syrup for the temporary relief of cough due to minor throat and bronchial irritation as may occur with common cold or with inhaled irritants.

Directions and dosage instructions

Directions: Adults – 1 to 2 teaspoonsful every 4 hours or 3 teaspoonsful every 6 to 8 hours, not to exceed 12 teaspoonsful in 24 hours, or as directed by a physician. Children 6 to under 12 years – $1/2$ to 1 teaspoonful every 4 hours or 1 $1/2$ teaspoonsful every 6 to 8 hours, not to exceed 8 teaspoonsful in 24 hours, or as directed by a physician. Children 2 to under 6 years – $1/4$ to $1/2$ teaspoonful every 4 hours or $3/4$ teaspoonful every 6 to 8 hours, not to exceed 3 teaspoonsful in 24 hours, or as directed by a physician. For children under 2 years, there is no recommended dosage except under the advice and supervision of a physician.

Warning, cautionary statements, and drug interaction precautions (if any)

Warnings: Keep this and all drugs out of the reach of children. In case of accidental overdose, seek professional assistance or contact a poison control center immediately. Do not take this product for persistent or chronic cough such as occurs with smoking, asthma, emphysema, or when cough is accompanied by excessive phlegm (mucus) unless directed by a physician. A persistent cough may be a sign of a serious condition. If cough persists for more than 1 week, tends to recur, or is accompanied by a high fever, rash, or persistent headache, consult a physician.

As with any drug, if you are pregnant or nursing a baby, seek the advice of a health professional before using this product.

Expiration date and lot or batch code

Expires 8/93, 09037L

BACK

Fig. 1-1, cont'd For legend see opposite page.

Table I-I
Possible Effects of OTC Drug Abuse

OTC drug	Intended effect	Possible side effects with large doses
Oral decongestants	Relieve nasal/sinus congestion	Hypertension, stroke?
Topical decongestants	Relieve nasal congestion	Rebound nasal congestion
Antihistamines	Relief of allergy symptoms, rhinorrhea	Excessive drowsiness, dry mouth, urinary retention
Stimulant laxatives	Relief of constipation	Cramping, abdominal discomfort
Analgesics	Pain relief	Abdominal discomfort, GI upset, gastritis, ulcers

Geriatric Patients

Geriatric patients present a challenge in recommending and dosing OTC drugs. There are a number of reasons for this including the following:

- Older patients are more likely to have comorbid conditions that increase the possibility of drug–disease state interactions (e.g., urinary retention or constipation caused by drugs with anticholinergic effects)
- Older patients generally take more drugs (both prescription and OTC), resulting in increased probability of significant drug–drug interactions
- Age-related declines in kidney and liver function

Diabetic Patients

Concerns relative to use of OTC drug products in diabetic patients include the following:

- Sugar content of drugs; brittle diabetics or those with difficult-to-control blood sugar must be aware of the sugar content of OTC products
- Oral decongestant products (sympathomimetics) such as pseudoephedrine and phenylpropanolamine can raise blood sugar in susceptible individuals

- Topical products that are capable of causing skin irritation/breakdown; because diabetics may have peripheral neuropathy and diminished peripheral circulation, products capable of skin irritation must be used cautiously because the risk of infection is higher than in nondiabetic patients

REFERENCES

Snyder K: The state of the OTC marketplace, *Drug Topics* June 2, 1997.

SUGGESTED READING

Cetaruk EW, Aaron CK: Hazards of nonprescription medications, *Emerg Med Clin North Am* 12(2):483-510, 1994.

PART II
GASTROINTESTINAL SYSTEM

Constipation

Drugs used to treat constipation include laxatives of the following types: saline, stimulant, bulk, lubricant, surfactant (stool softener), and hyperosmotic.

SALINE LAXATIVES (ORAL AND RECTAL)

MAGNESIUM SULFATE
MAGNESIUM HYDROXIDE
MAGNESIUM CITRATE
SODIUM PHOSPHATE
SODIUM BIPHOSPHATE

Pharmacology

Saline laxatives act primarily by drawing water into the lumen of the small intestine. The increased fluid accumulation produces distension in the bowel. Distension promotes peristalsis and evacuation. The release of cholecystokinin from the intestinal mucosa may also enhance the laxative effect.

Side Effects

A serious but rare side effect that can occur as a result of an acute overdose or chronic misuse of a saline laxative is electrolyte imbalance characterized by confusion, irregular heartbeat, muscle cramps, and/or unusual tiredness or weakness. In patients with compromised renal function, magnesium accumulation may occur and result in dizziness or lightheadedness. Other less serious side effects of saline laxatives include cramping, diarrhea, gas formation, and increased thirst.

Drug Interactions

Any laxative can interact with potassium-sparing diuretics and potassium supplements. Chronic or excessive use of laxatives may reduce serum potassium levels by promoting excessive potassium loss from the intestinal tract. The following drugs interact with magnesium-containing laxatives:

- **Warfarin, digoxin, and phenothiazines.** Interaction of these drugs with magnesium-containing laxatives has not been well-studied; however, reduced effectiveness of the interacting drugs has been observed when used with magnesium-containing antacids. Coadministration of magnesium-containing saline laxatives and magnesium-containing antacids should be avoided until further studies are conducted.
- **Ciprofloxacin.** Chelation of ciprofloxacin results in lower serum and urine concentrations of the antibiotic.
- **Etidronate.** Concurrent use prevents absorption of etidronate. A 2-hour interval between administration of drugs is recommended.
- **Sodium polystyrene sulfonate.** Magnesium binds sodium polystyrene sulfonate, preventing neutralization of bicarbonate ions, leading to systemic alkalosis. Rectal administration of sodium polystyrene may lessen risk.
- **Tetracyclines.** Use of tetracyclines and magnesium-containing laxatives may result in formation of nonabsorbable complexes. A 2-hour interval between administration of drugs is recommended.

Lifespan Considerations

Geriatric

Water intoxication or dilutional hyponatremia characterized by weakness, excessive perspiration, shock, seizures, and/or coma can occur in elderly patients with the use of rectal solutions.

Pediatric

Non-drug treatment is preferred in young children because constipation is frequently related to lack of dietary fiber or insufficient water intake. Before initiating drug therapy, a history should be elicited from the parents. A physical examination should be completed by a practitioner experienced with young children. A diagnosis should always precede the use of laxatives in children under the age of 6 years to avoid the complication of existing conditions. Water intoxication or dilutional hyponatremia characterized by weakness, excessive perspiration, shock, seizures, and/or coma can occur in children with the use of rectal solutions. Children receiving sodium phosphates rectally may suffer seizures as a result of hypocalcemia if too large an amount of phosphate is absorbed.

Pregnancy
Sodium-containing preparations may promote sodium retention and edema.

Patient Education
- The patient should drink at least 6 to 8 full glasses (8 oz each) of liquids each day when using any laxative.
- The anus should be lubricated with petroleum jelly before insertion of enema applicator, which should be inserted carefully to prevent damage to rectal wall.
- The patient should drink a full glass (8 oz) or more of liquid with each dose to prevent dehydration.
- Flavor can be improved if the patient follows a dose with juice or other beverage.
- When saline laxatives are taken orally, results should occur within 30 minutes to 3 hours.
- Faster results may be experienced when laxatives are taken on empty stomach.

STIMULANT LAXATIVES (ORAL AND RECTAL)
CASCARA
SENNA
BISACODYL
CASANTHRANOL
CASTOR OIL

Pharmacology
Although the exact mechanism of action is unknown, stimulant laxatives are thought to stimulate intramural nerve plexi, thereby increasing peristalsis by a direct effect on intestinal smooth muscle tissue.

Side Effects
A serious but rare side effect that can occur as a result of an acute overdose or chronic misuse of a stimulant laxative is electrolyte imbal-

ance characterized by confusion, irregular heartbeat, muscle cramps, and/or unusual tiredness or weakness. Cascara and senna can cause a pink, red, violet, or brown discoloration of alkaline urine or a brown discoloration of acidic urine. Other more frequent side effects include belching, cramping, diarrhea, and nausea. Rectal irritation can result when the suppository dosage form is used.

Drug Interactions

Any laxative can interact with potassium-sparing diuretics and potassium supplements. Chronic or excessive use of laxatives may reduce serum potassium levels by promoting excessive potassium loss from the intestinal tract. Interactions between bisacodyl laxatives and antacids, cimetidine, famotidine, nizatidine, ranitidine, and milk can result in gastric or duodenal irritation if the two items are administered within 1 hour of each other. The irritation is caused by premature dissolution of the enteric coating of the bisacodyl tablet.

Lifespan Considerations
Geriatric

When stimulant laxatives are used repeatedly to evacuate the colon in elderly patients, weakness, incoordination, and orthostatic hypotension may be exacerbated because of significant electrolyte loss. Keep in mind that laxative dependence is most often seen in elderly patients. When a stimulant laxative is used too frequently, elderly patients may lose the ability to move their bowels effectively without it.

Pediatric

Children are often unable to precisely describe the symptoms they feel. Therefore proper diagnosis should always precede the use of laxatives in children under the age of 6 years. This will avoid the complication of existing conditions. Children under the age of 6 years may have difficulty swallowing enteric-coated bisacodyl tablets without chewing them first, which will result in gastric irritation.

Pregnancy

Castor oil is contraindicated in pregnancy because of the risk of pelvic engorgement, which may stimulate the uterus.

Nursing Mothers

Cascara is reportedly distributed into the breast milk in an amount large enough to produce loose stools in the nursing infant, but this finding is controversial.

Patient Education

- The patient should drink at least 6 to 8 full glasses (8 oz each) of liquids each day when using any laxative.
- The anus should be lubricated with petroleum jelly before insertion of enema applicator, which should be inserted carefully to prevent damage to rectal wall.
- A suppository can be moistened by placing either under a stream of water for 30 seconds or in a cup of water for at least 10 seconds before insertion.
- Laxatives can be taken on an empty stomach for faster results.
- Enteric-coated bisacodyl tablets should not be chewed or crushed.
- Enteric-coated bisacodyl tablets should not be taken with milk or antacids.
- Castor oil should not be taken late in the day because results occur in 2 to 6 hours.
- The taste of castor oil can be improved by mixing it with cold orange juice.
- Results are usually obtained within 15 minutes to 1 hour after administration of rectal bisacodyl and within 30 minutes to 2 hours after use of rectal senna.
- Most oral products are taken at bedtime, causing a bowel movement to occur in the morning.

BULK LAXATIVES (ORAL)

METHYLCELLULOSE
PSYLLIUM
POLYCARBOPHIL

Pharmacology

Bulk laxatives absorb water and expand in the intestinal tract, providing increased bulk and moisture to the stool. The increased bulk promotes peristalsis and motility.

Side Effects

Two serious but rare side effects may be seen in patients using bulk laxatives. The first is an allergic reaction to vegetable components of natural products characterized by difficulty breathing, skin rash, or itching. The second is esophageal blockage or intestinal impaction, which is usually caused by insufficient fluid intake. Other more common and less serious side effects include gas formation and feeling bloated.

Drug Interactions

Any laxative can interact with potassium-sparing diuretics and potassium supplements. Chronic or excessive use of laxatives may reduce serum potassium levels by promoting excessive potassium loss from the intestinal tract. Interactions may also occur between laxatives made of cellulose derivatives and warfarin, digoxin, and salicylates, reducing the desired effect of the object drug because of physical binding or absorptive hindrance. A 2-hour interval between drugs is recommended. Laxatives containing calcium polycarbophil may interact with tetracyclines, decreasing absorption of the drug because of the formation of nonabsorbable complexes. A 2-hour interval between drugs is recommended.

Lifespan Considerations
Pediatric

Children are often unable to precisely describe the symptoms they feel. Therefore proper diagnosis should always precede the use of laxatives in children under the age of 6 years. This will avoid the complication of existing conditions.

Patient Education

- The patient should drink at least 6 to 8 full glasses (8 oz each) of liquids each day when using any laxative.
- Laxatives should not be swallowed in their dry form; mix with liquid.
- The patient should drink a full glass (8 oz) of liquid with every dose.
- Results are obtained in 12 hours to 3 days.

LUBRICANT LAXATIVES (ORAL AND RECTAL)

MINERAL OIL

Pharmacology

Lubricant laxatives ease the passage of the stool through the intestines by coating the stool and intestinal surfaces with a water-immiscible film.

Side Effects

Lubricant laxatives may cause a local skin irritation surrounding the rectal area.

Drug Interactions

Any laxative can interact with potassium-sparing diuretics and potassium supplements. Chronic or excessive use of laxatives may reduce serum potassium levels by promoting excessive potassium loss from the intestinal tract. For patients taking warfarin, oral contraceptives, or digoxin, mineral oil interferes with the absorption of these drugs, reducing their effectiveness. Mineral oil also causes decreased absorption of vitamin K, which could lead to increased anticoagulation. Concurrent use of docusate with mineral oil may cause increased absorption of mineral oil, resulting in the formation of tumorlike deposits in tissues.

Lifespan Considerations
Geriatric

Oral administration of mineral oil is generally not a good choice in elderly or bedridden patients because of potential for pneumonia caused by aspiration of oil droplets.

Pediatric

Children are often unable to precisely describe the symptoms they feel. Therefore proper diagnosis should always precede the use of laxatives in children under the age of 6 years. This will avoid the complication of existing conditions. Similar to geriatric patients, children under 6 years of age are also more prone to aspiration of oil droplets, making an oral lubricant laxative a poor choice because of the risk of lipid pneumonia.

Pregnancy

Repeated use of mineral oil during pregnancy may result in a decreased absorption of food, fat-soluble vitamins, and some other drugs. Chronic use increases the risk of the neonate developing hypoprothrombinemia and hemorrhagic disease.

Patient Education

- The patient should drink at least 6 to 8 full glasses (8 oz each) of liquids each day when using any laxative.
- The anus should be lubricated with petroleum jelly before insertion of enema applicator, which should be inserted carefully to prevent damage to rectal wall.
- Mineral oil laxatives should not be taken within 2 hours of meals because of potential for malabsorption of food nutrients and vitamins.
- Mineral oil laxatives are usually taken at bedtime, but not while reclining.
- When taken orally, results are obtained in about 6 to 8 hours.
- When administered rectally, results occur in 2 to 15 minutes.

SURFACTANT (ORAL STOOL SOFTENER)

Docusate

Pharmacology

Surfactant laxatives allow permeation of liquid into the stool by reducing surface tension of interfacing liquid contents. The result is a softer stool mass, hence the name *stool softeners*.

Side Effects

Allergies accompanied by an undetermined skin rash have been rarely noted with docusate. Stomach and/or intestinal cramping are more common. Local throat irritation is also seen with liquid dosage forms.

Drug Interactions

Any laxative can interact with potassium-sparing diuretics and potassium supplements. Chronic or excessive use of laxatives may reduce serum potassium levels by promoting excessive potassium loss from the intestinal tract. Concurrent use of docusate and mineral oil may cause increased absorption of mineral oil, resulting in the formation of tumorlike deposits in tissues.

Lifespan Considerations
Pediatric

Children are often unable to precisely describe the symptoms they feel. Therefore proper diagnosis should always precede the use of laxatives in children under the age of 6 years. This will avoid the complication of existing conditions.

Patient Education

- Docusate is not a laxative; it softens the stool, making bowel movements easier. Best results are obtained when docusate is taken daily.
- The patient should drink at least 6 to 8 full glasses (8 oz each) of liquids each day when using any laxative.
- The flavor of liquid preparations can be improved by mixing in milk or fruit juice.
- Results are usually obtained in 1 to 2 days after first dose.

HYPEROSMOTIC (ORAL AND RECTAL)

GLYCERIN

Pharmacology

Glycerin stimulates rectal contractions and softens and lubricates by attracting water to the stool. This produces an osmotic effect and, in turn, increased peristalsis and bowel evacuation.

Side Effects

Glycerin can cause some local skin irritation surrounding the rectal area.

Drug Interactions

Any laxative can interact with potassium-sparing diuretics and potassium supplements. Chronic or excessive use of laxatives may reduce serum potassium levels by promoting excessive potassium loss from the intestinal tract.

Lifespan Considerations
Pediatric

Children are often unable to precisely describe the symptoms they feel. Therefore proper diagnosis should always precede the use of laxatives in children under the age of 6 years. This will avoid the complication of existing conditions.

Patient Education

- The patient should drink at least 6 to 8 full glasses (8 oz each) of liquids each day when using any laxative.
- The anus should be lubricated with petroleum jelly before insertion of enema applicator, which should be inserted carefully to prevent damage to rectal wall.
- A suppository can be moistened by placing either under a stream of water for 30 seconds or in a cup of water for at least 10 seconds before insertion.
- Results are usually obtained with glycerin within 15 minutes to 1 hour.

Product Selection

The goal of product selection is to choose a product that will alleviate the discomfort of constipation while causing the fewest possible side effects and/or drug interactions. The age and coexisting conditions of the individual patient must be considered carefully. In the treatment of constipation, the advantage of using certain laxative combinations rather than a single laxative agent has not been established. In some instances, just as with the selection of a single-entity laxative, the improper selection of a laxative combination may turn constipation into a more serious condition. The following items should be considered when considering the use of a laxative:

- Surfactants (stool softeners) are safe in almost every situation and are an excellent choice when attempting to prevent constipation.
- Oral bulk, lubricant, and surfactant laxatives are indicated prophylactically in patients who should not strain during defecation.
- Oral bulk and stimulant laxatives are good choices to facilitate defecation in geriatric patients with diminished colonic motor response.
- Oral bulk laxatives and surfactants are good choices to use during pregnancy or postpartum to re-establish normal bowel function and prevent straining.
- In severe cases of constipation or fecal impaction, mineral oil administered orally or rectally is indicated to help soften the stool. To help evacuate the colon, a rectal stimulant or saline laxative may follow.
- Laxative dependency can be a problem, especially in elderly patients. Glycerin suppositories are indicated to re-establish normal bowel function in these patients.

Product Information: Oral Dosage Laxative Forms

Brand Name	Laxative Type	Ingredient	Adult Dose (Maximum Recommended Daily Dose)	Pediatric Dose
Alphamul emulsion	Stimulant	Castor oil 60% w/v	15-45 ml	*<2 years:* 1-5 ml *>2 years:* 5-15 ml
Bisacodyl tablets	Stimulant	Bisacodyl 5 mg	2-3 tablets (6 tablets)	*<6 years:* Not recommended *>6 years:* 1 tablet
Carter's Little Pills tablets	Stimulant	Bisacodyl 5 mg	1-3 tablets	*<6 years:* Not recommended *6-12 years:* 1 tablet
Casanthranol and Docusate capsules	Stimulant	Casanthranol 30 or 50 mg	1-2 capsules	*>6 years:* 1 capsule
Casanthranol and Docusate syrup	Stimulant	Casanthranol 10 mg/5 ml	7.5-30 ml	*>3 years:* 5-15 ml
Cascara tablets	Stimulant	Cascara sagrada 150 mg	1 tablet	Not recommended
Cascara aromatic fluidextract	Stimulant	Cascara sagrada 1 g/1 ml	5 ml (15 ml)	*>2 years:* 1-3 ml *<2 years:* 1-5 ml
Castor oil	Stimulant	Castor oil	15-60 ml	*>2 years:* 5-15 ml
Cillium powder	Bulk	Psyllium 4.94 g/full tsp	1 full tsp in 240 ml liquid 1-3 times/day	*>6 years:* ½ tsp in 120 ml liquid
Citrate of magnesia oral solution	Saline	Magnesium citrate 1.55-1.9 g/100 ml, citric acid 7.59 g/100 ml	240 ml	*2-6 years:* 4-12 ml *6-12 years:* 50-100 ml

Continued

HS, At bed time; *tbsp,* tablespoon; *tsp,* teaspoon; *w/v,* weight/volume.

Product Information: Oral Dosage Laxative Forms—cont'd

Brand Name	Laxative Type	Ingredient	Adult Dose (Maximum Recommended Daily Dose)	Pediatric Dose
Citroma oral solution	Saline	See citrate of magnesia oral solution	See citrate of magnesia oral solution	See citrate of magnesia oral solution
Citrucel Orange Flavor granules	Bulk	Methylcellulose 2 g/heaping tbsp or 19-g packet	1 heaping tbsp or 1 19-g packet in 240 ml liquid 1-3 times/day	*>6 years:* ½ tbsp in 120 ml liquid 3-4 times/day
Colace capsules	Surfactant (stool softener)	Docusate sodium 50 or 100 mg	50-200 mg	*> 6 years:* 100 mg
Colace solution	Surfactant (stool softener)	Docusate sodium 10 mg/ml	Intended for pediatric use	*<3 years:* 1-2 ml *3-6 years:* 2 ml 1-3 times/day
Colace syrup	Surfactant (stool softener)	Docusate sodium 20 mg/5 ml	15-45 ml	*3-6 years:* 5-15 ml/day *6-12 years:* 10 ml 1-2 times/day
Correctol Extra Gentle tablets	Surfactant (stool softener)	Docusate sodium 100 mg	1-2 tablets AM or HS	*>6 years:* 1 tablet AM or HS
Correctol tablets	Stimulant	Bisacodyl 5 mg	1-2 tablets AM or HS	*>6 years:* 1 tablet AM or HS
Dialose tablets	Surfactant (stool softener)	Docusate sodium 100 mg	1 tablet 1-2 times/day	*>6 years:* 1 tablet

Dialose Plus tablets	Surfactant (stool softener)	Docusate sodium 100 mg	1-2 tablets 2 times/day	*>6 years:* 1 tablet
Docusate calcium capsules	Surfactant (stool softener)	Docusate calcium 240 mg	1 capsule	Not available
Doxidan capsules	Stimulant Surfactant (stool softener)	Casanthranol 30 mg Docusate calcium 60 mg	1-2 capsules	*>6 years:* 1 capsule
Dulcolax tablets	Stimulant	Bisacodyl 5 mg	2-3 tablets (usually 2) AM or HS	*<6 years:* Not recommended *>6 years:* 1-2 tablets
Equalactin chewable tablets	Bulk	Calcium polycarbophil 500 mg (base)	2 tablets 1-4 times/day	*3-6 years:* 1 tablet 1-2 times/day *6-12 years:* 1 tablet 1-4 times/day
Ex-Lax tablets (chewable)	Stimulant	Sennosides 15 mg	1-2 tablets	*>6 years:* ½-1 tablet
Ex-Lax pills	Stimulant	Sennosides 15 mg	1-2 tablets	*>6 years:* ½-1 tablet
Ex-Lax Extra Gentle tablets	Surfactant (stool softener)	Docusate sodium 100 mg	1-2 tablets	*>6 years:* 1 tablet
Feen-a-Mint chewable tablets	Stimulant	Bisacodyl 5 mg	1-2 tablets	*>6 years:* 1 tablet

Continued

Product Information: Oral Dosage Laxative Forms—cont'd

Brand Name	Laxative Type	Ingredient	Adult Dose (Maximum Recommended Daily Dose)	Pediatric Dose
Fiberall powder	Bulk	Psyllium hydrophilic mucilloid 3.4 g/full tsp	1 full tsp in 240 ml liquid 1-3 times/day	*>6 years:* ½ tsp in 120 ml liquid 1-3 times/day
FiberCon tablets	Bulk	Calcium polycarbophil 500 mg (base)	2 tablets 1-4 times/day	*2-6 years:* 1 tablet 1-2 times/day *6-12 years:* 1 tablet 1-3 times/day
Fleet Flavored Castor Oil emulsion	Stimulant	Castor oil 67% w/v	45 ml	*<2 years:* 1-5 ml *2-12 years:* 5-15 ml
Fleet Laxative tablets	Stimulant	Bisacodyl 5 mg	2-3 tablets (6 tablets)	*<6 years:* Not recommended *>6 years:* 1 tablet
Fleet Phospho-Soda oral solution	Saline	Sodium biphosphate 2.4 g/5 ml, sodium phosphate 0.9 g/5 ml	20 ml diluted in 120 ml liquid	*6-9 years:* 5 ml *>10 years:* 10 ml diluted in 120 ml liquid
Fletcher's Castoria oral solution	Stimulant	Senna 675 mg/5 ml (135 mg/ml)	Intended for pediatric use	*1-6 months:* 0.125-2.5 ml *7-12 months:* 2.5-5 ml *1-5 years:* 5-10 ml *6-12 years:* 10-15 ml
Kondremul emulsion	Lubricant	Mineral oil (heavy) 2.75 ml	15-30 ml	*>6 years:* 5-10 ml
Kondremul with Cascara emulsion	Stimulant Lubricant	Cascara sagrada extract 220 mg Mineral oil (heavy) 2.75 ml	15 ml in 240 ml liquid	*>6 years:* 5-10 ml in 240 ml liquid

Continued

Konsyl powder	Bulk	Psyllium hydrophilic mucilloid 3.4 g/full tsp or 7-g packet	1 full tsp or 7-g packet in 240 ml liquid 1-3 times/day	>6 years: ½ tsp in 120 ml liquid 1-3 times/day
Maltsupex powder	Bulk	Malt soup extract 16 g/full tbsp	2 full tbsp 2 times/day for 3-4 days, then 1-2 tbsp HS	1 month-2 years: 1-2 tsp in 2-4 oz liquid 1-2 times/day; >2 years: 1-2 tbsp in 8 oz liquid 1-2 times/day
Maltsupex oral solution	Bulk	Malt soup extract 5.3 g (16 g/15 ml)	30 ml 2 times/day for 3-4 days, then 15-30 ml HS	1 month-2 years: 5-10 ml in 2-4 oz liquid 1-2 times/day; >2 years: 15-30 ml in 8 oz liquid 1-2 times/day
Metamucil powder	Bulk	Psyllium hydrophilic mucilloid 3.4 g/full tsp	1 full tsp in 240 ml liquid 1-3 times/day	>6 years: ½ tsp in 120 ml liquid 1-3 times/day
Mineral oil	Lubricant	Mineral oil	15-45 ml	>6 years: 5-15 ml
Nature's Remedy tablets	Stimulant	Aloe 100 mg and cascara sagrada 150 mg	1-2 tablets	>6 years: 1 tablet
Perdiem granules	Stimulant	Senna 0.74 g/full tsp; Psyllium 3.25 g/full tsp	1-2 full tsp 1-2 times/day (2 full tsp every 6 hours)	>7 years: 1 full tsp 1-2 times/day
Perdiem Plain granules	Bulk	Psyllium 4.03 g/full tsp	1-2 full tsp 1-2 times/day (2 full tsp every 6 hours)	>7 years: 1 full tsp 1-2 times/day
Peri-Colace capsules	Stimulant Surfactant (stool softener)	Casanthranol 30 mg; Docusate sodium 100 mg	1-2 capsules	>6 years: 1 capsule

Product Information: Oral Dosage Laxative Forms—cont'd

Brand Name	Laxative Type	Ingredient	Adult Dose (Maximum Recommended Daily Dose)	Pediatric Dose
Peri-Colace syrup	Stimulant Bulk	Casanthranol 10 mg/5 ml Docusate sodium 20 mg/5 ml	15-30 ml	*>3 years:* 5-15 ml
Senokot granules	Stimulant	Standardized senna concentrate 325 mg/level tsp	1 level tsp (2 level tsp 2 times/day)	*>6 years:* ½ tsp (1 level tsp 2 times/day)
Senokot syrup	Stimulant	Standardized extract of senna fruit	10-15 ml (15 ml 2 times/day)	*<1 year:* 1.25-2.5 ml (2.5 ml 2 times/day) *1-5 years:* 2.5-5 ml (5 ml 2 times/day) *5-15 years:* 5-10 ml (10 ml 2 times/day)
Senokot tablets	Stimulant	Senna concentrate 187 mg	2 tablets	*>6 years:* 1 tablet
Senokot-S tablets	Stimulant	Standardized senna concentrate 187 mg	2 tablets	*>6 years:* 1 tablet
Surfak capsules	Surfactant (stool softener)	Docusate calcium 50 mg or 240 mg	100-240 mg	*>6 years:* 50-150 mg

Product Information: Rectal Dosage Laxative Forms

Brand Name	Laxative Type	Ingredient	Adult Dose (Maximum Recommended Daily Dose)	Pediatric Dose
Bisacodyl suppositories	Stimulant	Bisacodyl 10 mg	1 suppository	*<2 years:* ½ suppository *>2 years:* 1 suppository
Dulcolax rectal solution	Stimulant	Bisacodyl 10 mg/5 ml	1 5-ml enema 1-2 hours before procedure	*<6 years:* ½ enema *>6 years:* See adult dose
Dulcolax suppositories	Stimulant	Bisacodyl 5 mg or 10 mg	1 10-mg suppository	*<6 years:* 1 5-mg suppository or ½ 10-mg suppository *>6 years:* See adult dose
Fleet Babylax rectal solution	Hyperosmotic	Glycerin 80% w/v	Intended for pediatric use	*>1 year:* Entire contents of applicator
Fleet Bisacodyl rectal solution	Stimulant	Bisacodyl 10 mg/37 ml	30 ml (delivered dose/bottle)	*<2 years:* Not recommended *>2 years:* See adult dose
Fleet Laxative suppositories	Stimulant	Bisacodyl 10 mg	1 suppository	*<2 years:* ½ suppository *>2 years:* 1 suppository
Fleet Bisacodyl Prep rectal solution	Stimulant	Bisacodyl 10 mg/10 ml aqueous hydroxy-propylmethylcellulose packet	1 packet in 1500 ml liquid or 1 packet into barium suspension	Not established

Continued

w/v, Weight/volume.

Page 28 — MOSBY'S OTC DRUGS

Product Information: Rectal Dosage Laxative Forms—cont'd

Brand Name	Laxative Type	Ingredient	Adult Dose (Maximum Recommended Daily Dose)	Pediatric Dose
Fleet Enema	Saline	Sodium biphosphate 19 g/118 ml, sodium phosphate 7 g/118 ml	118 ml (delivered dose/133 ml bottle)	*>2 years:* 60 ml
Fleet Enema Mineral Oil	Lubricant	Mineral oil	120 ml (delivered dose/130 ml bottle)	*>2 years:* 30-60 ml
Glycerin suppositories	Surfactant	Glycerin	1 adult-size suppository	*<6 years:* 1 pediatric-size suppository; *>6 years:* 1 adult-size suppository
Senokot suppositories	Stimulant	Senna concentrate 625 mg	1 suppository after meals	*>6 years:* ½ suppository after meals

Diarrhea

Diarrhea can be defined as an increase in frequency, volume, or fluidity of fecal discharges in comparison with the patient's normal stools. There are many causes of diarrhea, including food poisoning, viruses, medications, lactose intolerance, and diseases of the gastrointestinal tract. Diarrhea may be either chronic or acute. OTC agents may be utilized to combat the symptoms of diarrhea in mild, nonspecific cases. In cases in which high fever and dehydration are present, the underlying cause should be treated under the supervision of a health care professional. Drugs used to treat diarrhea include antiperistaltic and absorbent agents.

ANTIPERISTALTIC AGENTS

Pharmacology

Antiperistaltic agents (e.g., loperamide) work by slowing down the colon's propulsive movements. Loperamide acts directly on the musculature of the small and large intestines, which results in a delay of transit of the intestinal contents. This allows the body time to reabsorb the necessary water and nutrients, resulting in the formation of a normal stool. Loperamide has been shown to decrease the frequency and increase the consistency of stools and relieve associated symptoms.

Side Effects

Loperamide has very few side effects. Drowsiness and dizziness are possible but uncommon at recommended OTC doses. Dry mouth, constipation, nausea, and vomiting may also occur.

Drug Interactions

Loperamide has no serious clinical drug interactions.

Lifespan Considerations

Geriatric

Elderly patients with multiple medical problems should contact a health care professional immediately at onset of symptoms.

Pediatric

Antiperistaltic agents should be avoided in children under the age of 2. Loperamide should be used cautiously in children because of the greater variability of response. Parents of infants and young children should be educated about the signs of dehydration (e.g., thirst, dry mouth, concentrated urine) and should seek medical treatment if these signs are present with diarrhea.

Pregnancy

Loperamide is an FDA Pregnancy Category B drug. Because of the risk of dehydration, pregnant women with diarrhea should be evaluated by a health care professional.

Nursing Mothers

Small amounts of loperamide have been found to be excreted in breast milk, with no reports of adverse effects. The American Academy of Pediatrics considers the use of loperamide while nursing to be safe.

Patient Education

- If the diarrhea is severe, involves abdominal distension or fever, and/or lasts more than 1 to 2 days, the patient should seek medical help to replace necessary fluids and nutrients.
- Patients who are pregnant, have bloody stools, or weight loss of more than 5% of total body weight should contact a health care professional immediately.
- Diarrhea in infants and young children must be treated with caution. These patients may become seriously dehydrated fairly quickly. Parents should be informed to contact a health care professional immediately.
- Individuals experiencing diarrhea secondary to lactose intolerance must either avoid lactose or take a product such as Lactaid, which supplies the enzymes that the body is missing to digest lactose.
- The patient should drink plenty of clear liquids to prevent dehydration.
- Use of loperamide to treat acute diarrhea that is associated with an intestinal organism (*Escherichia coli*, *Salmonella*, *Shigella*) should be avoided. Loperamide may inhibit the excretion of the organism in a timely manner.
- Loperamide should be used cautiously in patients with ulcerative colitis. Agents, such as loperamide, that slow intestinal motility may induce toxic megacolon in these patients.

ABSORBENT AGENTS/BISMUTH SUBSALICYLATE

Pharmacology

Absorbent agents (e.g., attapulgite, polycarbophil, kaolin, and pectin) absorb excess water in the colon, thus allowing the formation of a normal stool. Absorbents are nonspecific and may bind to necessary nutrients, medications, etc. Attapulgite is a naturally occurring magnesium/aluminum salt that has the ability to absorb up to eight times its weight in water. Polycarbophil is a hydrophilic resin that is promoted as both a laxative and as an antidiarrheal agent; it is often referred to as a *stool normalizer*. It has a capacity for binding water and absorbs 60 times its original weight. Kaolin and pectin are naturally occurring adsorbent agents that are not absorbed into the systemic circulation. Bismuth subsalicylate may also be used to treat diarrhea; the exact mechanism of action of bismuth subsalicylate in the treatment of diarrhea is unknown. It is believed to work possibly by three mechanisms, including (1) normalizing fluid movement via an antisecretory mechanism, (2) binding bacterial toxins, and (3) antimicrobial activity. There are minimal to no data to support bismuth subsalicylate's efficacy as an antidiarrheal agent.

Three agents (attapulgite, polycarbophil, and loperamide) have been deemed safe and effective for treatment of diarrhea by the FDA. The FDA continues to review data concerning the kaolin-pectin combination and bismuth subsalicylate.

Side Effects

Absorbent agents work locally, with limited systemic activity; thus they have limited side effects. Constipation is the most common side effect. Dose-related abdominal pain and bloating may also occur. Bismuth subsalicylate may cause the mouth, tongue, and stool to appear darkened (gray-black or black) temporarily.

Drug Interactions

Absorbent agents may adhere to many nutrients and medications, decreasing their absorption. In general, other medications should be taken 1 hour before or 2 to 3 hours after using these products.

Pepto-Bismol contains nonaspirin salicylates. Salicylates should be used with caution in patients who take warfarin (Coumadin) because they may increase bleeding tendencies. Salicylates may interact with some medications for diabetes and gout (see Part IX, Fever and Internal Pain, p. 363).

Lifespan Considerations

Geriatric

Elderly patients with multiple medical problems should contact a health care professional immediately at onset of symptoms.

Pediatric

Diarrhea in infants and young children must be treated with caution. As a general rule, the American Academy of Pediatrics recommends that pharmacologic agents should not be used unless monitored by a health care professional.

Absorbent agents and bismuth subsalicylate should be avoided in children under the age of 3. Parents of infants and young children should be educated about the signs of dehydration (e.g., thirst, dry mouth, concentrated urine) and should seek medical treatment if these signs are present with diarrhea. Children and teenagers who have or are recovering from a viral illness should not take bismuth subsalicylate because of the possibility of developing Reye's syndrome. Aspirin-containing and aspirin-like medications have been linked to Reye's syndrome, a rare but serious illness associated with viral infections.

Pregnancy

Kaolin-pectin and bismuth subsalicylate are both FDA Pregnancy Category C drugs. Only limited data are available for attapulgite and polycarbophil. Although the risk of toxicity when using bismuth subsalicylate is relatively small, significant adverse effects to the fetus have resulted from chronic exposures to salicylates in general. The use of bismuth subsalicylate should be restricted to the first half of pregnancy in amounts that do not exceed the recommended doses.

Nursing Mothers

The American Academy of Pediatrics recommends that salicylates should be used cautiously while nursing. Absorbent agents should have no effect on lactation or the infant.

Patient Education

- If diarrhea is severe, involves abdominal distension or fever, and/or lasts more than 1 to 2 days, the patient should seek medical help to replace necessary fluids and nutrients.
- Infants and children may become seriously dehydrated fairly quickly. Parents of infants and children should contact a health care profes-

sional immediately if signs of dehydration (thirst, dry mouth, and concentrated urine) appear.

- Individuals with diarrhea secondary to lactose intolerance must either avoid lactose or take a product such as Lactaid, which supplies the enzymes that the body is missing to digest lactose.
- The patient should drink plenty of clear liquids to prevent dehydration.
- Full recommended dosages should be taken at the first sign of diarrhea and after each subsequent loose bowel movement.
- Polycarbophil may be used either as a laxative or as an antidiarrheal to normalize the stool's moisture content and produce bulk. Other bulk laxatives, such as psyllium, may also normalize stool content in patients with symptoms of diarrhea.
- Bismuth subsalicylate may cause the mouth, tongue, and stool to appear darkened (gray-black or black) temporarily. Patients should be aware of this darkening of the stool in comparison with that caused by melena.
- Kaopectate caplets should be swallowed whole with water and not chewed.
- Liquid Kaopectate should not be used with children under the age of 3 without the supervision of a health care professional.
- Donnagel tablets should be chewed thoroughly and swallowed.
- Polycarbophil (Mitrolan, Equalactin, FiberCon, Fiberall) tablets should be chewed thoroughly and not swallowed whole. Minimal fluid intake is encouraged.

Product Selection

Loperamide has a quicker onset of action than absorbent agents. Absorbent agents may take up to a day or so to work effectively.

SUGGESTED READINGS

Brownlee HJ: Family practitioner's guide to patient self-treatment of acute diarrhea, Am J Med 88(suppl 6A):6A, 27S-29S, 1990.

Dukes GE: Over-the-counter antidiarrheal medications used for self-treatment of acute nonspecific diarrhea, Am J Med 88(suppl 6A):6A,24S-26S, 1990.

Okhuysen PC, Ericsson CD: Travelers' diarrhea: prevention and treatment, Med Clin North Am 76(6):1357-1373, 1992.

Product Information: Antidiarrheal Drugs

Brand Name	Ingredient	Adult Dose	Pediatric Dose
Donnagel	Attapulgite liquid: 600 mg/15 ml; tablets: 600 mg	30 ml (2 tbsp) or 2 tablets after each bowel movement, up to 7 doses/day	*3-6 years:* 7.5 ml (½ tbsp) or ½ tablet *6-12 years:* 15 ml (1 tbsp) or 1 tablet Dose after each bowel movement, up to 7 doses/day
Equalactin (available in citrus flavor)	Polycarbophil chewable tablets 500 mg	1000 mg every 30 minutes, as needed, up to 6 g/day	*3-6 years:* 500 mg every 30 minutes, as needed, up to 1.5 g/day *6-12 years:* 500 mg every 30 minutes, as needed, up to 3 g/day
Fiberall (scored; available in lemon flavor)	Polycarbophil tablets 1000 mg	1000 mg every 30 minutes, as needed, up to 6 g/day	*3-6 years:* 500 mg every 30 minutes, as needed, up to 1.5 g/day *6-12 years:* 500 mg every 30 minutes, as needed, up to 3 g/day
FiberCon (sodium free)	Polycarbophil tablets 500 mg	1000 mg every 30 minutes, as needed, up to 6 g/day	*3-6 years:* 500 mg every 30 minutes, as needed, up to 1.5 g/day *6-12 years:* 500 mg every 30 minutes, as needed, up to 3 g/day
Fiber-Lax	Polycarbophil tablets 500 mg	1000 mg every 30 minutes, as needed, up to 6 g/day	3-6 years: 500 mg every 30 minutes, as needed, up to 1.5 g/day 6-12 years: 500 mg every 30 minutes, as needed, up to 3 g/day

Imodium	Loperamide capsules 2 mg	4 mg after first loose bowel movement, followed by 2 mg after each subsequent loose bowel movement, up to 8 mg/day	*6-8 years (48-59 lbs):* 1 mg after first bowel movement, followed by 1 mg after each subsequent loose bowel movement, up to 4 mg/day for no more than 2 days *9-11 years (60-95 lbs):* 2 mg after first bowel movement, followed by 1 mg after each subsequent loose bowel movement, up to 6 mg/day for no more than 2 days
Imodium A-D	Loperamide liquid 1 mg/5 ml; tablets 2 mg	4 mg after first loose bowel movement, followed by 2 mg after each subsequent loose bowel movement, up to 8 mg/day for no more than 2 days	*6-8 years (48-59 lbs):* 1 mg after first bowel movement, followed by 1 mg after each subsequent loose bowel movement, up to 4 mg for no more than 2 days *9-11 years (60-95 lbs):* 2 mg after first bowel movement, followed by 1 mg after each subsequent loose bowel movement, up to 6 mg/day for no more than 2 days

Continued

Product Information: Antidiarrheal Drugs—cont'd

Brand Name	Ingredient	Adult Dose	Pediatric Dose
Imodium Advanced (contains simethicone [antigas agent])	Loperamide tablets 2 mg; simethicone tablets 125 mg	4 mg after first loose bowel movement, followed by 2 mg after each subsequent loose bowel movement, up to 8 mg/day	*6-8 years (48-59 lbs)*: 2 mg after first bowel movement, followed by 1 mg after each subsequent loose bowel movement, up to 4 mg/day *9-11 years (60-95 lbs)*: 2 mg after first bowel movement, followed by 1 mg after each subsequent loose bowel movement, up to 6 mg/day
Kaopectate Advanced Formula (available in regular and peppermint flavors; alcohol free)	Attapulgite 600 mg/15 ml	30 ml (2 tbsp) after each bowel movement, up to 7 doses/day	*3-6 years*: 7.5 ml (½ tbsp) *6-12 years*: 15 ml (1 tbsp) Dose after each bowel movement, up to 7 doses/day
Children's Kaopectate (available in cherry flavor)	Attapulgite liquid: 600 mg/15 ml; chewable tablets: 300 mg	30 ml (2 tbsp) or 4 tablets after each bowel movement, up to 7 doses/day	*3-6 years*: 7.5 ml (½ tbsp) or 2 tablets *6-12 years*: 15 ml (1 tbsp) or 1 tablets Dose after each bowel movement, up to 7 doses/day

Kaopectate II	Loperamide tablets 2 mg	4 mg after first loose bowel movement, followed by 2 mg after each subsequent loose bowel movement, up to 8 mg/day *6-8 years (48-59 lbs):* 1 mg after first bowel movement, followed by 1 mg after each subsequent loose bowel movement, up to 4 mg for no more than 2 days *9-11 years (60-95 lbs):* 2 mg after first bowel movement, followed by 1 mg after each subsequent loose bowel movement, up to 6 mg/day for no more than 2 days
Kaopectate Maximum Strength Caplets	Attapulgite 750 mg	2 caplets after each bowel movement, up to 6 doses/day *6-12 years:* 1 caplet after each bowel movement, up to 6 doses/day
Kapectolin	Kaolin 90 g; pectin 2 g/30 ml	60-120 ml after each bowel movement *3-6 years:* 15-30 ml after each bowel movement *6-12 years:* 30-60 ml after each bowel movement
K-Pek (available in regular and peppermint flavors)	Attapulgite 600 mg/15 ml	30 ml (2 tbsp) after each bowel movement, up to 7 doses/day *3-6 years:* 7.5 ml (½ tbsp) *6-12 years:* 15 ml (1 tbsp) Dose after each bowel movement, up to 7 doses/day

Continued

Product Information: Antidiarrheal Drugs—cont'd

Brand Name	Ingredient	Adult Dose	Pediatric Dose
Maalox Anti-Diarrheal	Loperamide tablets 2 mg	4 mg after first loose bowel movement, followed by 2 mg after each subsequent loose bowel movement, up to 8 mg/day	*6-8 years (48-59 lbs):* 1 mg after first bowel movement, followed by 1 mg after each subsequent loose bowel movement, up to 4 mg for no more than 2 days *9-11 years (60-95 lbs):* 2 mg after first bowel movement, followed by 1 mg after each subsequent loose bowel movement, up to 6 mg/day for no more than 2 days
Mitrolan (available in citrus and vanilla flavors)	Polycarbophil chewable tablets 500 mg	1000 mg every 30 minutes, as needed, up to 6 g/day	*3-6 years:* 500 mg every 30 minutes, as needed, up to 1.5 g/day *6-12 years:* 500 mg every 30 minutes, as needed, up to 3 g/day
Parepectolin	Attapulgite 600 mg/15 ml	30 ml (2 tbsp) after each bowel movement; up to 7 doses/day	*3-6 years:* 7.5 ml (½ tbsp) *6-12 years:* 15 ml (1 tbsp) Dose after each bowel movement, up to 7 doses/day

Drug	Formulation	Adult dosage	Pediatric dosage
Pepto Diarrhea Control	Loperamide liquid 1 mg/5 ml	4 mg after first loose bowel movement, followed by 2 mg after each subsequent loose bowel movement, up to 8 mg/day	*6-8 years (48-59 lbs):* 1 mg after first bowel movement, followed by 1 mg after each subsequent loose bowel movement, up to 4 mg for no more than 2 days; *9-11 years (60-95 lbs):* 2 mg after first bowel movement, followed by 1 mg after each subsequent loose bowel movement, up to 6 mg/day for no more than 2 days
Pepto-Bismol Maximum Strength Liquid	Bismuth subsalicylate 525 mg/15 ml	30 ml (2 tbsp or 1 dose cup) Repeat dosage every 60 minutes, as needed, to maximum of 4 doses/day	*3-6 years:* 5 ml (1 tsp or ⅙ dose cup); *6-9 years:* 10 ml (2 tsp or ⅓ dose cup); *9-12 years:* 15 ml (1 tbsp or ½ dose cup) Repeat dosage every 60 minutes, as needed, to maximum of 4 doses/day
Pepto-Bismol original liquid	Bismuth subsalicylate 262 mg/15 ml	30 ml (2 tbsp or 1 dose cup); repeat dosage every 30-60 minutes, as needed, to maximum of 8 doses/day	*3-6 years:* 5 ml (1 tsp or ⅙ dose cup); *6-9 years:* 10 ml (2 tsp or ⅓ dose cup); *9-12 years:* 15 ml (1 tbsp or ½ dose cup) Repeat every 30-60 minutes, as needed, to a maximum of 8 doses/day
Pepto-Bismol tablets and caplets	Bismuth subsalicylate 262 mg	2 tablets/caplets Repeat dosage every 30-60 minutes, as needed, to maximum of 8 doses/day	*3-6 years:* ⅓ tablet/caplet; *6-9 years:* ⅔ tablet/caplet; *9-12 years:* 1 tablet/caplet

Hemorrhoids

A hemorrhoid is an enlarged vein in the mucous membrane in the anal area that may cause pain, itching, discomfort, and bleeding. The hemorrhoid may be either internal (located inside the rectum), external (located on the rim of the anus), or internal-external (mixed hemorrhoids). Internal hemorrhoids normally do not cause pain. The presence of blood after bowel movements may be the first sign of internal hemorrhoids. Internal hemorrhoids are classified on a grading system (first through fourth degree). Fourth degree is the most severe and may cause severe pain and bleeding. External hemorrhoids may cause extreme pain, itching, burning, inflammation, stool seepage, bleeding, and even thrombosis.

Pharmacology

There are many agents available to treat the symptoms of hemorrhoids. Nonprescription medications do not cure hemorrhoids. In addition, particular therapeutic agents/classes work more effectively on specific types of hemorrhoid. The following list includes therapeutic agents or classes, type of hemorrhoid treated, and the OTC agent involved:

- **Steroids** (external hemorrhoids) reduce inflammation, irritation, and itching, but do not relieve pain directly. OTC agent: hydrocortisone.
- **Local anesthetic agents** (external hemorrhoids) relieve pain, itching, discomfort, and irritation by reversibly blocking the transmission of nerve impulses. OTC agents: benzocaine, benzyl alcohol, dibucaine, dyclonine, lidocaine, pramoxine, and tetracaine.
- **Astringents** (external and internal hemorrhoids, depending on the agent) reduce the swelling and irritation caused by hemorrhoids. Astringents work by drying the area and coagulating proteins on the skin surface, thus protecting underlying tissue. OTC agents: calamine, witch hazel (hamamelis water), and zinc oxide.
- **Protectants** (external and internal hemorrhoids) form a physical barrier between fecal matter and the skin, thus limiting the irritation and itching. OTC agents: aluminum hydroxide gel, calamine, cocoa butter, cod liver oil, glycerin, shark liver oil, kaolin, lanolin, mineral oil, petrolatum, topical starch, and bismuth salts.
- **Vasoconstrictors** (external and internal hemorrhoids) work by promoting constriction of the blood vessels; therefore they decrease

swelling, itching, discomfort, and irritation. OTC agents: ephedrine sulfate, epinephrine, and phenylephrine.

- **Keratolytics** (external hemorrhoids) cause sloughing of the skin epidermal cells, allowing therapeutic agents to reach inflamed tissues. In addition, keratolytic agents may be helpful in reducing itching and discomfort. OTC agents: alcloxa and resorcinol.

Often, products that utilize a combination of these ingredients are preferred.

The most important step in hemorrhoid management is prevention. Avoiding constipation/straining during defecation; eating a balanced, high-fiber diet; drinking plenty of fluids; and exercising may not only prevent hemorrhoids but also help to shrink them.

Side Effects

Side effects are dependent on the agent(s) utilized. In general, hypersensitivities and allergic reactions, including burning and itching, may occur with all agents. Serious, but infrequent, adverse effects of vasoconstrictors include elevation of blood pressure, cardiac arrhythmias, tremor, insomnia, and aggravation of symptoms of hyperthyroidism. Use of vasoconstrictors should be avoided in patients with diabetes, hyperthyroidism, hypertension, and urination difficulties caused by an enlarged prostate. In general, the concentrations of vasoconstrictors used in OTC products are safe to use.

Drug Interactions

Interactions between vasoconstrictors and monoamine oxidase inhibitors can cause increased blood pressure. Interactions between vasoconstrictors and tricyclic antidepressants can result in decreased blood pressure.

Lifespan Considerations

Geriatric

There are no special recommendations for the use in the elderly.

Pediatric

These products are not recommended for children under 12 years of age. Children with hemorrhoids should be seen by a health care professional.

Pregnancy/Nursing Mothers

These agents are considered safe to use during pregnancy and lactation. Hemorrhoids may develop or worsen in pregnant patients; correction of constipation, use of stool softeners, and sitz baths may be helpful.

Patient Education

- OTC medicines do not cure hemorrhoids; they only relieve the symptoms. If symptoms worsen or do not improve after 7 days of self-treatment, or if bleeding, protrusion, or seepage occurs, a health care professional should be contacted.
- There are a variety of dosage forms available, including suppositories, creams, lotions, gels, ointments, wipes, pads, and foams. Some products have applicators or rectal pipes to allow easier intrarectal administration; caution should be used with these devices to avoid further irritation and trauma to the affected area.
- Proper cleaning of the rectal area is important in the management of hemorrhoids. The area should be cleaned with water and a gentle, unscented soap after each bowel movement.
- Patients with hemorrhoids should use unscented soaps and toilet paper; perfumes and fragrances can irritate hemorrhoids.
- Sitz baths help to relieve symptoms and cleanse the rectal area. A sitz bath involves sitting in warm water two or three times a day for 15 minutes at a time.
- Constipation and hard stools can cause and irritate hemorrhoids. Use of fiber-containing products or stool softeners and drinking plenty of fluids should be considered to avoid constipation. Excessive laxative use should be avoided.
- For maximum effect, hemorrhoidal agents should be used after, rather than before, bowel movements.
- If use of a product causes an increase in irritation, redness, or swelling, discontinue the use of that agent. Certain individuals may develop allergic reactions or hypersensitivity to agents in the product.
- Patients should not sit for prolonged periods, but should take short walks or stand periodically. In addition, patients should avoid heavy lifting.
- Some foods and beverages that may worsen the symptoms of hemorrhoids include spicy foods, nuts, coffee, and alcohol. Patients should avoid these products if possible.

Product Selection

- For internal hemorrhoids, OTC products that contain a vasoconstrictor, astringent, or protectant are the only FDA-approved agents for treatment. For external hemorrhoids, the symptoms dictate the appropriate therapy.
- Foams have a more rapid onset of action; however, these products are often difficult to apply and have erratic absorption because of bubble consistency.
- Patients with diabetes, hypertension, hyperthyroidism, or difficult urination, and those who are taking antidepressants should avoid products containing vasoconstrictors.

SUGGESTED READINGS

Cocchiara JL: Hemorrhoids: a practical approach to an aggravating problem, *Postgrad Med* 89(1):149-152, 1991.

Pfenninger JL: Nonsurgical treatment options for internal hemorrhoids, *Am Fam Phys* 52(3):821-834, 1995.

Product Information: Hemorrhoidal Drugs

Brand Name (Use as Directed)	Product Type	Ingredient
Americaine Ointment	Anesthetic	Benzocaine 20%
Anusol Ointment	Anesthetic	Pramoxine 1%
	Astringent	Zinc oxide 12.5%
	Protectant	Mineral oil, cocoa butter
*Anusol Suppositories**	Anesthetic	Benzyl benzoate 1.2%
	Astringent	Zinc oxide 11%
	Protectant	Bismuth salts
Anusol HC-1	Steroid	Hydrocortisone 1%
BiCozene Cream	Anesthetic	Benzocaine 6%
	Protectant	Castor oil, glycerin
	Keratolytic	Resorcinol 1.67%
Cortizone-10 External Anal Itch Relief	Steroid	Hydrocortisone 1%
Fleets Pain Relief Pads	Anesthetic	Pramoxine 1%
	Protectant	Glycerin 12%
Fleets Medicated Wipes†	Astringent	Hamamelis water 50%
	Protectant	Glycerin 10%
Hemorid Cream	Anesthetic	Pramoxine 1%
	Protectant	White petrolatum, mineral oil
	Vasoconstrictor	Phenylephrine 0.25%
Hemorid Suppositories	Astringent	Zinc oxide 11%
	Protectant	Hard fat
	Vasoconstrictor	Phenylephrine 0.25%
Hem-Prep Ointment	Astringent	Zinc oxide 11%
	Protectant	White petrolatum
	Vasoconstrictor	Phenylephrine 0.025%
Hem-Prep Suppositories	Astringent	Zinc oxide 11%
	Vasoconstrictor	Phenylephrine 0.25%
Medicore Ointment	Anesthetic	Benzocaine 20%
	Protectant	Mineral oil, white petrolatum
Nupercainal Suppositories	Astringent	Zinc oxide 0.25 mg
	Protectant	Cocoa butter
Nupercainal Ointment	Anesthetic	Dibucaine 1%
	Protectant	Lanolin, mineral oil, white petrolatum

* Contains balsam Peru, which is claimed to be a wound-healing agent.
† For external hemorrhoids only.
‡ Contains camphor, which is a counterirritant; it provides a cooling or tingling sensation.
§ For external hemorrhoids only.   *Continued*

Product Information: Hemorrhoidal Drugs—cont'd

Brand Name (Use as Directed)	Product Type	Ingredient
Pazo Ointment‡	Astringent	Zinc oxide 5%
	Protectant	Lanolin, petrolatum
	Vasoconstrictor	Ephedrine 0.2%
Pazo Suppositories	Astringent	Zinc oxide 96.5 mg
	Vasoconstrictor	Ephedrine 3.8 mg
Preparation H Cream, Ointment, or Suppositories	Protectant	Glycerin, shark liver oil, lanolin, petrolatum, mineral oil
	Vasoconstrictor	Phenylephrine 0.25%
ProctoFoam NS	Anesthetic	Pramoxine 1%
Tronolane Cream	Anesthetic	Pramoxine 1%
	Astringent	Zinc oxide
Tronolane Suppositories	Astringent	Zinc oxide 11%
	Protectant	Hard fat
Tucks Pads§	Astringent	Witch hazel 50%
	Protectant	Glycerin

Indigestion/Gas

Indigestion and gas are common disorders that are caused by a variety of culprits. Common causes include food and beverage indiscretions or overindulgences, ulcers (either duodenal or gastric), gastroesophageal reflux disease (GERD), and medications. Symptoms range from belching, bloating, and passing gas to severe abdominal pain. There are many OTC agents that are safe and effective in the treatment of indigestion and gas symptoms.

Drugs used in the treatment of indigestion and gas include H_2 antagonists, antacids, and antiflatulents.

H_2 ANTAGONISTS

CIMETIDINE
FAMOTIDINE
NIZATIDINE
RANITIDINE

Pharmacology

H_2 receptor antagonists competitively inhibit the interaction of gastric histamine with H_2 receptors. They are highly selective and have little or no effect on H_1 receptors (the receptors blocked by antihistamines). H_2 receptor antagonists inhibit gastric acid secretion stimulated by gastric histamine, gastrin, food, caffeine, and distension of the stomach. The H_2 antagonists both reduce the volume of gastric juice secreted and raise its pH. They inhibit all phases of gastric acid secretion and inhibit fasting, meal-stimulated, and nocturnal secretions. Heartburn and acid indigestion can be caused by excess gastric acid, which in turn causes gastrointestinal discomfort. Reducing the amount of stomach acid may relieve the symptoms of heartburn and indigestion. When acid is continually excessive and protective mechanisms such as prostaglandins are inhibited, the incidence of ulcer formation is increased. At prescription strengths and doses, H_2 antagonists are effective in preventing and treating peptic ulcer disease, GERD, and erosive esophagitis. The lower-strength nonprescription H_2 receptor antagonists are indicated only for prevention of heartburn and indigestion. Taken before bothersome foods are ingested, they reduce the formation of gastric acid, minimizing or preventing indigestion.

Side Effects

H_2 antagonists are remarkably free of side effects. Headache is the most common side effect, but occurs rarely. Confusion can occur in the elderly or in patients with renal impairment.

Drug Interactions

H_2 antagonists are strikingly free of drug interactions with the exception of cimetidine. Cimetidine inhibits the cytochrome P-450 enzyme system, inhibiting the metabolism of a number of drugs. Consequently, blood levels of the affected drugs can increase dramatically, leading to side effects. Additional drug interactions include the following:

- **H_2 antagonists and ketoconazole.** Decreases absorption of ketoconazole because of increase in gastric pH.
- **Cimetidine and warfarin.** Increased bleeding potenial, as evidenced by an increase in International Normalized Ratio (INR).
- **Cimetidine and metoprolol/propanolol.** Possible increase in metoprolol/propranolol effects and side effects.
- **Cimetidine and tricyclic antidepressants.** Possible increase in blood levels and side effects of tricyclic antidepressants.
- **Cimetidine and phenytoin (Dilantin).** Possible increase in phenytoin blood levels and toxicity.
- **Cimetidine and theophylline.** Possible increase in theophylline levels and toxicity.

Lifespan Considerations
Geriatric

Confusion can occur in older patients (particularly with cimetidine or ranitidine). This is most likely related to higher blood levels of these drugs secondary to age-related reduction in renal function. Confusion is unlikely at nonprescription doses.

Pediatric

OTC H_2 antagonists are not recommended in children younger than 12 years of age.

Pregnancy

Cimetidine, famotidine, and ranitidine are FDA Pregnancy Category B drugs. Nizatidine is a Category C drug.

Nursing Mothers

These drugs are excreted in breast milk at very low concentrations. The American Academy of Pediatrics considers these drugs to be safe for use while nursing.

Patient Education

- Patients should avoid use of foods, drinks (alcohol), or medications that cause heartburn.
- Encourage the patient to stop smoking. Smoking aggravates symptoms of gastritis and delays healing of ulcers in patients taking prescription strengths of these products.
- Because these drugs are used to prevent heartburn, they should be taken 30 to 60 minutes before eating. If immediate relief is needed, antacids should be taken.
- These drugs are excreted by the renal system. Dosage must be reduced in patients with renal impairment.
- H_2 antagonists may possibly interfere with acid secretion tests and should not be used for 24 hours preceding the test.

Product Selection

If the patient is on multiple chronic medications and cimetidine, check for possible drug–drug interactions.

ANTACIDS

ALUMINUM SALTS
MAGNESIUM SALTS
CALCIUM CARBONATE
SODIUM BICARBONATE
OTHERS

Pharmacology

Antacids neutralize gastric acid, resulting in increased pH of the stomach and duodenum. Additionally, by increasing the gastric pH to 4 or greater, antacids inhibit the conversion of pepsinogen to pepsin and pepsin activity. Antacids do not coat the mucosal lining. However, they may stimulate components of the gastric mucosal barrier, including bicarbonate and mucus secretion, mucosal cell regeneration, and mucosal blood flow, and may also increase the release of gastric-protective prostaglandins. Because of antacids' rapid onset, they are useful in the treatment of heartburn, acid indigestion, and "sour" stomach. In addition, they may used as a nutritional supplement (e.g., Tums for calcium replacement) or to treat GERD, peptic ulcer disease, and hyperphosphatemia (specifically, aluminum-containing products).

Side Effects

Aluminum-Containing Products
Constipation frequently occurs with use of aluminum-containing antacids; osteomalacia and hypophosphatemia are possible with high doses or prolonged use.

Magnesium-Containing Products
Diarrhea is most common; hypermagnesemia can occur with prolonged use or in patients with renal impairment.

In general, antacids may cause rebound hyperacidity, especially with calcium carbonate, because of the local effect of calcium on the gastric lining and the possibility of an increase in gastric secretion. Milk-alkali syndrome, consisting of headache, nausea, and weakness, can develop in renally impaired patients while using calcium carbonate and sodium bicarbonate products.

Drug Interactions

Antacids may impair the absorption of many drugs because of the increase of gastric pH, binding of the medications, and/or increasing urinary pH. In general, patients should avoid taking medications within 1 to 2 hours of antacid administration. Common drug interactions with antacids include the following:

- **Tetracycline antibiotics.** Decreases absorption and effectiveness of the antibiotic.
- **Quinolone antibiotics (e.g., Cipro, Levaquin, Trovan, Floxin).** Decreases absorption and effectiveness of the antibiotic.
- **Alendronate (Fosamax).** Decreases absorption and effectiveness of Fosamax.
- **Ketoconazole (Nizoral).** Decreases absorption of ketoconazole because of increased gastric pH.

Lifespan Considerations

Geriatric

Antacids contain a significant amount of sodium. Patients on low-sodium diets, such as those with congestive heart failure, might need to restrict antacid use. Riopan contains a unique aluminum-magnesium complex that is low in sodium.

Pediatric

Many products are not approved for children younger than 12 years of age. Children's Mylanta is approved for use in children ages 2 to 11.

Pregnancy

It is unlikely that occasional use of antacids would be harmful to a developing fetus; however, this has not been studied sufficiently to make a recommendation. Antacid use in pregnant/nursing women is generally considered safe as long as chronic high doses are avoided.

Nursing Mothers

Aluminum, magnesium, and calcium are excreted in breast milk. It is unlikely that toxicity would result, but data are lacking.

Patient Education

- Patients should stagger administration times of antacids and other oral medications by 1 to 2 hours to avoid possible interactions.
- Aluminum-magnesium combination products are designed to balance the constipating effects of aluminum salts and the laxative effects of magnesium salts.
- The onset of action of antacids is generally much quicker than H_2 antagonists. Liquid antacids work best because their small particle size increases the surface area between the antacid and the acid. Chewable tablets are more convenient, but should be chewed thoroughly before being swallowed.
- Patients should not take maximum doses for longer than 2 weeks unless under the supervision/direction of a trained medical professional.
- Hypermagnesemia may occur in renally impaired individuals. Patients should avoid doses greater than 50 mEq of magnesium daily.

Product Selection

- Gas is formed as a by-product of acid neutralization. Use of antacid products containing simethicone helps to neutralize gas that is formed.

- Sodium content of antacids may be significant; check individual products for sodium content if patient is currently on a restricted or low-sodium diet. Riopan is low in sodium.
- Patients complaining of reflux symptoms might benefit from using Gaviscon. This product contains alginic acid in addition to antacids. When chewed and followed by water as directed, a layer of foam forms on top of the gastric contents, forming a barrier against acid.

ANTIFLATULANTS

SIMETHICONE
CHARCOAL

Pharmacology

Simethicone changes the surface tension of gas bubbles in the stomach and intestines, eliminating and preventing formation of gas pockets and allowing the gas formed to be freely and more easily released by belching or passing flatus. Charcoal acts as an adsorbent and soothing agent. It reduces the amount and volume of gas, thus providing relief from intestinal discomfort. Both agents are useful in treatment of the painful symptoms of excess gas and/or gas retention. Simethicone is particularly useful in infants suffering from colic.

Side Effects

There are no clinically significant side effects with either simethicone or charcoal at normal doses.

Drug Interactions

Charcoal may reduce absorption of many drugs, thus decreasing their effectiveness. Therefore it should be taken 2 hours before or 1 hour after other oral medications. There are no clinically significant drug interactions with simethicone.

Lifespan Considerations
Geriatric
There are no unique considerations for the use of antiflatulents in the elderly population.

Pediatric

Simethicone is useful in the treatment of colic. Colic pain is at least partially the result of the presence of trapped gas in the colon. Simethicone drops added to formula can help relieve colic pain. Do not use charcoal in children younger than 3 years of age.

Pregnancy

Because simethicone and charcoal are inert, nonabsorbed substances, it is reasonable that occasional use should not pose substantial risk to a developing fetus. Studies are lacking, however.

Nursing Mothers

Because simethicone and charcoal are inert, nonabsorbed substances, it is reasonable that occasional use should not pose substantial risk to a nursing infant.

Patient Education/Product Selection

- For best results, simethicone tablets should be chewed thoroughly before being swallowed. For children younger than 2 years old, simethicone drops may be mixed with water, formula, or other liquids.
- Simethicone is effective in relieving intestinal gas associated with infant colic. However, nonpharmacologic measures to prevent or resolve colic (e.g., feeding in an upright position to facilitate burping, or limiting feeding times to 10 minutes) may need to be utilized.

SUGGESTED READINGS

Agreus L, Talley NJ: Dyspepsia: current understanding and management, *Annu Rev Med* 49:475-493, 1998.
Colon AR, Dipalma JS: Colic, *Am Fam Phys* 40:122-124, 1989.

Product Information: H$_2$ Antagonists

Brand Name	Ingredient	Dose	Comments
Axid AR	Nizatidine 75 mg	*Indigestion relief:* 75 mg 30-60 minutes before eating, up to 150 mg daily	
Mylanta AR and Pepcid AC	Famotidine 10 mg	*Indigestion relief:* 10 mg with water *Prevention:* 10 mg 1 hour before eating, up to 20 mg daily	Mylanta AR does **not** contain an antacid; the active ingredient is famotidine
Tagamet HB	Cimetidine 200 mg	*Indigestion relief:* 200 mg with water *Prevention:* 200 mg 30 minutes before eating, up to 400 mg daily	If patients have any questions on potential drug interactions, they can call 1-800-482-4394
Zantac 75	Ranitidine 75 mg	*Indigestion relief:* 75 mg with water, up to 150 mg daily	

Product Information: Antacids

Brand Name	Ingredient	Comments
Alka-Mints tablets	Calcium carbonate 850 mg	
Original Alka-Seltzer effervescents	Sodium bicarbonate 1916 mg	Aspirin 325 mg, citric acid 1000 mg
Extra Strength Alka-Seltzer effervescents	Sodium bicarbonate 1985 mg	Aspirin 500 mg, citric acid 1000 mg
Alu-Cap capsules	Aluminum hydroxide 400 mg	
Alu-Tab tablets	Aluminum hydroxide 500 mg	
Aludrox liquid	Aluminum hydroxide 307 mg	
	Magnesium hydroxide 103 mg	
Amphojel liquid and tablets	Aluminum hydroxide 300 mg, 600 mg, 320 mg/5 ml	
Basaljel capsules and liquid	Aluminum carbonate 500 mg, 400 mg/5 ml	
BromoSeltzer effervescents	Sodium bicarbonate 2781 mg	Acetaminophen 325 mg, citric acid 2224 mg
Children's Mylanta liquid and tablets	Calcium carbonate 400 mg/5 ml	
Chooz gum	Calcium carbonate 500 mg	
Advanced Formula	Calcium carbonate 280 mg	
Di-Gel tablets	Magnesium hydroxide 128 mg	
	Simethicone 20 mg	
Di-Gel liquid	Aluminum hydroxide 200 mg/5 ml	
	Magnesium hydroxide 200 mg/5 ml	
	Simethicone 20 mg/5 ml	
Gaviscon tablets	Aluminum hydroxide 80 mg	
	Magnesium trisilicate 20 mg	
	Sodium bicarbonate	

Continued

Product Information: Antacids—cont'd

Brand Name	Ingredient	Comments
Double Strength Gaviscon-2 tablets	Aluminum hydroxide 160 mg Magnesium trisilicate 40 mg Sodium bicarbonate	
Gaviscon Extra Strength Relief Formula tablets and liquid	Aluminum hydroxide 160 mg, 254 mg/5 ml Magnesium trisilicate 105 mg, 237.4 mg/5 ml Sodium bicarbonate (tablet only) Simethicone (liquid only)	
Gelusil tablets and liquid	Aluminum hydroxide 200 mg, 200 mg/5 ml Magnesium hydroxide 200 mg, 200 mg/5 ml Simethicone 25 mg, 25 mg/5 ml	
Maalox tablets and liquid	Aluminum hydroxide 200 mg, 225 mg/5 ml Magnesium hydroxide 200 mg, 200 mg/5 ml	
Extra Strength Maalox and *Extra Strength Maalox Plus* tablets and liquid	Aluminum hydroxide 350 mg, 500 mg/5 ml Magnesium hydroxide 350 mg, 450 mg/5 ml Simethicone 30 mg, 40 mg/5 ml	
Mag-Ox 400 tablets	Magnesium oxide 400 mg	
Phillips' Milk of Magnesia tablets and liquid	Magnesium hydroxide 311 mg, 400 mg/5 ml	
Concentrated Phillips' Milk of Magnesia liquid	Magnesium hydroxide 800 mg/5 ml	

Mylanta tablets and liquid	Aluminum hydroxide 200 mg, 200 mg/5 ml Magnesium hydroxide 200 mg, 200 mg/5 ml Simethicone 20 mg, 20 mg/5 ml
Mylanta gelcap	Calcium carbonate 311 mg Magnesium hydroxide 232 mg
Mylanta Double Strength tablets and liquid	Aluminum hydroxide 400 mg, 400 mg/5 ml Magnesium hydroxide 400 mg, 400 mg/5 ml Simethicone 40 mg, 40 mg/5 ml
Fast-Acting Mylanta tablets	Calcium carbonate 350 mg Magnesium hydroxide 150 mg
Maximum Strength Fast Acting Mylanta tablets	Calcium carbonate 700 mg Magnesium hydroxide 300 mg
Riopan liquid	Magaldrate (aluminum magnesium hydroxide sulfate) 540 mg/5 ml
Riopan Plus liquid	Magaldrate 540 mg/5 ml Simethicone 40 mg/5 ml
Riopan Plus tablets	Magaldrate 480 mg Simethicone 20 mg
Riopan Plus Double Strength tablets	Magaldrate 1080 mg Simethicone 20 mg
Rolaids tablets	Calcium carbonate 550 mg Magnesium hydroxide 110 mg

Continued

Product Information: Antacids—cont'd

Brand Name	Ingredient	Comments
Tempo tablets	Calcium carbonate 414 mg	
	Aluminum hydroxide 133 mg	
	Magnesium hydroxide 81 mg	
	Simethicone 20 mg	
Titralac tablets	Calcium carbonate 420 mg	
Titralac Plus tablets and liquid	Calcium carbonate 420 mg, 500 mg/5 ml	
	Simethicone 21 mg, 20 mg/5 ml	
Titralac Extra Strength tablets	Calcium carbonate 750 mg	
Tums tablets	Calcium carbonate 500 mg	
Extra Strength *Tums E-X* tablets	Calcium carbonate 750 mg	
Tums Ultra tablets	Calcium carbonate 1000 mg	
*Tums Anti-	Calcium carbonate 50 mg	
Gas/Antacid* tablets	Simethicone 20 mg	

Product Information: Usual Antacid Doses by Indication

Therapeutic Use	Ingredient	Adult Dose	Pediatric Dose	Comments
Heartburn/indigestion	Products listed in the Antacid product table	1-2 tablets or 5-15 ml as needed	*Children's Mylanta:* *Children 2-5 years (24-47 lbs):* 1 tablet or 5 ml (1 tsp) as needed, up to three doses/day *Children 6-11 years (48-95 lbs):* 2 tablets or 10 ml (2 tsp) as needed, up to three doses/day	See individual product directions for the exact dosage
Calcium supplementation (prevention of osteoporosis)	Calcium carbonate	*Postmenopausal women:* 1000-1500 mg elemental calcium daily in divided doses between meals *Others:* Up to 1500 mg daily		500 mg calcium carbonate = 200 mg elemental calcium

Product Information: Antiflatulents

Brand Name	Ingredient / Strength	Adult Dose	Pediatric Dose
Charcoal Plus	Charcoal 200 mg and simethicone 40 mg	2 tablets three times daily after meals	
CharcoCaps	Charcoal 260 mg	520 mg after meals or with discomfort, up to 2080 mg (8 capsules)/day	
Flatulex	Charcoal 250 mg and simethicone 80 mg	1 tablet three times daily and HS	
Gas-X	Simethicone 80 mg	80-160 mg after meals and HS, up to 480 mg (6 tablets)/day	
Extra-Strength Gas-X	Simethicone 125 mg	125 mg after meals and HS, up to 500 mg (4 tablets)/day	
Maalox Anti-Gas Extra Strength	Simethicone 150 mg	150-300 mg daily after meals and HS	
Maximum Strength Mylanta Gas Relief	Simethicone 125 mg	125 mg four times daily after meals and HS	
Mylanta Gas Relief	Simethicone 62.5 mg (gelcaps) or simethicone 80 mg (tablets)	80 mg (tablets) four times daily after meals and HS, up to 480 mg (6 tablets)/day or 125-250 mg (2-4 gelcaps) as needed after meals and HS, up to 500 mg (8 gelcaps)/day	

Mylicon Drops	Simethicone 40 mg/0.6 ml	40 mg (0.6 ml) four times daily after meals and HS, no more than 12 doses/day	*Infants <2 years:* 20 mg (0.3 ml) four times daily after meals and HS *Children >2 years:* 40 mg (0.6 ml) four times daily after meals and HS
Phazyme	Simethicone 95 mg	95 mg four times daily after meals and HS, up to 475 mg (5 tablets)/day	
Phazyme Infant Drops	Simethicone 40 mg/0.6 ml	80 mg (1.2 ml) four times daily after meals and HS, no more than 6 doses/day	*Children <2 years:* 20 mg (0.3 ml) four times daily after meals and HS *Children 2-12 years:* 40 mg (0.6 ml) four times daily after meals and HS
Phazyme Maximum Strength	Simethicone 125 mg (chewable tablet) or 62.5 mg/5 ml Simethicone 166 mg (soft gel)	125 mg four times a day after meals and HS, up to 500 mg (4 tablets)/day or 125 mg (10 ml) four times daily after meals and HS, up to 4 doses/day 166 mg four times a day after meals and HS, up to 4 doses/day	

HS, At bedtime.

Motion Sickness

Motion sickness is a common cause of nausea and vomiting and is the result of irregular and abnormal motions that disturb the organs of balance located in the inner ear. In addition to motion sickness induced by moving vehicles, infections of the inner ear can also cause nausea and vomiting. Specialized structures within the cochlea of the inner ears are responsible for maintaining balance. These structures contain fluid that moves as the head moves. When the flow of this fluid is moved or disturbed, balance is lost, resulting in dizziness, nausea, and vomiting.

Certain antihistamines are effective in the treatment of motion sickness.

ANTIHISTAMINES

MECLIZINE
CYCLIZINE
DIMENHYDRINATE

Pharmacology

Antihistamines (meclizine, cyclizine, and dimenhydrinate) are utilized to *prevent* motion sickness by controlling the overstimulation of the balance center in the inner ear. They work by depressing the excitability and impulse conduction in the inner ear. The anticholinergic and central nervous system (CNS) depressant properties of these antihistamines also contribute to its anti–motion-sickness action as an antiemetic.

Side Effects

Drowsiness is the most common side effect of antihistamines. Dry mouth, blurred vision, and constipation may also occur with these agents. Disorientation and confusion may occur, especially in the elderly, who are more sensitive to the effects of these agents.

Drug Interactions

Antihistamines may cause additional drowsiness when used with other agents that cause sedation (including alcohol, tranquilizers, hypnotics, and sedatives). Antihistamines may aggravate narrow-angle glaucoma, asthma, urinary retention or incontinence, or benign prostatic hypertrophy; use with caution in patients with these conditions.

Lifespan Considerations

Geriatric

The elderly may be more sensitive to the side effects of these medicines. These effects, namely disorientation and confusion, may lead to falls, which can be serious and debilitating.

Pediatric

Only cyclizine (Marezine) and dimenhydrinate (Dramamine, but not Dramamine II) are recommended in children younger than 12 years. Infants (younger than 2 years) are less likely to experience motion sickness.

Pregnancy

Cyclizine, dimenhydrinate, and meclizine are all FDA Pregnancy Category B drugs. Therapeutic doses of these agents are unlikely to pose a substantial risk to the fetus.

Nursing Mothers

Small amounts of dimenhydrinate are excreted in breast milk. Safety for use in nursing mothers has not been established for cyclizine or meclizine.

Patient Education

- Antihistamines are effective only in the prevention of motion sickness, not in the treatment of the symptoms. Therefore it is important to use these agents 30 to 60 minutes before traveling, to ensure effectiveness, and to continue to take them during the entire period of travel.
- These agents may cause drowsiness; therefore individuals should be cautioned not to drive a vehicle, operate hazardous machinery, or engage in tasks that require high mental alertness while on these agents. In addition, alcohol and other CNS depressants (e.g., hypnotics and sedatives) should be avoided.
- Elevating a child's car seat or allowing the child to peer outside the automobile's windows may reduce or eliminate motion sickness.

SUGGESTED READINGS

Rascol O et al: Antivertigo medications and drug-induced vertigo: a pharmacological review, *Drugs* 50(5):777-791, 1995.
Ruckenstein MJ, Harrison RV: Motion sickness, *Postgrad Med* 89:139-144, 1991.

Product Information: Motion Sickness

Brand Name	Ingredient	Adult Dose	Pediatric Dose
Bonine	Meclizine chewable tablets 25 mg	25-50 mg daily, not to exceed 50 mg/day	
Dizmiss	Meclizine chewable tablets 25 mg	25-50 mg daily, not to exceed 50 mg/day	
Dramamine	Dimenhydrinate tablets and chewable tablets: 50 mg Children's liquid: 12.5 mg/5 ml	50-100 mg every 4-6 hours, not to exceed 400 mg/day	2-6 years: 12.5-25 mg every 6-8 hours, not to exceed 75 mg/day 6-12 years: 25-50 mg every 6-8 hours, not to exceed 150 mg/day
Dramamine II	Meclizine tablets 25 mg	25-50 mg daily, not to exceed 50 mg/day	
Marezine	Cyclizine tablets 50 mg	50 mg every 3-4 hours, not to exceed 200 mg/day	6-12 years: 25 mg, three times daily

Nausea and Vomiting

Nausea and vomiting may be caused by stomach irritation, medications, inner ear imbalance/motion sickness, or stomach flu or virus. Agents utilized to treat nausea and vomiting work locally by adjusting the gastric pH and coating gastric mucosa. Antihistamines modulate the excessive over-stimulation in the balance center (see Motion Sickness, p. 63). Phosphorated carbohydrate solution and bismuth subsalicylate are used to treat nausea and vomiting.

PHOSPHORATED CARBOHYDRATE SOLUTION AND BISMUTH SUBSALICYLATE

Pharmacology

Phosphorated carbohydrate solution works locally by adjusting the gastric pH. Bismuth subsalicylates work by coating the gastric mucosa. Both products can relieve nausea associated with the stomach upset caused by the stomach flu or overindulgence or indiscretions with food or beverage. There are limited data documenting the effectiveness of these agents in the treatment of nausea and vomiting.

Side Effects

Diarrhea is the main side effect, often occurring with large doses of either phosphorated carbohydrate solution or bismuth subsalicylate. Bismuth subsalicylate may cause the mouth, tongue, and stool to appear darkened (gray-black or black) temporarily.

Drug Interactions

Pepto-Bismol contains nonaspirin salicylates. Salicylates should be used with caution in patients who take warfarin (Coumadin), because they may increase bleeding tendencies. Salicylates can also interact with some medications used in the treatment of diabetes and gout (see p. 368).

Lifespan Considerations

Geriatric

There are no special considerations for the use of these agents in the elderly.

Pediatric

Emetrol is considered safe for use in children. Pepto-Bismol can be given to children 3 years of age and older. However, Pepto-Bismol should be avoided in children (of any age) and teenagers who have or are recovering from chickenpox or flu. Aspirin-like medications have been linked to Reye's syndrome, a rare but serious illness associated with viral infections.

Pregnancy

Bismuth subsalicylate is an FDA Pregnancy Category C drug. There are no data on phosphorated carbohydrate. Although the risk of toxicity when using bismuth subsalicylate is relatively small, significant adverse effects to the fetus have resulted from chronic exposure to salicylates in general.

Nursing Mothers

The American Academy of Pediatrics recommends that salicylates be used cautiously during nursing. There are limited or no data concerning the use of bismuth subsalicylate while nursing.

Patient Education

- Patients should seek professional medical advice for continuous (more than 2 days) stomach discomfort and/or nausea and vomiting.
- Patients should consult a health care professional if symptoms are accompanied by a high fever.
- If the patient is disorientated or confused, complains of a headache, or experienced a recent trauma and is experiencing nausea and vomiting, contact medical help immediately.
- Nonpharmacologic measures should be taken to prevent nausea and vomiting, including avoidance of excessive or disagreeable foods or beverages and sudden motion changes (e.g., roller coaster rides).
- The patient should never dilute phosphorated carbohydrate solution or drink fluids of any kind immediately before or 15 minutes after taking a dose.
- Bismuth subsalicylate may cause the mouth, tongue, and stool to appear darkened (gray-black or black) temporarily. Inform patients to

be aware of this darkening of the stool compared with the changes that occur with melena.

Product Selection

- Phosphorated carbohydrate solution has a high sugar content. Patients who are diabetic and/or intolerant to fructose/glucose items should be closely monitored.
- Antacids may be used to provide gastrointestinal relief of symptoms associated with hyperacidity caused by nausea and vomiting.

Product Information: Nausea and Vomiting

Brand Name	Ingredient	Adult Dose	Pediatric Dose
Emetrol*	Phosphorated carbohydrated solution; each 5 ml contains dextrose 1.87 g, levulose 1.87 g, phosphoric acid 21.5 mg	15-30 ml (1-2 tbsp) at 15-minute intervals, as needed, until symptoms subside	5-10 ml (1-2 tsp) at 15-minute intervals, as needed, until symptoms subside; do not take for more than 1 hour (5 doses total)
Pepto-Bismol Maximum Strength liquid	Bismuth subsalicylate 525 mg/15 ml	30 ml (2 tbsp or 1 dose cup) Repeat dosage every 60 minutes, as needed, to maximum of 4 doses/day	3-6 years: 5 ml (1 tsp or ⅙ dose cup) 6-9 years: 10 ml (2 tsp or ⅓ dose cup) 9-12 years: 15 ml (1 tbsp or ½ dose cup) Repeat dosage every 60 minutes, as needed, to maximum of 4 doses/day
Pepto-Bismol original liquid	Bismuth subsalicylate original liquid 262 mg/15 ml	30 ml (2 tbsp or 1 dose cup) Repeat dosage every 30-60 minutes, as needed, to maximum of 8 doses/day	3-6 years: 5 ml (1 tsp or ⅙ dose cup) 6-9 years: 10 ml (2 tsp or ⅓ dose cup) 9-12 years: 15 ml (1 tbsp or ½ dose cup) Repeat every 30-60 minutes, as needed, to a maximum of 8 doses/day
Pepto-Bismol tablets and caplets	Bismuth subsalicylate 262 mg	2 tablets/caplets Repeat dosage every 30-60 minutes, as needed, to maximum of 8 doses/day	3-6 years: ⅓ tablet/caplet 6-9 years: ⅔ tablet/caplet 9-12 years: 1 tablet/caplet

*Contains high sugar content.

Pinworms

Pinworm (*Enterobius vermicularis*) infections are considered the most frequent helminth infections in humans. Pinworm infestation occurs most often in preschool- and school-age children. The route of transmission is fecal-oral, and perineal pruritus is a common manifestation of this infection. Although pinworm infestation is often considered to be more bothersome than a cause of serious disease, treatment of infected individuals, as well as family members, is necessary for eradication. Anthelmintics are used to treat pinworms.

ANTHELMINTICS

PYRANTEL PAMOATE

Pharmacology

Pyrantel pamoate is used for the self-medication of pinworm infection. Pyrantel pamoate is a neuromuscular blocking agent and exerts its anthelmintic (worm killing) effect by spastic paralysis of the worm. The paralyzed worms are subsequently expelled from the gastrointestinal tract. The use of pyrantel pamoate for helminthic infections other than pinworm should be done only under the instruction/supervision of a health care professional.

Side Effects

The most frequent side effects are nausea, vomiting, diarrhea, and abdominal cramping. Less frequent side effects include headache, dizziness, rash, drowsiness, and transient increases in transaminase concentrations.

Drug Interactions

Pyrantel pamoate and piperazine have antagonistic mechanisms of action and should not be used concomitantly.

Lifespan Considerations

Geriatric
There are no unique recommendations for the elderly population.

Pediatric
Safety and efficacy of pyrantel pamoate have not been established for children younger than 2 years of age. Consider risk versus benefit when treating a patient younger than 2 years of age.

Pregnancy
Pyrantel pamoate is an FDA Pregnancy Category C drug. Treatment with pyrantel pamoate should be delayed until after delivery unless the benefit clearly outweighs the risk to the fetus. Pregnant women should not consider self-medication with pyrantel pamoate without first consulting a health care professional.

Nursing Mothers
There are no data available in this population.

Patient Education

- Pyrantel pamoate may be taken with or without food at any time of the day.
- The liquid forms of the drug may be mixed in milk or juice. If the suspension form is selected, the patient should be sure to shake well before use.
- Before patients self-medicate with pyrantel pamoate, visual presence of pinworms should be confirmed.
- For self-medication of pinworm infections, one dose only is necessary. A repeat dose 14 days later should be undertaken only under the instruction of a health care professional.
- Other family members are likely to become infected if one child is infected, therefore it is necessary to treat the entire family simultaneously.
- Because the primary route of infection is fecal-oral, careful handwashing after defecation is necessary. Eggs can remain infective in an indoor environment for 2 to 3 weeks and can be spread from infested clothes and bedding. Laundering bed clothes and linens daily disinfects them and helps reduce the incidence of reinfection.
- Families should understand the importance of hygienic measures, but excessive attention in this area may induce feelings of guilt and will be counterproductive.

SUGGESTED READINGS

Hamblin J, Connor PD: Pinworms in pregnancy, J Am Board Fam Pract 8(4):321-323, 1995.

Hospital for Tropical Disease, London: Enterobius vermicularis infection, Gut 35: 1159-1162, 1994.

Product Information: Pinworms

Brand Name*	Dosage Form	Adult/Pediatric Dosage
Antiminth	50 mg/ml (suspension)	11 mg/kg once; max dose is 1 g
Pin-Rid	50 mg/ml (liquid)	11 mg/kg once; max dose is 1 g
	180 mg (capsule)	
Pin-X	50 mg/ml (liquid)	11 mg/kg once; max dose is 1 g
Reese's Pinworm	50 mg/ml (liquid)	11 mg/kg once; max dose is 1 g
	180 mg (capsule)	

*The ingredient in each product listed is pyrantel pamoate.

Acne

In response to the rising hormone levels occurring at puberty, the sebaceous glands increase in size and activity, causing increased production of sebum. Sebum is carried to the skin surface through pores. When pores become clogged with oils, skin, and dirt, the outflow of sebum is obstructed. Bacteria, particularly *Propionibacterium acnes* (P. *acnes*) produce enzymes that break sebum down into short-chain fatty acids. These fatty acids cause irritation and "pimples."

Keratolytics and benzoyl peroxides are used in the treatment of mild to moderate acne.

KERATOLYTICS AND BENZOYL PEROXIDE

Pharmacology

Keratolytics remove keratin and dry, dead skin, helping to get rid of comedones (whiteheads and blackheads) and preventing new pimples from forming by unblocking pores. Salicylic acid, sulfur, and resorcinol are examples of keratolytics. Keratolytics used in products in combinations may have synergistic activity. Benzoyl peroxide has antibacterial activity, especially against P. *acnes*, the most common organism found in comedones. In addition to its antibacterial effect on P. *acnes*, benzoyl peroxide causes irritation and sloughing of dry, dead skin and has a drying action that helps remove excess oil.

Side Effects

These products can cause itching, dryness, and reddening of the skin, especially when used simultaneously with other topical agents. Benzoyl peroxide may also cause bleaching of the hair, clothes, and linens.

Drug Interactions

There are no clinically significant drug interactions with either keratolytics or benzoyl peroxide.

Lifespan Considerations

Pediatric

Acne is primarily associated with patients ≤18 years of age. The onset of puberty is associated with the onset of acne.

Pregnancy

Benzoyl peroxide and keratolytics are considered safe for use in pregnant women because the drugs are not absorbed in appreciable amounts.

Nursing Mothers

Data are not available regarding the presence of these agents in breast milk, but given the fact that they are topical agents, their use during breastfeeding should not pose a risk to the infant.

Patient Education

- An important step in preventing/treating acne is proper skin cleansing. The affected areas should be washed at least twice daily using soap, warm water, and a soft washcloth. The area should be patted dry, and the product used to treat acne should be applied.
- These products should be kept away from the eyes, mouth, lips, and nose because these mucous tissues can become irritated.
- These products are for external use only.
- Individuals may need to be counseled on proper scalp and hair care.
- Cosmetics may contribute to blocking of pores, aggravating acne. If cosmetics are to be used on the affected area, water-based cosmetics are preferred.
- Avoid other sources of skin irritation, such as excessive sunlight, sunlamps, or application of facial products containing perfumes.
- These products may cause a feeling of warmth or stinging when initially applied.
- The patient should allow 4 to 6 weeks of continued treatment before evaluating the therapeutic effects of these agents. Patients may even notice an exacerbation of acne with the initiation of therapy.
- Use of benzoyl peroxide should be initiated beginning with lower concentrations for short periods (15 to 30 minutes), gradually increas-

ing the concentration and time (by 15-minute increments) the product is kept on the affected areas. When it can be tolerated for 2 hours, it can be left on the skin overnight.

- Benzoyl peroxide may bleach hair and colored fabric.

Product Selection

- If acne is severe or is associated with scarring, use of nonprescription products should be discontinued in favor of more potent prescription medications as directed by a health care professional.
- Benzoyl peroxide is widely used and effective in the treatment of acne. However, in 1991, the Advisory Review Panel of the OTC Antimicrobial Drug Panel of the FDA labeled benzoyl peroxide as being under "nonmonograph conditions" or Category III. The "nonmonograph conditions" label is attributed to either lack of sufficient data or documented information concerning efficacy and safety. Benzoyl peroxide received this label as a result of reports and studies that identified a safety concern regarding benzoyl peroxide as a tumor promoter in mice. The final determination of benzoyl peroxide safety requires further investigation.
- Medicated products are available as creams, lotions, gels, liquid cleansers, and bar soaps. Creams and lotions are recommended for use in patients with dry or sensitive skin. Gels, in general, have the ability to remain on the skin for a longer duration. Water-based gels dry slowly and completely, whereas gels and liquids containing alcohol dry rapidly.
- If these nonprescription products are not producing the desired results, prescription products, such as oral or topical antibiotics and/or isotretinoin, may be necessary.

SUGGESTED READINGS

Stern RS: Acne therapy: medication use and sources of care in office-based practices, *Arch Dermatol* 132:776-780, 1996.

Sykes NL Jr, Webster GF: Acne: a review of optimum treatment, *Drugs* 48(1):59-70, 1994.

Product Information: Acne*

Brand Name	Ingredient	Dosage	Comments
Acnomel	Sulfur 8% and resorcinol 2%	Use once or twice daily	
Benoxyl	Benzoyl peroxide 5% or 10%	Use once or twice daily	
Clearasil	Salicylic acid 1.25% or 2%	Use one to three times daily as tolerated	Available as *Clearstick Regular Strength, Clearstick Maximum Strength,* or *Double Clear Maximum Strength Pads*
Clearasil Adult Care	Sulfur and resorcinol	Use once or twice daily	
Clearasil Maximum Strength	Benzoyl peroxide 10%	Use once or twice daily	Available as a cream, lotion, and cleanser
Fostex 10%	Benzoyl peroxide 10%	Use once or twice daily	
Neutrogena	Benzoyl peroxide 2.5%	Use once or twice daily	
Neutrogena Acne Mask	Benzoyl peroxide 5%	Initially apply once daily, gradually increase to two or three times daily as needed	
Noxema Pads	Salicylic acid 2%	Use one to three times daily as tolerated	
Oxy 10	Benzoyl peroxide 10%	Use once or twice daily	
Oxy 10 Balance	Benzoyl peroxide 10%	Use once or twice daily	

Product	Ingredient	Directions	Notes
Oxy 10 Maximum Strength Advanced	Benzoyl peroxide 10%	Use once or twice daily	Oxy Medicated Cleanser and Pads contains salicylic acid
Oxy 5 Advanced Formula for Sensitive Skin	Benzoyl peroxide 5%	Use once or twice daily	Gel
Oxy Balance	Benzoyl peroxide 5%	Use once or twice daily	Available as pads and face-cleansing wash
Oxy Balance	Salicylic acid 2%	Use one to three times daily as tolerated	
Oxy Balance (Deep Action Night Formula)	Benzoyl peroxide 2.5%	Use once or twice daily	
Persa	Benzoyl peroxide 5% or 10%	Use once or twice daily	
PROPA pH	Salicylic acid 0.5% or 2%	Use one to three times daily as tolerated	Available as *Cleansing Lotion for Normal/Combination Skin, Cleansing Pads, Cleansing for Oily Skin Lotion,* or *Acne Maximum Strength Cream*
Stridex Clear Gel	Salicylic acid 2%	Use one to three times daily as tolerated	Available as pads in different strengths

*This product table does not contain liquid cleansers or bar soaps. NOTE: Generic benzoyl peroxide products available; please read individual product ingredients and directions for proper use.

Alopecia

Alopecia (hair loss) can be divided into two types, scarring or nonscarring. Scarring is associated with a loss of hair follicles and is often irreversible. In nonscarring alopecia, the hair shafts are gone but the hair follicles are preserved and hair growth may recur. In addition, alopecia may be due to a variety of causes. OTC products used to treat alopecia focus on the alopecia subtype known as *androgenetic alopecia*, defined as male pattern baldness (baldness of the vertex of the scalp) and in females as thinning or hair loss of the frontoparietal areas.

The nonprescription drug used in the treatment of androgenetic alopecia is minoxidil.

MINOXIDIL

Pharmacology

Minoxidil was originally marketed as an oral prescription medication for treatment of hypertension, possessing activity as a vasodilator. When it was discovered that minoxidil also causes hair growth, the drug was subsequently marketed as a topical product for the treatment of androgenetic alopecia. Although the exact mechanism of minoxidil in the treatment of alopecia is unknown, the vasodilating effects may be the mechanism by which it is effective.

Side Effects

When taken orally, minoxidil causes tachycardia and fluid/salt retention, which require concurrent use of diuretics and sympatholytics. The systemic bioavailability of topical minoxidil is not typically sufficient to cause cardiovascular side effects. Absorption may be increased in cases where the scalp is injured, such as sunburn or psoriasis. Minoxidil may cause irritation to the scalp in the form of dryness, itching, and erythema. The 5% solution may be more irritating than the 2% solution, and this may be caused by an increased concentration of propylene glycol in the 5% solution versus less in the 2% solution. Irritant contact dermatitis occurs more frequently than allergic dermatitis. Hypertrichosis, the growth of vellus hair in areas where it is not wanted (such as the face), may occur if the drug comes in contact with these areas. This side effect may take months to subside when it occurs and may be particularly bothersome for women.

Drug Interactions

Some topical agents, including topical steroids, retinoids, and petrolatum, may increase the absorption of minoxidil and could potentially lead to systemic effects involving the cardiovascular system (e.g., hypotension and tachycardia). This would be more significant in patients with preexisting cardiovascular disease and those receiving drugs for treatment of hypertension.

Lifespan Considerations

Geriatric

Patients with preexisting cardiovascular disease should be monitored for evidence of systemic effects of minoxidil (i.e., tachycardia, fluid and water retention), although these effects would be expected to be rare.

Pediatric

Minoxidil is not recommended for use in patients under the age of 18 years.

Pregnancy

Topical minoxidil is an FDA Pregnancy Category C drug and is not recommended for use during pregnancy.

Nursing Mothers

Topical minoxidil is not recommended for use in women who are breastfeeding. Minoxidil is excreted in breast milk.

Patient Education

- The usual dose of minoxidil is 1 ml of solution applied twice daily to the scalp. Applying the product more frequently or in large doses does not speed up hair growth and may increase the chance of side effects.
- Minoxidil will not work for everyone. It is not effective in patients with hair loss caused by severe nutritional problems, drug-induced hair loss (including both prescription and nonprescription medications), low thyroid states, or diseases that cause scarring of the scalp.

- Hair should be shampooed once daily. Minoxidil is applied after shampooing and when the hair and scalp are completely dry.
- At first, the hair growth may be soft, colorless hairs. After continued minoxidil use, the new hair should be the same color and thickness as the other hairs on the scalp.
- Patients should avoid having minoxidil come into contact with the eyes, nose, and mouth, as well as areas where hair growth is not desired.
- After applying the drug, patients should wash hands thoroughly to remove any excess drug so that unintentional exposure can be minimized. The solution should also be allowed to dry after application and before going to bed.
- For maximal effects, minoxidil should remain on the scalp for about 4 hours before wetting the hair, washing the hair, and/or swimming.
- Minoxidil is not a cure for hair loss and will not support hair growth if use is discontinued. If treatment is discontinued before therapy is completed, the new hair will be lost within a few months.
- Irritation and inflammation of the scalp, such as occurs with sunburn, could cause increased minoxidil penetration and thus increase the possibility of systemic side effects.
- If the 5% solution of minoxidil causes scalp irritation, treatment may be resumed with the 2% solution provided the reaction was not of an allergic nature.
- Use of larger doses or more frequent applications has not shown any quicker results; on the contrary, side effects may be more prevalent.
- It is not known if the effects of minoxidil will persist after completing the therapy course. There are some reports that indicate hair loss and balding return 3 to 4 months after cessation of minoxidil application.

Product Selection

- Use of 5% minoxidil may achieve more rapid hair growth compared with use of 2% minoxidil (8 weeks versus 16 weeks, respectively). The 5% strength is approved by the FDA for use only by men, though it is marketed for use by women in other countries.
- 2% minoxidil should be used in patients unable to tolerate 5% minoxidil (e.g., if irritation occurs). If skin irritation is severe, use of the 5% solution should be discontinued before resumption of therapy with the weaker strength.
- Rogaine Regular Strength for Men and Rogaine for Women contain the same concentration (2%) of minoxidil.

SUGGESTED READING

Roberts JL: Androgenetic alopecia in men and women: an overview of cause and
treatment, *Dermatol Nurs* 9:379-386, 1997.

Product Information: Alopecia

Brand Name*	Ingredients	Comments
Rogaine Regular Strength for Men	Minoxidil 2%	May take up to 4 months to see results; up to 12 months may be needed to see best results
Rogaine Extra Strength For Men	Minoxidil 5%	May take up to 2 months to see results; may take up to 4 months to see best results
Rogaine for Women	Minoxidil 2%	May take up to 4 months to see results; up to 8 months may be needed to see best results

*Directions for use: Apply 1 ml twice daily, every day, directly onto the scalp in the
hair-loss area.

Bacterial Infections

OTC topical antibiotics are useful treatment options for infections that involve the epidermis or papillary dermis. The antibiotic is applied directly to the infection, thus providing high local concentrations with minimal systemic effects. For infections that involve the lower dermis or subcutis, topical antibiotics may not penetrate these areas sufficiently, requiring the use of prescription systemic antibiotics.

ANTIBIOTICS

BACITRACIN
NEOMYCIN
POLYMYXIN B

Pharmacology

Three topical antibiotics are used widely in OTC combinations: bacitracin, neomycin, and polymyxin B. Bacitracin is a polypeptide antibiotic and works by inhibiting cell-wall synthesis. Bacitracin's spectrum of activity is primarily limited to gram-positive organisms, such as staphylococci, streptococci, corynebacteria, and clostridia. Neomycin is an aminoglycoside antibiotic. Neomycin inhibits protein synthesis by binding to the bacteria ribosome, leading to misreading of the genetic code. Neomycin may also be involved with the inhibition of the bacterial DNA polymerase. Neomycin's spectrum of activity includes gram-positive organisms, including some species of staphylococci, and gram-negative organisms, including *Escherichia coli* (E. *coli*) and *Haemophilus influenzae* (H. *influenzae*). Polymyxin B is a branched cyclic decapeptide that destroys bacterial membranes. The spectrum of activity of polymyxin B is mainly limited to gram-negative organisms. Combinations of bacitracin, neomycin, and/or polymyxin B are often used because they provide broad coverage against most topical bacterial infections.

Side Effects

Side effects of topical antibiotics are most often local and can include skin irritation, pruritus, and edema. Contact sensitization may occur. Chronic application of neomycin, especially on damaged skin or wounds in patients with contact dermatitis and chronic dermatoses, may increase the risk of sensitization and systemic toxicity. Although rare, patients with renal dysfunction may develop further nephrotoxicity and/or ototoxicity if large quantities of topical neomycin are absorbed systemically.

Drug Interactions

Because of limited systemic absorption, there are no clinically significant drug interactions with topical antibiotics.

Lifespan Considerations

Geriatric
There are no unique recommendations in the elderly population.

Pediatric
There are no unique recommendations for the pediatric population.

Pregnancy
Bacitracin and neomycin are FDA Pregnancy Category C drugs. Polymyxin B is a category B drug. There have been reported cases of teratogenicity when these agents are used topically in pregnant women.

Nursing Mothers
There are no data available on the distribution of these agents in breast milk.

Patient Education

- Proper cleansing of the affected area is important for eradicating the infection. Proper cleansing includes using soap and water, with or without hydrogen peroxide, and covering the affected area with clean bandages if necessary.
- OTC topical antibiotics should only be used in superficial and uncomplicated infections. If the infection involves lower dermis and/or does not show improvement within 3 to 7 days, the patient should be referred to a health care professional.
- These agents should not be used for more than 7 days.
- A health care professional should be contacted if the affected area becomes inflamed or painful, or if pus is present.

- Topical antibiotics should not be used in the eyes, nose, mouth, or mucous membranes unless instructed on the individual product label.
- Patients should wash their hands before applying the topical antibiotic to the affected area; touching the tip of the medication apparatus to the affected area should also be avoided to prevent contamination of the medication.
- Topical antibiotics should not be used with deep or puncture wounds, animal bites, or serious burns without seeking the advice of a health care professional.

Product Selection

- Neomycin should not be used for an extended length of time, on large affected areas, or in patients with damaged skin. Bacitracin and polymyxin B are in general more widely recommended than neomycin.
- Comparative studies showing the efficacy of topical antibiotics are limited. These agents should be used for minor cuts, scrapes, and burns. For serious skin infections, contact a health care professional.

SUGGESTED READINGS

Tunkel AR: Topical antibacterials. In Mandell GL, Bennett JE, Dolin R, editors: *Principles and practice of infectious diseases*, ed 4, New York, 1995, Churchill Livingstone, pp. 381-389.

Winkleman W, Gratton D: Topical antibacterials, *Clin Dermatol* 7:156-162, 1989.

Product Information: Topical Antibiotics

Brand Name	Dosage Form	Ingredient	Comments
Baciguent	Ointment	Bacitracin 500 units/g	Available from various manufacturers
Bacitracin	Ointment	Bacitracin 500 units/g	Contains 10 mg diperodon
Bactine First Aid Antibiotic Plus Anesthetic	Ointment	Bacitracin 400 units/g; neomycin 3.5 mg/g; polymyxin B 5000 units/g	
Campho-Phenique Antibiotic Plus Pain Reliever	Ointment	Bacitracin 500 units/g; neomycin 3.5 mg/g; polymyxin B 5000 units/g	Contains 40 mg lidocaine
Clomycin	Ointment	Bacitracin 500 units/g; neomycin 3.5 mg/g; polymyxin B 5000 units/g	Contains 40 mg lidocaine
Lanabiotic	Ointment	Bacitracin 500 units/g; neomycin 3.5 mg/g; polymyxin B 10,000 units/g	Contains 40 mg lidocaine
Maximum Strength Mycitracin Triple Antibiotic	Ointment	Bacitracin 500 units/g; neomycin 3.5 mg/g; polymyxin B 5000 units/g	
Maximum Strength Neosporin	Ointment	Bacitracin 500 units/g; neomycin 3.5 mg/g; polymyxin B 10,000 units/g	
Medi-Quick	Ointment	Bacitracin 400 units/g; neomycin 3.5 mg/g; polymyxin B 5000 units/g	
Myciguent	Ointment and cream	Neomycin 3.5 mg/g	
Mycitracin	Ointment	Bacitracin 500 units/g; neomycin 3.5 mg/g; polymyxin B 5000 units/g	
Mycitracin Plus	Ointment	Bacitracin 500 units/g; neomycin 3.5 mg/g; polymyxin B 5000 units/g	Contains 40 mg lidocaine

Product	Form	Composition	Notes
N.B.P.	Ointment	Bacitracin 400 units/g; neomycin 3.5 mg/g; 5000 units/g	
Neomixin	Ointment	Bacitracin 400 units/g; neomycin 3.5 mg/g; 5000 units/g	Available from various manufacturers
Neomycin	Ointment	Neomycin 3.5 mg/g	
Neosporin	Cream	Neomycin 3.5 mg/g; polymyxin B 10,000 units/g	
Neosporin	Ointment	Bacitracin 400 units/g; neomycin 3.5 mg/g; polymyxin B 5000 units/g	
Neosporin Maximum Strength Plus Pain Relief	Cream and ointment	Neomycin 3.5 mg/g; polymyxin B 10,000 units/g	Contains 10 mg pramoxine
Polysporin	Ointment and powder	Bacitracin 500 units/g; polymyxin B 10,000 units/g	
Polysporin	Spray	Bacitracin 111 units/ml; polymyxin B 2222 units/ml	
Septa	Ointment	Bacitracin 400 units/g; neomycin 3.5 mg/g; polymyxin B 5000 units/g	
Spectrocin Plus	Ointment	Bacitracin 400 units/g; neomycin 3.5 mg/g; polymyxin B 5000 units/g	Contains 5 mg lidocaine
Triple Antibiotic	Ointment	Bacitracin 400 units/g; neomycin 3.5 mg/g; polymyxin B 5000 units/g	Available from various manufacturers

*Directions for use: Clean affected area and apply a small amount (equal to the surface area of a fingertip) to the area 1 to 3 times daily. Cover with sterile bandage if desired. Do not use for longer than 1 week.

Contact Dermatitis

Dermatitis is a general term referring to inflammation or irritation of the skin. When dermatitis is induced by contact with an external agent, it is called *contact dermatitis*. Basically, an external agent, such as an allergen, insect bite, poison ivy, or sunburn, may trigger the skin to become irritated and itch. Avoidance of the external causative factors is important in the treatment of contact dermatitis. However, once contact dermatitis has occurred, OTC agents may be helpful in the treatment of symptoms associated with contact dermatitis. This chapter will focus on general contact dermatitis and poison ivy. Sunburn will be discussed in more detail beginning on p. 150.

Drugs used to treat contact dermatitis include antihistamines, local anesthetics, topical steroids, and astringents.

TOPICAL ANTIHISTAMINES

DIPHENHYDRAMINE

Pharmacology

Antihistamines competitively inhibit histamine receptors, which prevents histamine from stimulating the receptor and causing an allergic reaction. Pruritus must be histamine mediated for antihistamines to work. Topical antihistamines are poorly absorbed and exhibit some local anesthetic activity. See Allergy, p. 187 for complete information on oral antihistamines.

Side Effects

In general, these products are well tolerated. Side effects of topical antihistamines can include local irritation and sensitization. Sensitization from topical antihistamine use occurs from repeated application of the antihistamine and can result in eczema, inflammation, photosensitivity, and pruritus at the site of application. Sensitization reactions are more likely to occur with prolonged use of topical antihistamines. Toxic psychosis has been reported, specifically in children.

Drug Interactions

No clinically significant drug interactions have been noted.

Lifespan Considerations

Geriatric

There are no unique recommendations for use of topical antihistamines in the elderly population.

Pediatric

Topical antihistamines should be used cautiously in children and are not recommended for children under the age of 6 years without first consulting a health care professional. Toxic psychosis, particularly in children, has been reported when topical antibiotics are used to treat certain skin disorders.

Patient Education

- Topical antihistamines are for external use only. Patients should avoid using these products around the eyes and other mucous membranes and on raw, oozing, or blistered areas on the skin.
- Topical antihistamines should not be used for more than 7 days. If symptoms persist or recur, or if a hypersensitivity reaction results, a physician should be consulted.

Product Selection

- Use of topical antihistamines is generally discouraged because of the potential for sensitivity (eczema, inflammation, photosensitivity, and pruritus) reactions.
- Topical and oral antihistamines used in combination should be discouraged.
- Oral antihistamines are more effective for histamine-mediated pruritus and are less likely to cause sensitivity reactions than topical antihistamines.
- Oral antihistamines should be considered for the treatment of severe contact dermatitis.

Product Information: Topical Antihistamines

Brand Name	Dosage Form	Active Ingredient	Adult Dose	Pediatric Dose	Comments
Benadryl Original	Cream, spray	Diphenhydramine 1%, zinc acetate 0.1%	Apply to affected area 3-4 times daily	For children <2 years of age, consult a physician	May cause sensitization reactions
Benadryl Extra Strength	Cream, spray, gel, stick	Diphenhydramine 2%, zinc acetate 0.1%	Apply to affected area 3-4 times daily	For children <6 years of age, consult a physician	May cause sensitization reactions
Dermarest Plus	Gel	Diphenhydramine 2%, menthol 1%	Apply to affected area 3-4 times daily	For children <2 years of age, consult a physician	

LOCAL ANESTHETICS

BENZOCAINE

BUTAMBEN PICRATE

DIBUCAINE

LIDOCAINE

TETRACAINE

PRAMOXINE

Pharmacology

Local anesthetics reversibly inhibit conduction of nerve impulses from sensory nerves by altering cell membrane permeability to sodium ions. This results in a temporary loss of feeling or sensation near the site of application of the drug on the body.

Side Effects

Side effects are rare; however, when they do occur they often result from excessive application of the drug, rapid absorption, decreased tolerance, or hypersensitivity. Minor local skin irritation, stinging, or burning can occur on application. Adverse events resulting from excessive application of the drug or rapid absorption may affect the central nervous system (CNS) or cardiovascular system. Though rare, systemic symptoms may include dizziness, nausea, drowsiness, speech disturbances, perioral numbness, muscle twitching, confusion, vertigo, and tinnitus.

Drug Interactions

No clinically significant drug interactions have been noted.

Lifespan Considerations

Geriatric

There are no unique recommendations for use in the elderly population.

Pediatric

Benzocaine is not indicated for infants under the age of 1 year, and the safety and efficacy of tetracaine has not been determined in children under the age of 12 years.

Pregnancy

Benzocaine, dibucaine, pramoxine, and tetracaine are all FDA Pregnancy Category C drugs. Lidocaine is a category B drug. The use of topical local anesthetics is only recommended when the potential benefits clearly outweigh the risks to the fetus.

Nursing Mothers

Some topical anesthetics have been excreted in breast milk; therefore nursing mothers should exercise caution when using these medications.

Patient Education

- Topical anesthetics are for external use only. They should not be used in or around the eyes.
- These products will provide pain relief for 15 to 45 minutes.
- Patients need to wash their hands thoroughly after applying topical anesthetics.
- Scratching, rubbing, or irritating the affected area should be avoided.
- The patient should use only the minimum dose necessary to achieve the desired effect to avoid potential side effects.
- Any patient who experiences a hypersensitivity reaction to any of these products should discontinue treatment and consult a health care professional immediately.

Product Selection

- Long-term use of any of these products is not recommended. If symptoms persist, worsen, or clear up but return after 7 days, the patient should consult a health care professional.
- Frequent application of lidocaine may result in systemic absorption and toxicity.
- Patients who experience benzocaine sensitivity may try either lidocaine or dibucaine as an alternative treatment. Benzocaine is an ester anesthetic, whereas lidocaine and dibucaine are amide anesthetics. Cross-sensitivity between the amide and ester anesthetics is rare. If sensitivity to an amide anesthetic occurs, use of that product should be discontinued immediately.

Product Information: Topical Local Anesthetics

Brand Name*	Dosage Form	Active Ingredient	Comments
Bicozene	Cream	Benzocaine 6%	
Americaine	Spray	Benzocaine 20%	
Americaine	Ointment	Benzocaine 20%	
Caladryl	Lotion, cream	Calamine 8%, pramoxine 1%	For clear lotion, SHAKE WELL
Medi-Quik	Spray	Benzocaine 20%	
Solarcaine	Spray	Benzocaine 20%	
Itch-X	Gel	Benzyl alcohol 10%, pramoxine HCL 1%	Not for application to open wounds or damaged skin
	Spray	Benzyl alcohol 10%, pramoxine HCL 1%	

*Adult and pediatric doses/instructions are the same. Apply to affected area 3 to 4 times daily.

TOPICAL CORTICOSTEROIDS

HYDROCORTISONE

Pharmacology

Inflammation occurs from the release of inflammatory mediators such as prostaglandins, kinins, histamines, and liposomal enzymes. These inflammatory mediators increase vascular permeability and vasodilation. Topical corticosteroids induce phospholipase A_2 inhibitory proteins, which diminish the activity of the inflammatory mediators. Topical application of corticosteroids to inflamed skin reverses vascular dilation and permeability, thus inhibiting leukocytes and macrophage accumulation. The inhibition results in decreased inflammation and decreased pruritus.

Side Effects

In general, topical corticosteroids are well-tolerated. Local side effects are primarily dermatologic. Some of these effects include pruritus, burning, erythema, irritation, secondary infection, dryness, and tightening of the skin. Occlusion of the affected area enhances corticosteroid absorption but also increases the risk of local and systemic adverse events. Side effects occur less frequently when low-potency versus high-potency corticosteroids are used. Side effects are more likely to occur with prolonged use. Nonprescription corticosteroids are of low potency; therefore side effects are rare with their use.

Drug Interactions

There are no clinically significant drug interactions.

Lifespan Considerations

Geriatric

Patients with liver failure may be at greater risk for systemic effects of topical corticosteroids; however, in general, dosages do not need to be altered in the elderly population.

Pediatric

Diaper rash is a common type of contact dermatitis seen in infants. Topical corticosteroids should not be used to treat diaper rash except under the guidance of a health care professional. The use of tight-fitting diapers or plastic pants should be avoided while topical corticosteroids are used in the diaper area because of their occlusive potential and increased risk of hydrocortisone absorption.

Pregnancy

Topical corticosteroids are FDA Pregnancy Category C drugs. When topical corticosteroid use is necessary in pregnancy, it should be limited to small amounts for short periods.

Nursing Mothers

It is unknown whether topical corticosteroids are systemically absorbed enough to be excreted in breast milk. Systemic corticosteroids have not been shown to be excreted in breast milk.

Patient Education

- Patients should sparingly apply enough topical corticosteroid to cover the affected area, but should not over apply. Use of more topical corticosteroid has not been shown to be any more effective in treating pruritus.
- Cleansing the affected area before application of a topical corticosteroid may help prevent infection from occurring and may increase drug penetration. If infection occurs, topical corticosteroid use should be

discontinued and topical antiinfective therapy considered. For serious infections, a health care professional should be consulted.

- Patients should avoid using occlusive dressings with topical corticosteroids unless directed to do so by a health care professional.
- Topical corticosteroids should not be used in the eyes; prolonged use around the eyes or other mucous membranes should be avoided.
- Topical corticosteroid use must be discontinued if edema, burning, or worsening of the affected site occurs after application, and a health care professional should be consulted.
- Long-term use of any of these products is not recommended. If symptoms persist, worsen, or clear up but return after 7 days, the patient should consult a health care professional.

Product Selection

- Topical hydrocortisone is the drug of choice for contact dermatitis covering a small surface area of skin because nonprescription-strength hydrocortisone is relatively safe and effective.
- For severe contact dermatitis, higher-potency topical prescription corticosteroids, such as fluocinonide, betamethasone, and clobetasol propionate, may be prescribed by a health care professional.
- Ointments are preferred for dry lesions, whereas creams are preferred for use on oozing lesions because creams tend to have a drying effect. Ointments are usually more potent than creams; however, some products have equal potency.
- Topical corticosteroid potency is also determined by the concentration of the drug used. This is expressed as a percentage (e.g., hydrocortisone 1%) and indicates the amount of drug distributed throughout the medication. The maximum strength of hydrocortisone available without a prescription is 1%.

Product Information: Topical Corticosteroids

Brand Name*	Dosage Form	Active Ingredient
Bactine Hydrocortisone	Cream	Hydrocortisone 0.5%
Cortagel	Gel	Hydrocortisone 1%
Cortaid	Ointment, cream, fast stick	Hydrocortisone 1%
Cortaid with Aloe	Ointment, cream	Hydrocortisone 0.5%
Corticaine (greaseless)	Cream	Hydrocortisone 0.5%
Cortisone 10	Ointment, cream	Hydrocortisone 1%
Cortisone 5	Ointment, cream	Hydrocortisone 0.5%
Cortisone for Kids	Cream	Hydrocortisone 0.5%
Dermolate (greaseless, vanishing)	Cream	Hydrocortisone 0.5%
Dermtex HC with Aloe	Cream	Hydrocortisone 0.5%
Hydro-Tex	Cream	Hydrocortisone 0.5%
Kericort	Cream	Hydrocortisone 1%
Lanacort 10 Creme	Cream	Hydrocortisone 1%
Lanacort 5	Ointment	Hydrocortisone 0.5%
Lanacort 5 Creme	Cream	Hydrocortisone 0.5%
Maximum Strength Bactine	Cream	Hydrocortisone 1%
Maximum Strength Cortaid	Ointment, cream, spray	Hydrocortisone 1%
Tegrin-HC	Ointment	Hydrocortisone 1%

*Apply to affected area 2 to 4 times daily.

ASTRINGENTS

Witch hazel

Aluminum acetate

Tannic acid

Zinc and iron oxides/calamine

Pharmacology

Astringents bind over the surface of lesions and remove debris while they promote drying and relief of pain and itch. These agents are often applied in tepid baths or in cool compresses. Astringents are particularly effective in the treatment of symptoms associated with poison ivy.

Side Effects

Side effects are rare; local irritation may occur.

Drug Interactions

There are no clinically significant drug interactions.

Lifespan Considerations

Geriatric

There are no unique recommendations for use in the elderly population.

Pediatric

There are no unique recommendations for use in the pediatric population.

Patient Education

- Astringents should be diluted and completely dissolved before application to avoid skin irritation or damage.
- For dressings, a clean, soft, white cloth should be saturated in solution and loosely applied to the affected area.
- Dressings should not be covered with plastic. When dressings begin to dry, they may be soaked again and reapplied.
- A new solution should be prepared for each application.
- Cool or warm water provides the greatest relief from itching. Use of hot water increases itching as a result of vasodilation and blood flow to the area.
- The affected area may be soaked for 15 to 30 minutes in the astringent solution; after soaking, the solution must be discarded.
- If symptoms persist or recur after 7 days, the patient should discontinue therapy and consult a health care professional.
- Astringents are for external use only. Use in or around the eyes should be avoided.

Product Selection

Aluminum acetate (Burow's) solution is diluted with water to a 1:10 or 1:40 dilution. The solution must be properly diluted to avoid skin irritation. Use of Burow's solution for more than 7 days may result in inflammation.

Product Information: Other Products

Category	Product Information
Colloidal oatmeal	Soothes pruritic skin through emollient properties; effective in treatment of moderate contact dermatitis with bullae and edematous swelling
Counterirritants	Camphor, phenol, and menthol produce a mild local inflammatory reaction at the application site, which decreases sensation and relieves itch
"Shake lotions"	Calamine lotion, which is a combination of zinc oxide and ferrous oxide, relieves itch by absorbing fluid from weeping lesions as it dries to the skin.

POISON IVY

Poison ivy is the name given to the acute skin reaction caused by contact with poison ivy, poison oak, or poison sumac. Urushiol is the chemical contained in the stems, leaves, and roots of these plants that induces an allergic reaction. Very small amounts of urushiol can cause symptoms to occur. Symptoms of poison ivy include erythema, irritation, swelling, and pruritus.

Patient Education

- Contrary to common belief, poison ivy is not spread by scratching.
- Patients should learn to identify and avoid poison ivy and related plants. This is the primary method for prevention of contact with poison ivy.
- Barrier creams may aid in reducing the risk of poison ivy dermatitis; however, their effectiveness is questionable.
- Individuals prone to poison-ivy exposure should wear protective clothing during outings (i.e., long-sleeve shirts and long pants).
- Clothes should be thoroughly laundered with detergent to remove urushiol.
- Any objects that come into contact with poison ivy or related plants should be disinfected with alcohol or other disinfectant product.
- Exposed skin areas should be thoroughly washed with soap and water as soon as possible after exposure to poison ivy has occurred. Washing the affected area within 10 to 15 minutes after contact can reduce the likelihood of developing poison ivy dermatitis.

- Patients should avoid scratching the affected area because this can lead to secondary bacterial infections.
- If oozing is present, greasy ointments should be avoided.
- If the reaction is severe, a health care professional should be consulted.
- None of the products used to treat poison-ivy exposure is indicated for long-term use. If the rash does not improve or recurs after 7 days, a health care professional should be consulted.

SUGGESTED READINGS

Beltrani VS, Beltrani VP: Contact dermatitis, *Ann Allergy Asthma Immunol* 78(2):160-175, 1997.

Drake LA et al: Guidelines of care for contact dermatitis, *J Am Acad Dermatol* 32(1):109-113, 1995.

Williford PM, Sheretz EF: Poison ivy dermatitis: nuances to treatment, *Arch Fam Med* 3(3):184-188, 1994.

Product Information: Poison Ivy

Brand Name*	Ingredient Type	Ingredient
Aveeno Anti-Itch (cream, lotion)	Counterirritant	Camphor 0.3%
	Local anesthetic	Pramoxine 1%
	Astringent	Calamine 3%
Aveeno Bath Powder	Other	Colloidal oatmeal
Caladryl (lotion, spray)	Local anesthetic	Pramoxine 1%
	Astringent	Calamine 8%
Calagel (lotion)	Antihistamine	Diphenhydramine 1.8%
	Astringent	Zinc acetate
Calamatum (spray)	Counterirritant	Camphor, menthol
	Local anesthetic	Benzocaine 1%
	Astringent	Calamine
	Other	Zinc oxide
Calamine Lotion	Astringent	Calamine 8%
	Other	Zinc oxide 8%
Cortaid/Cortaid Maximum Strength & others† (lotion, spray)	Corticosteroid	*Regular strength:* hydrocortisone 0.5%; *maximum strength:* hydrocortisone 1%
Ivarest (cream, lotion)	Antihistamine	Cream: diphenhydramine HCL 2%
	Local anesthetic	Benzocaine 5%
	Astringent	Calamine 14%
Ivy Block	Counterirritant	Bentoquotam 5%
Ivy Dry (cream, liquid)	Counterirritant	*Cream:* menthol, camphor
	Local anesthetic	Cream: Benzocaine 5 mg/g
	Astringent	Tannic acid, zinc acetate
Ivy-Chex	Counterirritant	Methyl salicylate
	Other	Benzalkonium chloride
Resinol (ointment)	Astringent	Calamine 6%
	Other	Zinc oxide 12%, resorcinol 2%
Rhuli (cream, gel, spray)	Counterirritant	*Cream:* camphor 0.3% *Gel:* camphor 0.3%; menthol 0.3%, benzyl alcohol 2% *Spray:* camphor 0.7%
	Local anesthetic	*Cream:* pramoxine HCL 1% *Spray:* benzocaine 5%
	Astringent	*Cream:* calamine 3% *Spray:* calamine 13.8%

*Directions for use: *Adults:* Apply to affected area 3 to 4 times daily; for children <2 years of age, consult a health care professional.

†See more products in the Topical Corticosteroids product information table, p. 99.

Corns, Calluses, and Warts

Friction and pressure increase mitotic activity in the basal cell layer of the skin and lead to a thicker stratum corneum and the eventual development of a corn or callus. Infection of the skin and mucous membranes with human papillomaviruses results in the development of warts. Only common warts (those on the hands, fingers, and face) and plantar warts (on the soles of the feet) should be treated with OTC products. Other types of warts require evaluation and treatment by a health care professional.

Salicylic acid is used to treat corns, calluses, and warts.

Pharmacology

Salicylic acid is a keratolytic agent thought to have two main mechanisms of action: (1) it decreases keratinocyte adhesion and (2) increases water binding, leading to hydration of keratin. Soaking the area in a warm bath before application of the medication is thought to enhance efficacy.

Side Effects

Burning and stinging may occur when salicylic acid is applied to normal skin and may increase in intensity with higher concentrations. It should not be applied to irritated, reddened, or infected skin. Salicylic acid is absorbed through the skin; however, salicylate toxicity is unlikely with use on corns, calluses, or warts. Prolonged use over large areas, especially in children and patients with significant renal and hepatic dysfunction, may result in salicylate toxicity. Signs and symptoms of salicylate toxicity include nausea, vomiting, dizziness, tinnitus, loss of hearing, lethargy, diarrhea, and psychic disturbances. Patients with hypersensitivity reactions to systemic salicylates may experience allergic reactions to topical salicylic acid.

Drug Interactions

Interactions have been reported with both topical and oral salicylates (see pp. 356, 360, 368).

Lifespan Considerations

Geriatric

Geriatric patients often have multiple, concomitant health conditions or organ system impairment. Because of the risks associated with potential tissue damage, salicylic acid should not be applied to the extremities of patients with diabetes mellitus or peripheral vascular disease. Patients with significant renal and hepatic impairment have a greater risk of having salicylate toxicity with extensive use of salicylic acid.

Pediatric

Use of salicylic acid preparations should be avoided in children under the age of 2 years. Prolonged use in large areas may result in systemic absorption and salicylate toxicity, particularly in children.

Pregnancy

Salicylic acid is an FDA Pregnancy Category C drug. There are no adequate well-controlled trials in pregnant women. Because salicylates readily cross the placenta, they should be used during pregnancy only if the potential benefits outweigh the potential risks to the fetus.

Nursing Mothers

Salicylates are distributed into breast milk. However, the extent of distribution is not clearly established, and salicylates should be used with caution in nursing mothers.

Patient Education

- Diabetic patients should receive professional foot care rather than self-treat foot problems.
- Elimination of the initiating environmental factors (pressure and friction) is essential for the treatment and prevention of corns and calluses. Patients should wear well-fitting shoes to reduce unnecessary pressure and friction. Excessive skin should be removed gently with a rough towel or callus file. Sharp objects should not be used to shave or cut away dead tissue.
- Salicylates should not be applied to open skin. Application to the eyes, mouth, and other mucous membranes should be avoided.
- Patients should soak the area in warm water for 5 minutes before application of the salicylate to enhance its efficacy.
- For proper use, salicylic acid lotions, creams, and gels should be applied in a thin layer to the affected area once or twice daily. Plaster or medicated pads should be cut to a size that will cover the corn,

callus, or wart, applied to the affected area, and left in place for 48 hours. The patient should not exceed five applications in a 2-week period. Salicylic solutions should be applied 1 drop at a time to form a thin layer over the affected area once or twice daily.

- Resolution of the corn, callus, or wart may take several days to several months. Improvement may be noted within the first few days to weeks, but complete remission may take longer. For corns and calluses, treatment should continue until resolution, up to a maximum of 14 days. Warts should be treated until resolution, up to a maximum of 12 weeks.

- These agents are keratolytic and will cause tissue to slough off. A pinkish tinge to the skin is normal. Use of the product should be discontinued if extreme inflammation (swelling, reddening), irritation, or pain on application occurs.

Product Selection

- Product selection is affected by the type, location, and size of the lesions.

- Solutions are the easiest to apply but may require longer treatment duration.

- Medicated discs or pads provide direct and prolonged contact of the medication and affected area.

Product Information: Corns, Calluses, and Warts

Brand Name	Dosage Forms Available	Salicylic Acid Concentration	Adult Dose
Compound W wart remover	Gel, liquid, medicated disks	17%	*Gel:* Squeeze tube and apply one drop at a time to cover affected area; use once or twice daily for up to 12 weeks *Liquid:* Using rod provided, apply one drop at a time to cover the wart once or twice daily for up to 12 weeks *Medicated discs:* Cut the disc to cover wart and apply to wart for 48 hours; repeat every 48 hours for up to 12 weeks
Dr. Scholl's Clear Away	Liquid Medicated disks	17% 40%	*Liquid:* Apply one drop at a time with applicator to the wart once or twice daily for up to 12 weeks *Medicated discs:* Cut the disc to fit wart; apply and keep in place for 48 hours; repeat every 48 hours for up to 12 weeks
Dr. Scholl's Clear Away Gel with Aloe	Gel	17%	Apply thin layer to cover the wart once or twice daily for up to 12 weeks
Dr. Scholl's Clear Away One Step Callus Remover	Medicated disc	40%	Apply medicated disc to the callus; remove after 48 hours; repeat every 48 hours for up to 14 days

Dr. Scholl's Clear Away One Step Corn Remover	Medicated disc	40%	Apply medicated disc to the corn; remove after 48 hours; repeat every 48 hours for up to 14 days
Dr. Scholl's Clear Away One Step Wart Remover System	Medicated disc	40%	Apply medicated disc to the wart; remove after 48 hours; repeat every 48 hours for up to 12 weeks
Dr. Scholl's Clear Away Plantar Wart Remover System	Medicated disc	40%	Apply a thin layer to the plantar wart once or twice daily for up to 12 weeks
Dr. Scholl's Callus Removers	Medicated disc	40%	Apply the medicated disc to the callus; remove after 48 hours; repeat every 48 hours for up to 14 days
Dr. Scholl's Corn Removers	Medicated disc	40%	Apply the medicated disc to the corn; remove after 48 hours; repeat every 48 hours for up to 14 days
Dr. Scholl's Liquid Corn/Callus Remover	Liquid	12.6%	Apply one drop at a time to cover the corn or callus once or twice daily for up to 14 days
Dr. Scholl's Wart Remover Kit	Liquid	17%	Apply one drop at a time with the applicator to cover the wart; repeat once to twice a day for up to 12 weeks
Duofilm	Liquid	17%	Apply a thin layer with the applicator brush once or twice daily for up to 12 weeks

Continued

Product Information: Corns, Calluses, and Warts—cont'd

Brand Name	Dosage Forms Available	Salicylic Acid Concentration	Adult Dose
Duofilm Patch for Kids	Medicated discs	40%	Cut the pad to size, and apply to the wart; remove after 48 hours; repeat every 48 hours for up to 12 weeks
Duoplant Wart Remover for Feet	Gel	17%	Apply a thin layer to cover the wart once or twice daily; may use for up to 12 weeks
Freezone Corn & Callus Remover	Liquid	13.6%	Apply one drop at a time to cover the corn or callus once or twice daily; may use up to 14 days
Gordofilm	Solution	16.7%	Apply one drop at a time to cover once or twice daily
Mosco Corn & Callus Remover	Liquid	17.6%	Apply a thin layer to cover the corn or callus once or twice daily; may use up to 14 days
Occlusal-HP	Liquid	17%	Using brush applicator, apply a small amount at a time to cover the wart once or twice daily; may use for up to 12 weeks
Off-Ezy Corn and Callus Remover Kit	Liquid	17%	Apply one drop a time to the corn or callus once or twice daily, for up to 14 days

Off-Ezy Wart Remover Kit	Liquid	17%	Apply one drop a time to the wart once or twice daily for up to 12 weeks
PediSilk Corn & Callus Remover	Liquid	17%	Apply one drop at a time to cover the corn or callus; may use once or twice daily for up to 14 days
Sal-Plant	Gel	17%	Apply a small amount to the wart once or twice daily for up to 12 weeks
Tinamed Plantar Patch	Medicated patch	40%	Trim the patch to size; apply center to wart; cover up disc provided; remove after 48 hours; repeat every 48 hours for up to 12 weeks
Tinamed Wart Remover	Liquid	17%	
Trans-Ver-Sal Adult Patch (12-mm wart remover kit)	Medicated patch	15% in karaya gum base	Apply medicated patch to the wart and remove after 48 hours; repeat every 48 hours
Trans-Ver-Sol Pedia Patch (6-mm wart remover kit)	Medicated patch	15% in karaya gum base	Apply medicated patch to the wart and remove after 48 hours; repeat every 48 hours
Trans-Ver-Sal Plantar Patch (20-mm wart remover kit)	Medicated patch	15% in karaya gum base	Apply medicated patch to the wart and remove after 48 hours, repeat every 48 hours.
Wart-Off	Liquid	17%	Apply one drop at a time to cover the wart once or twice daily; may be used for up to 12 weeks

Dandruff

Dandruff is a chronic scalp condition that is characterized by accelerated epidermal cell turnover, irregular keratin breakup pattern, and the shedding of the cells in large flakes. The specific cause of the accelerated cell turnover is unknown. Elevated microorganism levels on the scalp may be associated with dandruff. Dandruff is more prominent at puberty and early adulthood.

Drugs used to treat dandruff include cytostatic agents, keratolytic agents, and tar derivatives.

Pharmacology

Cytostatic agents (pyrithione zinc and selenium sulfide) reduce cell turnover rate. Keratolytic agents (salicylic acid and sulfur) and tar derivatives help correct abnormalities of keratinization by decreasing epidermal cell proliferation and skin infiltration. *Regardless of the agent used, frequent washing and thorough rinsing are important with all medicated and nonmedicated shampoos.*

Side Effects

Side effects related to the use of dandruff shampoos occur locally and include skin irritation, hair/skin discoloration (avoided or minimized by thorough rinsing after treatment), and oiliness or dryness of hair and scalp.

Drug Interactions

No clinically significant drug interactions have been noted.

Lifespan Considerations
Geriatric
Dandruff conditions normally decline in advancing years. There are no unique recommendations for use in the elderly population.

Pediatric

Generally, use of dandruff shampoos should be avoided in children under the age of 2 years. Safety and efficacy in infants has not been established.

Pregnancy/Nursing Mothers

Dandruff shampoos are considered safe when used in accordance with recommended directions and duration in pregnant/nursing women.

Patient Education

- Washing hair and scalp frequently (3 to 7 days a week) with nonmedicated shampoo may control the dandruff.
- Patients should massage medicated shampoo onto the wet scalp and allow the shampoo to remain on the hair for 5 to 10 minutes before rinsing. Increasing the contact time of shampoo on the scalp increases the effectiveness.
- These shampoos are for external use only. Patients should avoid contact between shampoos and eyes and should not use shampoos on irritated, inflamed skin or on open skin lesions.
- Patients should rinse thoroughly after using medicated shampoos because these products may cause skin or hair discoloration.
- If the dandruff persists for more than 6 months, a health care professional should be consulted.
- If using selenium sulfide products before or after hair bleaching, tinting, or permanent waving, patients should rinse hair for more than 5 minutes in cool, running water.
- Selenium sulfide may damage jewelry; remove before using.
- Tar derivatives may increase tendency to sunburn up to 24 hours after use; patients should use proper protection in sunlight or artificial light.
- Dosage/directions for use: Patients should initially use medicated shampoos once to twice weekly (depending on the severity) and less frequently thereafter to maintain dandruff control. Many products are safe to use every day.

Product Selection

- Cytostatic agents (pyrithione zinc and selenium sulfide) are considered agents of choice in the treatment of dandruff. These agents should be used first.

- Products that contain higher concentrations of active ingredients may be preferred.

SUGGESTED READING

Dolnick E: A flaky concern, H*ippocrates* 3(1);28-30, 1989.

Product Information: Dandruff

Brand Name	Ingredients	Comments
Danex	Pyrithione zinc 1%	
Denorex	Coal tar 9%, menthol 1.5%, alcohol 7.5%	Regular, herbal, or with conditioner
Denorex Advanced Formula	Pyrithione zinc 2%	
DHS Tar	Coal tar 0.5%	
DHS Zinc	Pyrithione zinc 2%	
Doctar	Coal tar 0.5%	With conditioner
Extra Strength Denorex	Coal tar 12.5%, menthol 1.5%, alcohol 10.4%	
Head & Shoulders	Pyrithione zinc 1%	Varieties include *Normal to oily* and *Normal to dry*
Head & Shoulders Dry Scalp	Pyrithione zinc 1%	Regular or with conditioner
Head & Shoulders Intensive Treatment Dandruff Shampoo	Selenium sulfide 1%	
Ionil T Plus	Coal tar 2%	
Neutrogena T/Gel	Coal tar 2%	Regular and with conditioner; conditioner contains coal tar 1.5%
Pentrax	Coal tar 4.3%	With conditioner
Sebulon	Pyrithione zinc 2%	
Selsun Blue	Selenium sulfide 1%	Varieties include *2 in 1 Treatment, Balanced Treatment, Medicated Treatment,* and *Moisturizing Treatment*
T/Gel Extra Strength	Coal tar 4%	
Tegrin Medicated	Coal tar 5%, alcohol 4.6%	Regular or herbal
Tegrin Medicated Extra Conditioning	Coal tar 7%, alcohol 6.4%	
Theraplex T	Coal tar 1%	
Theraplex Z	Pyrithione zinc 2%	
Zetar	Coal tar 1%	
Zincon	Pyrithione zinc 1%	

Fungal Infections

Tinea pedis (athlete's foot) is the most common fungal infection of the skin. Other topical fungal infections include tinea corporis (ringworm), tinea capitis (fungal infection of the scalp), and tinea cruris (jock itch). All of these topical fungal infections are responsive to topical treatment with antifungal products. The information provided regarding tinea pedis is applicable to the other topical fungal infections as well. Onychomycosis (fungal infection of the nails) is not addressed in this book because it is not responsive to OTC topical therapy.

Drugs used to treat tinea pedis include imidazole-derivative antifungals, tolnaftate, undecylenic acid–zinc undecylenate, and clioquinol.

IMIDAZOLE-DERIVATIVE ANTIFUNGALS

CLOTRIMAZOLE

MICONAZOLE

Pharmacology

Tinea pedis afflicts millions of people annually. The most common causative organisms include *Trichophyton rubrum*, *Trichophyton mentagrophytes*, or *Epidermophyton floccosum*. Environmental factors, such as climatic conditions, foot hygiene, and footwear affect the likelihood of developing athlete's foot. Imidazole-derivative antifungal agents, such as clotrimazole and miconazole, affect the integrity of the fungal cell membrane and its cellular components. They inhibit biosynthesis of ergosterol, resulting in damage to the fungal cell membrane, loss of essential intracellular components, and cell death. Clotrimazole and miconazole have high cure rates in the treatment of tinea pedis, 80% to 100% and 90%, respectively.

Side Effects

Rare cases of mild skin irritation, burning, stinging, erythema, pruritus, and urticaria have occurred with the use of these agents.

Drug Interactions

Systemic absorption of clotrimazole and miconazole through intact skin is negligible (<1%), rendering these products unlikely to interact with other systemic medications.

Lifespan Considerations

Geriatric

Elderly patients often have concomitant chronic health conditions. In patients with diabetes or peripheral vascular disease, it is important to exclude the possibility of bacterial infections or other serious complications before self-treatment with OTC antifungal products.

Pediatric

Children under the age of 2 years should use imidazole-derivative agents only under the direction and supervision of a health care professional. These agents should be kept out of reach of children to avoid the risk of accidental ingestion.

Pregnancy

Imidazole-derivative antifungals are FDA Pregnancy Category B drugs. Clotrimazole has been used vaginally in the second and third trimester without associated adverse effects on the fetus. However, adequate, well-controlled studies in pregnant women in the first trimester are not available. During the first trimester, these agents should be used only when the potential benefits outweigh the potential risks.

Nursing Mothers

It is not known whether these agents are excreted in breast milk. Therefore it is impossible to make a firm statement about their absolute risks. Despite the fact that only small amounts are absorbed systemically with topical application, these agents should be used with caution in nursing mothers.

TOLNAFTATE

Pharmacology

Tolnaftate is the only antifungal currently available that is indicated for both *prevention* and *treatment* of athlete's foot. Its exact mechanism of action has not been described. However, it is thought to distort the hyphae and impair growth of susceptible fungal cells. It is active against T. *rubrum*, T. *mentagrophytes, and* E. *floccosum*, the most common causative organisms of tinea pedis. Tolnaftate has a cure rate in the treatment of tinea pedis of approximately 80%.

Side Effects

Overall, tolnaftate is well tolerated, including when applied to broken skin. Mild skin irritation, burning, and pruritus may occur. Delayed hypersensitivity reactions are rare.

Drug Interactions

Tolnaftate is intended for external use only. Because systemic absorption is minimal, it is unlikely to interact with other systemic medications.

Lifespan Considerations

Geriatric

No specific concerns or precautions with tolnaftate exist. However, as with the imidazole-derivative antifungals, patients with diabetes and/or peripheral vascular disease should be evaluated by a health care professional before instituting self-treatment to rule out other potential complications.

Pediatric

Use in children under the age of 2 years is recommended only with the supervision and guidance of a health care professional. The product should be kept out of reach of children to avoid accidental ingestion.

Pregnancy

Tolnaftate is an FDA Pregnancy Category C drug. Because systemic absorption is minimal, risk to a developing fetus is low. However, data are insufficient to state there is no risk to the fetus.

Nursing Mothers

Small amounts, if any, are absorbed systemically with topical application, and entry into the breast milk is unlikely. However, because information regarding distribution into breast milk is unavailable, the benefits and risks should be considered before using in nursing mothers.

UNDECYLENIC ACID–ZINC UNDECYLENATE

Pharmacology

The combination of undecylenic acid and its salts is primarily fungistatic. Fungicidal activity may be seen with long exposure to high concentrations. Because undecylenic acid only retards fungal growth, the infection commonly persists despite treatment, with a cure rate of 50% at best. Zinc undecylenate also has astringent properties that may assist in reducing inflammation and irritation associated with the infection.

Side Effects

Application of ointment, powder, or diluted solution to the skin results in minimal adverse effects. Because alcohol is used as the vehicle, mild, transient stinging or burning may be noted when the solution is applied to broken skin. Undecylenic acid has a strong odor, which may be undesirable for some patients and result in noncompliance.

Drug Interactions

There are no clinically significant drug interactions.

Lifespan Considerations

Geriatric

No specific concerns or precautions exist. However, as with the imidazole-derivative antifungals, patients with diabetes and/or peripheral vascular disease should be evaluated by a health care professional before instituting self-treatment to rule out other potential complications.

Pediatric

Undecylenic acid–zinc undecylenate should not be used in children under the age of 2 years except with advice of a health care professional.

Pregnancy

No information is available about the risks for a developing fetus.

Nursing Mothers

Adequate information about the systemic absorption and excretion of undecylenic acid–zinc undecylenate in breast milk is lacking.

CLIOQUINOL

Pharmacology

The exact mechanism of clioquinol's antifungal properties has not been described.

Side Effects

Incidence of side effects are rare, but itching, redness, and irritation have been reported with clioquinol use. Clioquinol can stain the skin, hair, and fabric.

Drug Interactions

Systemic absorption of clioquinol with topical application is low. However, it may still result in alteration of thyroid function tests. Patients who are on thyroid replacement products and undergoing this testing must be evaluated for prior use of clioquinol, which contains iodine. Clioquinol should be discontinued for 1 month before thyroid function testing.

Lifespan Considerations

Geriatric

As with the other antifungal agents, in patients with diabetes or peripheral vascular disease, bacterial infections or other complications must be excluded before self-treatment. Elderly patients on thyroid supplementation should be evaluated for interaction (see Drug Interactions above).

Pediatric

Use in children under the age of 2 years is not recommended.

Pregnancy

Adequate information regarding the use of clioquinol in pregnant women and the risk for the fetus is not available.

Nursing Mothers

It is not known whether clioquinol is excreted in breast milk. Therefore caution should be exercised with use in nursing mothers.

Patient Education

- Patients should apply clioquinol twice daily to the affected area after washing and drying thoroughly. With application, special attention should be paid to the area between the toes.
- These products are intended for external use only. Contact with the eyes should be avoided.
- Adverse effects and hypersensitivity reactions are rare. However, if a patient should notice itching, swelling, or worsening of the condition, the product should be discontinued.
- Resolution of the infection may require several weeks. A trial of continued use for 2 to 4 weeks is needed. If no improvement is noted after 4 weeks, a health care professional should be consulted for further evaluation. The presence of oozing or purulent material may indicate a bacterial infection requiring evaluation and either topical or oral antibiotic therapy.
- Strict compliance to the recommended dosing regimen is necessary for topical therapy to be effective.
- Eliminating or controlling environmental factors predisposing the foot to fungal infections is imperative to the overall efficacy of therapy. Local hygiene measures are crucial.
- The foot should be cleansed with soap and water and thoroughly dried daily. Shoes and light cotton socks should allow ventilation and reduce heat and perspiration. Occlusive footwear should be avoided or minimized. Shoes should be alternated to allow adequate drying.
- Foot powders and insoles can be used to absorb moisture.
- Contaminated clothing, socks, and towels should be washed thoroughly and regularly in hot water.

Product Selection

- Most antifungal agents are available in a variety of dosage forms, including creams, ointments, solutions, powders, and various aerosol products. Because compliance is greatly affected by the product selected, recommendations should be individualized.
- Creams, ointments, or solutions should be used as *primary* therapy. Powders and aerosol products are recommended for use as *adjunctive* therapy, particularly for patients with excessive perspiration.
- Imidazole-derivative antifungal agents and tolnaftate may be preferred over other therapies because of their fungicidal action and higher cure rates. Tolnaftate is useful primarily in the dry, scaly type of athlete's foot. For weeping or inflamed lesions, treatment with tolnaftate should be delayed until weeping and inflammation have subsided.

- In patients predisposed to recurrent tinea pedis, powders or powder aerosols containing tolnaftate are indicated for use once or twice daily to prevent infection.
- Patients should keep in mind that product extensions with the same brand name may not have the same active ingredient. For example, traditional Desenex ointment and powder contain undecylenic acid–zinc undecylenate, but Prescription Strength Desenex AF cream contains clotrimazole and Prescription Strength Desenex Powder Spray contains miconazole.
- Fungal infections of the scalp are usually treated with topical antifungal solutions because solutions allow the best contact between the drug and the scalp. Creams and powders tend to become attached to the hair and not reach the scalp.

Product Information: Fungal Infections

Brand Name	Dosage Forms Available	Active Ingredient	Adult Dose	Comments
Absorbine Jr. Antifungal Foot Care	Cream, powder, liquid (pump spray)	Tolnaftate 1%	Apply twice daily	*Pump spray:* Shake well, hold can approximately 2 inches from the affected area
Absorbine Jr. Antifungal Foot	Powder spray	Miconazole nitrate 2%	Apply twice daily	Alcohol 10%; shake well
Aftate Antifungal	Gel, liquid spray, powder, powder spray	Tolnaftate 1%	*Treatment:* Apply twice daily *Prevention:* Apply once to twice daily	Shake well before using aerosol products
Cruex	Aerosol powder, squeeze powder, cream	Undecylenic acid–zinc undecylenate	*Treatment:* Apply twice daily *Prevention:* Apply once to twice daily	*Spray powder:* Shake well before spraying; promoted primarily for jock itch
Desenex	Ointment, powder, powder spray	Undecylenic acid–zinc undecylenate	Apply twice daily	*Spray powder:* Shake well, hold the can approximately 4 to 6 inches from the affected area
Prescription Strength Desenex AF	Cream	Clotrimazole 1%	Apply twice daily	

Product	Form	Active Ingredient	Directions	Notes
Prescription Strength Desenex Powder Spray	Powder spray	Miconazole nitrate 2%	Apply twice daily	Alcohol 10% / *Spray powder:* Shake well; hold the can approximately 4 to 6 inches from the affected area
Dr. Scholl's Athletes Foot	Powder, spray powder	Tolnaftate 1%	Apply twice daily	*Spray powder:* Alcohol 14%, shake well
Dr. Scholl's Athletes Foot Spray Liquid	Aerosol spray liquid	Tolnaftate 1%	Apply twice daily	Alcohol 36%, shake well
Fungi-Care	Gel	Tolnaftate 1%	Apply twice daily	
Fungi-Care	Liquid	Undecylenic acid 10%	Apply twice daily	
Johnson's Odor-Eaters Antifungal spray	Spray powder	Tolnaftate 1%	Apply twice daily	Ethanol 14.9%; shake well, spray, and apply thin layer
Johnson's Odor-Eaters Foot & Sneaker Spray Powder	Spray powder	Tolnaftate 1%	Apply twice daily	Shake well, hold 4 to 6 inches away from the affected area
Lotrimin AF	Cream, topical solution	Clotrimazole 1%	Apply twice daily	*Spray powder:* Alcohol 10%
	Powder, spray powder, spray liquid	Miconazole nitrate 2%	Apply twice daily	*Spray liquid:* Alcohol 17%; shake well, hold approximately 6 inches away from the affected area when applying
Micatin	Cream, powder, spray liquid, spray powder	Miconazole nitrate 2%	Apply twice daily	*Spray powder:* Alcohol 10% / *Spray liquid:* Alcohol 16.8%; shake well, hold approximately 6 inches away from the affected area when applying

Continued

Product Information: Fungal Infections—cont'd

Brand Name	Dosage Forms Available	Active Ingredient	Adult Dose	Comments
Mycelex OTC	Cream	Clotrimazole 1%	Apply twice daily	
NP-27	Cream, solution, powder, spray powder	Tolnaftate 1%	Apply twice daily	Spray powder: Alcohol 14%
The Original Fungi-Nail Antifungal Solution	Solution	Undecylenic acid	Apply twice daily	
Pro-Clearz	Liquid	Tolnaftate 1%	Apply twice daily	
Quinsana Plus Antifungal Powder	Powder	Tolnaftate 1%	Treatment: Apply twice daily Prevention: Apply once to twice daily	
Tinactin	Cream, liquid spray, ointment, solution	Tolnaftate 1%	Apply twice daily	Liquid spray: Alcohol 36%
Tinactin Deodorant Powder spray	Powder spray	Tolnaftate 1%	Apply twice daily	Alcohol 14%
Tinactin Super Absorbent Powder	Powder	Tolnaftate 1%	Apply twice daily	

Insect Bites

Insect repellents can help prevent bites from ticks, mosquitoes, and other biting insects, reducing irritation and risk of diseases spread via these insects. To be effective, repellents must be applied before contact with the insect. Insect repellents are not effective in eliminating the sensitivities (e.g., itching, redness, burning) caused by contact with the insect.

Diethyltoluamide (DEET) is the main ingredient used in insect repellents.

DIETHYLTOLUAMIDE

Pharmacology

Insect repellents do not kill insects; rather, their vapors discourage insects from landing on or biting the skin. Most insect repellents contain DEET in various strengths. Other compounds (e.g., ethohexadiol, dimethyl phthalate, dimethyl ethyl hexanediol carbate, butopyronoxyl) may be combined with DEET to make the product effective against a larger variety of insects.

Side Effects

All insect repellents are toxic if taken internally. Some patients may develop a contact dermatitis from use of products containing DEET. Reactions include itching, burning, bullous eruptions, swelling, and anaphylaxis. Care should be taken when insect repellents are applied around the eyes, broken skin, or mucous membranes, because they may cause burning and stinging. Products containing less than 50% DEET are almost devoid of side effects on adults. However, encephalopathy has followed repeated and extensive use of up to 20% DEET in children. Toxicity may occur one half to 1 hour after exposure or days to months after chronic exposure. Children may be more susceptible to the toxic effects of DEET compared with adults. In relationship to DEET poisonings, the route of exposure may be more important than age or DEET concentration.

Drug Interactions

There are no clinically significant drug interactions with DEET.

Lifespan Considerations

Geriatric

There are no unique recommendations for use in the elderly population.

Pediatric

DEET is not recommended for use in children under the age of 2 years because of an increased risk of absorption and CNS toxicity (including ataxia, confusion, insomnia, tremor, and seizures). DEET-containing products should be kept in a safe place out of reach of children.

Pregnancy/Nursing Mothers

There are no data with regards to use of DEET in pregnant or nursing women.

Patient Education

- Insect repellents may damage rayon, fingernail polish, artificial nails, some plastics (plastic watch crystals), paints, and varnishes.
- All exposed skin areas should be treated with the insect repellent.
- DEET is not recommended for use in children under the age of 2 years.
- Patients should avoid applying DEET to their hands, and especially to children's hands, to minimize accidental ingestion.
- Patients should wash their hands after application of DEET to minimize accidental ingestion. Liquid, cream, gel, lotion, and stick forms of insect repellents should be used whenever possible to avoid inhalation.
- Contact should be avoided between insect repellents and the eyes, mucous membranes, or broken skin.
- Application will last 4 to 8 hours.
- Chronic use or total body use should be avoided.
- Insect repellents should be removed with soap and water when the exposure period has passed.
- When a sunscreen is also used, insect repellent should be applied at least 30 minutes to 1 hour after sunscreen application.
- Patients should wash insect repellents off with soap and water if a skin reaction is suspected.

Product Selection

- No oral product including thiamine (vitamin B_1) has been shown to be an effective insect repellent.
- The higher the concentration of DEET, the longer the duration of protection the insect repellent will provide. Lower concentrations are appropriate when exposure is minimal or in persons more susceptible to DEET toxicity.
- Products containing 40% or less DEET are recommended for adults. Higher concentrations of DEET have a greater potential for adverse effects.
- Products containing 20% or less DEET should be used on children.
- Spray products will provide more even coverage and will cover a large area more quickly. Sprays also minimize contact with the hands.
- Liquid, cream, gel, lotion, and stick forms of insect repellents can be applied with more control and precision.
- Avon *Skin So Soft* enjoys "folk medicine" status as an insect repellent. There are no scientific studies to confirm its effectiveness.
- Insect repellents containing DEET, epecially those with higher concentrations, may be more effective in repelling ticks.
- Permethrin (discussed in more detail in the next section on Pediculosis [lice]) applied to clothing may be effective in repelling ticks.

SUGGESTED READING

Swanson LN, Byrd TC: Insect repellents, US *Pharm* 21:16-31, 1996.

Product Information: Insect Repellents

Brand Name	Type	DEET Percentage
Ben's Backyard	Lotion	23
Cutter Outdoorsman	Aerosol, stick, lotion	28.5
Cutter Pleasant Protection	Gel, pump, aerosol	9.5
Cutter Stick	Stick	30
Deep Woods Off! Outdoor Fresh Scent and Unscented	Aerosol	25
Deep Woods Off! Sportsman	Pump spray	95
Deeps Woods Off with Sunscreen (SPF 15)	Lotion	20
Muskol Maximum Strength	Pump spray	100
Off!	Aerosol	15
Off! Skintastic for Kids	Liquid	5
Off! Skintastic Lotion	Lotion	7.125
Off! Skintastic with Sunscreen (SPF 30)	Lotion	10
Repel Family Formula	Aerosol	27
Skedaddle! Insect Protection for Kids	Lotion	10
Ultra Muskol	Aerosol	40
Ultrathon	Aerosol	24

Pediculosis (Lice)

Pediculosis is a parasitic infestation of lice. Lice are wingless and have no ability to fly or jump. Lice are passed between individuals through direct physical contact or contact with the individual infested articles of clothing or grooming materials (e.g., combs, brushes). Pediculosis includes three types of infestations: head lice (*Pediculus humanus capitis*), body lice (*Pediculus humanus corporis*), and pubic lice (*Phthirus pubis*). Head lice is the most common type of lice infestation. Infestation causes itching that may lead to a secondary skin infection.

Drugs used to treat lice are permethrin and pyrethrum extract.

PERMETHRIN AND PYRETHRUM EXTRACT

Pharmacology

Permethrin and pyrethrum disrupt the neuronal membrane of the lice, resulting in paralysis of the affected organisms. The action of permethrin results in the death of lice and their eggs. Its residual action on hair follicles prevents reinfestation. Piperonyl butoxide decreases the metabolism of pyrethrum extract in lice. It is added to pyrethrum extract to enhance its activity.

Side Effects

Permethrin has been reported to cause pruritus, burning, stinging, and irritation. Pyrethrum extract may cause contact dermatitis, but systemic absorption is low and adverse effects are rare. Piperonyl butoxide may cause contact dermatitis.

Drug Interactions

There are no clinically significant drug interactions with agents in this class.

Lifespan Considerations
Geriatric

There are no unique recommendations for use in the elderly population.

Pediatric

These agents should not be used in children under the age of 2 years.

Pregnancy

Permethrin is an FDA Pregnancy Category B drug. An assessment of the benefits and risks should be considered before use of these products.

Nursing Mothers

It is unknown if the drug is excreted in breast milk.

Patient Education

- Patients should avoid contact between these agents and the eyes and mucous membranes; these products should not be used in eyelashes or eyebrows.
- Some patients require a second treatment in 7 days.
- A health care professional should be notified if itching, redness, or swelling occurs after use of these agents.
- Patients should wash their hair or body before applying permethrin or pyrethrin/piperonyl butoxide. Hair should be towel dried after washing.
- A special comb included with the product is used to remove nits.
- Patients should see individual products for instructions on use. Generally, permethrin 1% creme rinse or pyrethrin/piperonyl butoxide is applied to the affected area and rinsed after 10 minutes.
- To prevent reinfestation, clothes, bedding, and personal items should be washed in hot, soapy water. Items that cannot be washed should be sealed in a plastic bag for 2 weeks.

Product Selection

- Permethrin is the OTC drug of choice for treatment of scabies and pediculosis.
- Permethrin or pyrethrin may cause an anaphylactic reaction in patients with a ragweed allergy.
- All household members and close contacts should be checked for infestation.
- Permethrin cream rinse and pyrethrin shampoo are used for scalp infestations.
- Pyrethrin liquid and gel are used for lice infestation of the skin.

SUGGESTED READING

Bergus GR: Topical treatments for head lice, J *Fam Pract* 42:21-22, 1996.

Product Information: Pediculosis (Lice)

Brand Name	Product Type	Active Ingredient
A-200 Pronto	Shampoo	Pyrethrins 0.33% Piperonyl butoxide 4%
Barc	Liquid	Pyrethrins 0.18% Piperonyl butoxide 2.2%
Blue	Gel	Pyrethrins 0.3% Piperonyl butoxide 3%
Control-L	Liquid	Pyrethrins 0.3% Piperonyl butoxide 3%
End Lice	Liquid	Pyrethrins 0.3% Piperonyl butoxide 3%
Lice Treatment	Liquid	Pyrethrins 0.3% Piperonyl butoxide 3%
Lice-Enz	Shampoo	Pyrethrins 0.3% Piperonyl butoxide 3%
Licide Shampoo	Shampoo	Pyrethrins 0.3% Piperonyl butoxide 3%
Nix	Creme rinse	Permethrin 1%
Pyrinex Pediculicide	Shampoo	Pyrethrins 0.2% Piperonyl butoxide 2%
Pyrinyl	Liquid	Pyrethrins 0.2% Piperonyl butoxide 2%
Pyrinyl II	Liquid	Pyrethrins 0.3% Piperonyl butoxide 3%
Pyrinyl Plus	Shampoo	Pyrethrins 0.3% Piperonyl butoxide 3%
R & C	Shampoo	Pyrethrins 0.3% Piperonyl butoxide 3%
Rid	Shampoo	Pyrethrins 0.3% Piperonyl butoxide 3%
Tisit	Liquid	Pyrethrins 0.3% Piperonyl butoxide 2%
	Shampoo	Pyrethrins 0.3% Piperonyl butoxide 3%
Tisit Blue	Gel	Pyrethrins 0.3% Piperonyl butoxide 3%
Triple X	Shampoo	Pyrethrins 0.3% Piperonyl butoxide 3%
Triple X Kit	Liquid	Pyrethrins 0.3% Piperonyl butoxide 3%

Psoriasis

Psoriasis causes a shortening of the cell cycle of corneocytes in the epidermis. Normal epidermal turnover takes 25 to 30 days, but in psoriasis it is shortened to 3 to 4 days. The result is a thickened epidermis with immature nucleated cells and the appearance of scales. Psoriatic skin lesions can be described as erythematous, sharply circumscribed plaque covered by loosely adherent, silvery-white scales. If scales are removed, there may be evidence of pin-point bleeding. Any area of the body may be involved, but commonly affected sites include the scalp, elbows, knees, genitalia, and gluteal cleft. If the disease is severe (covering more than 20% of body surface area), more intensive therapy and the use of medications available only by prescription may be required. These more severe cases should be managed by a health care professional.

OTC drugs used topically in the treatment of psoriasis include hydrocortisone, salicylic acid, and coal tar.

HYDROCORTISONE

Pharmacology

Hydrocortisone has antiinflammatory, antimitotic, antipruritic, vaso-constrictive, and immunosuppressive properties. Topical corticosteroids induce phospholipase A2 inhibitory proteins, which diminishes the activity of the inflammatory mediators. Topical application of corticosteroids to inflamed skin reverses vascular dilation and permeability, thus inhibiting leukocytes and macrophage accumulation. The inhibition results in decreased inflammation and decreased pruritus.

Along with emollients, hydrocortisone would be a reasonable choice early in the onset of psoriatic lesions because, unlike salicylic acid and coal tar, it is nonirritating.

Side Effects

In general, hydrocortisone products are well-tolerated. Local side effects from topical corticosteroids are primarily dermatologic. Some of these include pruritus, burning, erythema, irritation, secondary infection, dryness, and tightening of the skin. Occlusion of the affected area enhances corticosteroid absorption and increases the risk of local and systemic adverse effects. Ointment dosage forms may cause problems such as maceration in intertriginous areas.

Drug Interactions

There are no clinically significant drug interactions.

Lifespan Considerations

Geriatric

In general, dosages do not need to be altered in the elderly population.

Pediatric

This patient population has a larger body surface area:weight ratio, which could result in systemic side effects if excessive amounts of topical steroid are used or conditions exist (e.g., occlusive dressings) that increase absorption.

Pregnancy

Hydrocortisone is an FDA Pregnancy Category C drug. When topical hydrocortisone use is necessary in pregnancy, it should be limited to small amounts for short periods.

Nursing Mothers

It is not known if topically applied hydrocortisone is excreted in breast milk in amounts sufficient enough to cause deleterious effects to an infant. Topical corticosteroids should be used cautiously in nursing mothers. Systemic corticosteroids have not been shown to be excreted in breast milk.

Patient Education

- When hydrocortisone is used for more than 2 to 3 weeks, the effectiveness may be decreased and rebound could occur. Hydrocortisone is a reasonable choice for treatment of new lesions because coal tar and salicylic acid may be too irritating. After inflammation decreases, other agents should be employed.
- Creams may be preferred over ointments for intertriginous areas because of problems such as maceration.
- Patients should not use occlusive dressings unless directed to do so by a health care professional.

- Tight-fitting diapers or plastic pants could act as an occlusive dressing if hydrocortisone is applied to the diaper area, resulting in increased absorption of hydrocortisone.
- Hydrocortisone should be applied as a thin film to affected areas and rubbed in gently 2 to 4 times a day.
- If lesions do not respond after 2 or 3 weeks of treatment, a health care professional should be consulted.

Product Selection

- Hydrocortisone may be a good choice for treatment of early-onset psoriatic lesions because of its nonirritating effects.
- Ointments are recommended for treatment of areas other than intertriginous areas. Lotion and gel forms may be used for treatment of psoriatic scalp lesions.

Product Information (Hydrocortisone): Psoriasis*

Brand Name†	Dosage Form
Cortizone 10	Ointment
Extra Strength Cortagel	Gel
Maximum Strength Bactine	Cream
Scalpicin	Liquid
T/Scalp	Liquid
Tegrin-HC	Ointment

*This product table contains hydrocortisone items that are indicated for the treatment of psoriasis and psoriasis-related conditions. For a more complete listing of hydrocortisone products, please refer to the Topical Corticosteroid product information table in the Contact Dermatitis chapter, p. 99.
†All of the products listed contain hydrocortisone 1%.

SALICYLIC ACID

Pharmacology

Salicylic acid at concentrations of 2% to 6% acts as a keratolytic. Keratolytics loosen the epidermis and facilitate its removal. Results may be seen within 7 to 10 days at these concentrations.

Side Effects

Salicylic-acid products may be irritating to the skin. Application of large amounts of salicylic acid could result in salicylate toxicity as evidenced by tachypnea, tinnitus, nausea, and vomiting.

Drug Interactions

Interactions typical of salicylates may occur if serum levels of the drug are elevated as a result of prolonged use on large areas (see p. 360). Although the concentrations of salicylic acid in shampoos are higher, the contact time is minimal; thus significant absorption of the agent is very low.

Lifespan Considerations

Geriatric

There are no unique recommendations in the elderly population.

Pediatric

Small children and patients with renal or hepatic impairment may be at risk for salicylism if large areas are treated for prolonged periods. Signs and symptoms of salicylism include nausea, vomiting, tinnitus, and tachypnea.

Pregnancy

Salicylic acid is an FDA Pregnancy Category C drug. There is limited information concerning its use in pregnant women.

Nursing Mothers

There is no information on salicylic-acid absorption or concentrations in milk.

Patient Education

- Patients should avoid contact between salicylic acid and normal skin, genitalia, eyes, and mucous membranes. If lesions are present in these areas, salicylic acid– and coal tar–containing products should be avoided; hydrocortisone-containing products should be used in these situations.
- Application of salicylic acid over large areas of skin and use of occlusive dressings may increase the likelihood of toxic effects such as

salicylism. Signs and symptoms of salicylism include nausea, vomiting, tachypnea, and tinnitus.

- For scalp psoriasis, medicated shampoos may not be necessary. Proper and frequent shampooing is the key to effective control of psoriasis.
- Patients should shampoo by wetting hair thoroughly with water, massaging shampoo into hair for several minutes, rinsing shampoo out, then repeating once.
- Ointments, creams, and lotion should be applied several times a day without removing the product.
- If possible, soaking the affected area in warm water for 5 to 20 minutes before use may enhance the effect of the salicylic acid.
- Salicylic acid may cause redness, peeling, and irritation. If this is severe, patients should discontinue use of the product and consult a health care professional.

Product Selection

- Ointments, creams, and lotions with 3% or less salicylic acid are used for treatment of psoriasis. Shampoos may contain higher concentrations of salicylic acid.
- Products containing salicylic acid are a reasonable choice when thick scales of psoriasis are present.

  For product information, see the table at the end of the Coal Tar section, p. 142.

COAL TAR

Pharmacology

The exact mechanism of coal-tar derivatives in psoriasis is unknown. Coal tar has been attributed with being an antiseptic, antipruritic, and keratoplastic. Coal tar has also been shown to reduce the size and number of epidermal cells and disperse scales.

Side Effects

Coal-tar products may possess an unpleasant odor; cause stains to skin, clothing, etc.; darken/alter hair color; and tarnish silver. Skin problems such as acneform eruptions, folliculitis, and allergic dermatitis may occur. Coal-tar products may be irritating and should not be used in active or inflamed psoriasis, weeping eczema, or erythrodermic and generalized pustular psoriasis.

Drug Interactions

Use of methotrexate and ultraviolet light with coal tar may result in skin ulcerations. Both methotrexate and UV radiation are used in the treatment of psoriasis. Concurrent use should be monitored closely by a health care professional.

Lifespan Considerations

Geriatric

There are no unique recommendations in the elderly population; however, when elderly patients use coal-tar products, they may be more prone to sunburn because of their sensitive skin.

Pediatric

Safety and efficacy of coal tar in children has not been established, and these products should not be used in children under the age of 2 years except under the direction of a health care professional.

Pregnancy

Coal tar is an FDA Pregnancy Category C drug. No data are available from human or animal studies.

Nursing Mothers

The amount of coal tar that may be present in breast milk is unknown.

Patient Education

- Patients should avoid application of coal-tar products to infected, blistering, or oozing areas of skin. Dosage forms other than bath emulsions should not be used in the genital area.
- Coal-tar products may cause photosensitivity; exposure of treated areas to sunlight or sunlamps should be avoided for at least 24 hours after application of the drug.
- Concurrent ultraviolet light therapy should be used only under the supervision of a health care professional.
- These products may temporarily discolor blond, bleached, or tinted hair.
- Coal tar may stain clothing and skin.

- Patients should keep these products away from the eyes; if accidental exposure to the eyes occurs, the eyes should be flushed with water at once.
- A health care professional should be contacted if irritation or rash occurs that was not present before use of a product.
- Ointments and creams should be applied in an amount sufficient to cover the area and rubbed in gently.
- Gels should be applied in an amount sufficient to cover the area, then rubbed in gently. Gels should remain on the affected area 5 minutes; excess gel can then be removed with a clean tissue.
- Patients should rub shampoo into the scalp after wetting the hair with lukewarm water. After the shampoo is rinsed out, patients should reapply shampoo, lather, and allow shampoo to remain on the scalp for 5 minutes and then rinse thoroughly.
- Liquids may be of several types. Some are intended to be applied to dry or wet skin. Others are intended to be added to lukewarm bath water. Still other products can be used by applying to wet or dry skin, or adding to bath water. If the product is intended for application to the skin, the patient should apply enough of the product to cover the affected area and rub in gently.
- Alcohol-containing products should not be used near heat or open flames, or while smoking.

SUGGESTED READINGS

Phillips TJ: Current treatment options in psoriasis, *Hosp Pract* 31:155-157, 161-164, 1996.

Seal R: Treatment options for the management of psoriasis, *Community Nurse* 3:57-59, 1997.

Product Information (Salicylic Acid and Coal Tar): Psoriasis *

Brand Name	Dosage Form	Ingredients
AquaTar	Gel	Coal tar 2.5%
Carbonis Detergens	Solution	Coal tar 20%
EsTar	Gel	Coal tar 5%
Fostex	Cream	Salicylic acid 2%
Fototar	Cream	Coal tar 2%
Ionil Plus	Shampoo	Salicylic acid 2%
Ionil T	Shampoo	Coal tar 4.25%
Ionil T Plus	Shampoo	Coal tar 2%
Medotar	Ointment	Coal tar 1%
MG 217	Shampoo	Coal tar 3%
Neutrogena T/Derm	Oil	Coal tar 5%
Neutrogena T/Gel	Shampoo	Coal tar 0.5-1%
Neutrogena T/Sal	Shampoo	Salicylic acid 3%
Oxipor VHC	Liquid Lotion	Coal tar 48.5%
		Salicylic acid 1%
		Benzocaine 2%
P & S	Shampoo	Salicylic acid 2%
P & S Plus	Gel	Coal tar 8%
		Salicylic acid 2%
Panscol	Ointment Lotion	Salicylic acid 3%
Pentrax	Shampoo	Coal tar 5%
PsoriGel	Gel	Coal tar 7.5%
Scalpicin	Shampoo	Salicylic acid 3%
Sebex-T	Shampoo	Coal tar 5%
		Salicylic acid 2%
Sebutone	Shampoo	Coal tar 0.5%
		Salicylic acid 2%
Tarsum	Shampoo Gel	Coal tar 10%
		Salicylic acid 5%
Tegrin for Psoriasis	Cream, lotion	Coal tar 5%
Vanseb-T	Shampoo	Coal tar 5%
		Salicylic acid 1%
X-Seb	Shampoo	Salicylic acid 4%
X-Seb T	Shampoo	Coal tar 10%
		Salicylic acid 4%
X-Seb T Plus	Shampoo	Coal tar 10%
		Salicylic acid 3%
		Menthol 1%

*Directions for use: Apply to affected area as necessary (for all products except shampoos). For shampoos, massage into scalp after wetting the hair and allow shampoo to remain on the scalp for 5 minutes.

Sunscreens/Sunburn

Ultraviolet radiation (UVR) causes both acute reactions (tanning, erythema, sunburn) and chronic reactions (premature aging, skin cancer). Acute reactions are related to the duration of UVR exposure that an individual can tolerate. Chronic reactions result from cumulative lifetime exposure. UVR, sometimes called *ultraviolet light*, is composed of ranges (UVC, UVB, and UVA) that are arranged according to the following wavelengths and activity on tissue:

- UVC has a wavelength of 200 to 290 nm. It is screened out by ozone in the atmosphere. UVC does not stimulate tanning and may cause erythema and cataracts.
- UVB has a wavelength of 290 to 320 nm. It is the most active UVR as a cause of erythema (suntan and sunburn). UVB is responsible for vitamin D_3 synthesis. It is the primary UVR responsible for causing skin cancer. UVB is also partially filtered by the ozone layer. The most intense exposure to UVB occurs during late morning to early afternoon.
- UVA has a wavelength of 320 to 400 nm. UVA is further divided into UVA I (340 to 400 nm) and UVA II (320 to 340 nm). UVA II is second to UVB in damage to skin. It contributes about 15% of the erythemal response. UVA has a fairly constant exposure throughout day.

A suntan is caused by gradual exposure to UVR, which stimulates the production of melanin. Sunburn is an inflammatory process caused by a duration of exposure to UVR greater than what the skin can tolerate.

SUNSCREENS

Pharmacology

Sunscreens work either by physically blocking the UVR or absorbing UVR in specific wavelengths. Physical sunscreens are opaque compounds with a wide band of absorption that scatter or reflect light.

Side Effects

Sunscreens, particularly paraaminobenzoic acid (PABA) and PABA esters, can cause photosensitivity and contact dermatitis. Benzophenones, cinnamates, homosalate, avobenzone, and methyl anthranilate are less

143

likely to cause photosensitivity and contact dermatitis. Patients who have had a phototoxic reaction or an allergic reaction to thiazide, benzocaine, or sulfonamides may be more prone to reactions with PABA or its esters. Sunscreens can occlude skin to produce miliaria (prickly heat) and folliculitis, particularly products with a high oil content. Products that contain ethyl and isopropyl alcohol can cause or exacerbate dry skin.

Drug Interactions

No clinically significant drug interactions have been reported with sunscreen products.

Lifespan Considerations

Geriatric

Elderly patients are more sensitive to the adverse effects of drugs. Because the incidence of chronic disease increases with age, geriatric patients tend to receive more medications than younger patients. It is therefore important to do a thorough drug and allergy history to determine a patient's potential for a photosensitivity reaction.

Pediatric

Use of sunscreens on infants younger than 6 months is not recommended because the agents could be absorbed and cause a systemic effect. An SPF of 15 or greater should be used in children ages 6 months to 18 years. Higher SPFs are preferable for extended sun exposure. Lifetime risk of skin cancer can be dramatically reduced with routine use of sunscreen.

Pregnancy/Nursing Mothers

Sunscreens are considered safe during pregnancy and for nursing mothers when used in accordance with recommended directions and duration.

Patient Education

Many misconceptions about UVR exposure that patients may need to be educated about include the following:
• On cloudy days, 60% to 80% of UVR will penetrate clouds.
• The closer you are to the equator, the greater the UVR exposure.
• Each 1000-ft increase in altitude increases exposure by 4%.

- Snow reflects 85% to 100% of UVR, so skiers should be take extra precautions because of the combination of altitude and reflection.
- Sand and white paint also reflect UVR, but less than snow. However, patients may not realize they are not fully protected by a beach umbrella because of the UVR reflection off the sand.
- Water reflects only 5% of UVR, so swimmers are not protected while in the water.
- Wet clothes will transmit 50% of UVR.
- Sunscreen should be reapplied as specified by the type of base used. Sweat-resistant products offer protection for up to 30 minutes of heavy sweating. Water-resistant products protect the user for up to 40 minutes of continuous water exposure. Waterproof products offer up to 80 minutes of protection with continuous water exposure.
- Sunscreens should be liberally applied as often as required.
- To prevent staining, sunscreens should be allowed to dry before the patient puts on clothing or comes into contact with other objects. This is especially true with PABA- and DHA-containing products.
- Patients should be encouraged to use a total block product (SPF >15 to 30) to minimize the risk of skin cancer and photoaging.
- Some people may develop a skin reaction or rash from the sunscreen. The sunscreen can be removed with soap and water.
- The patient's medication should be reviewed for drugs that may cause a photosensitivity reaction. These reactions may include an acute or unexpected sunburn (erythema), bullae or vesicles, macules, papules, edema, and acute eczematous or urticarial reactions.
- Photosensitivity reactions are generally induced by UVA. The reaction can happen hours to days after UVR exposure. The most common agents that may cause a reaction include sulfonamides, tetracyclines, nalidixic acid, sulfonylureas, thiazides, phenothiazines, procaine group of anesthetics, quinolones (more common with lomefloxacin and sparfloxacin), and coal tars.

Product Selection

- To select a product, the skin type of the patient should be determined (Table 3-1). The patient should also be asked about past sun exposure/tanning history. Patients who spend long periods of time outdoors should use a product with an SPF of 30. An SPF of at least 15 should be used on areas exposed to the sun to reduce the incidence of skin cancer or photoaging. If a patient insists on developing a gradual tan, the recommended minimum SPF in

Table 3-1
Skin Types

Type of complexion	Skin type	Sun exposure characteristic	Recommended minimum SPF
Very fair	I	Always burns easily, never tans	15
Fair	II	Always burns easily, tans minimally	15
Light	III	Burns moderately, tans gradually	10-15
Medium	IV	Burns minimally, always tans well	6-10
Dark	V	Rarely burns, tans profusely	4-6
Very Dark	VI	Never burns, deeply pigmented	Usually not required

Table 3-1 may be used. Even though an SPF of 15 completely blocks UVR, patients who burn easily will need a higher SPF for prolonged exposure to the sun.

- A drug and allergy history should be done to determine if there is additional risk for a photosensitivity reaction to occur.
- Maximal protection can be achieved with a sunscreen product that is a combination of a PABA derivative and a benzophenone, blocking a broad spectrum of UVA and UVB.
- DHA is used for sunless tans; it is a skin dye and provides no sun protection by itself.
- There are over 150 sunscreen products available. Some common brand names are Bain de Soleil, Banana Boat, Bug and Sun, Club Bronze, Coppertone, Neutrogena, Sea and Ski, and Sun Tropic. The ingredients of these products frequently change, so product labels should be checked to determine if the product meets requirements.
- Drug-induced photosensitivity reactions occur in the UVA range. Therefore a combination product will be required to provide protection against drug-induced photosensitivity reactions. For a list of medications causing photosensitivity, see Box 3-1.

Product Information: Sunscreens*

Sunscreen	UVR Absorbance Range (nm)	UVA Absorbance (320-400 nm)	UVB Absorbance (290-320 nm)
Benzophenones			
Oxybenzone	270-350	—	X
Dioxybenzone	250-390	—	X
Sulisobenzone	260-375	—	X
Cinnamates			
Ethyl hexyl p-methoxycinnamate	290-320	—	X
Diethanolamine p-methoxycinnamate	280-310	—	X
Octocrylene	250-360	—	X
PABA and Derivatives			
PABA	260-313	—	X
Padimate O	290-315	—	X
Glyceryl PABA	264-315	—	X
Salicylates			
Ethylhexyl salicylate	280-320	—	X
Homosalate	295-315	—	X
Triethanolamine salicylate	260-320	—	X
Miscellaneous			
Methyl anthranilate	260-380	X	—
Avobenzone	320-400	X	—
Phenylbenzimidazole sulfonic acid	290-340	—	X
Red petrolatum	290-365	—	X
Titanium dioxide	290-700	X	X
Zinc oxide	290-700	X	X

*Because sunscreens are clinically effective on a portion of their UVR band, the table indicates what type of UVR the sunscreens are effective in blocking. Because the ingredients of these sunscreens frequently change, consult the product label to determine if it meets requirements.

Box 3-1 Drug Photosensitizers

Acenocoumarol	Dantrolene
Acetazolamide	Dapsone
Acetophenazine	Decarbazine
Alprazolam	Demeclocycline
Amiloride	Desipramine
Amiodarone	Desoximetasone
Amitriptyline	Dibucaine
Amoxapine	Dichlorphenamide
Anesthetics (procaine group)	Diethylstilbestrol
Antimalarials	Diflunisal
Aspirin	Disopyramide
Astemizole	Doxepin
Auranofin	Doxycycline
Aurothioglucose	Enalapril
Barbiturates	Enoxacin
Benoxaprofen	Erythromycin
Benzocaine	Estrogens
Benzthiazide	Ethionamide
Bithionol	Fenofibrate
Buclosamide	Fluorouracil
Captopril	Flutamide
Carbamazine	Formaldehyde
Carbinoxamine	Furosemide
Carprofen	Ganciclovir
Ceftazidime	Glibenclamide
Chlordiazepoxide	Glipizide
Chlorhexidine	Glisoxepide
Chloroquine	Glyburide
Chlorothiazide	Gold Salts
Chlorphenoxamine	Green soap
Chlorpromazine	Grepafloxacin
Chlorpropamide	Griseofulvin
Chlorprothixene	Haloperidol
Chlortetracycline	Hexachlorophene
Cholestyramine	Hydralazine
Ciprofloxacin	Hydrochlorothiazide
Clinafloxacin	Hydroflumethiazide
Clofazimine	Hydroxychloroquine
Clozapine	Hypericum
Coal tar	Ibuprofen
Cyclobenzaprine	Isoniazid
Cyclothiazide	Isotretinoin
Cyproheptadine	Ketoprofen

Box 3-1	Drug Photosensitizers—cont'd

Lincomycin	PuvaTherapy
Lomefloxacin	Pyrazinamide
Losartan	Pyridoxine
Maprotiline	Pyrimethamine
Mefloquine	Quinethazone
Mesoridazine	Quinidine
Methacycline	Ranitidine
Methazolamide	Risperidone
Methdilazine	Ritonavir
Methotrexate	Salicylates
Methoxsalen	Saquinavir
Methyclothiazide	Secobarbital
Methyldopa	Selegiline
Methylene blue	Sertraline
Minocycline	Sotalol
Mirtazapine	Sparfloxacin
Moexipril	Sulbentine
Mupirocin	Sulfacytine
Nalidixic acid	Sulfamethizole
Naproxen	Sulfamethoxazole
Nifedipine	Sulfisoxazole
Nortriptyline	Sulfonamides
Ofloxacin	Tacrolimus
Olsalazine	Terfenadine
Omeprazole	Tetracycline
Oral contraceptives	Thioridazine
Oxolinic acid	Tolazamide
Oxytetracycline	Tolbutamide
Pentobarbital	Trandolapril
Perazine	Tretinoin
Perphenazine	Triamterene
Phenothiazines	Trichlormethiazide
Phenylbutazone	Triflupromazine
Phenytoin	Trifluoperazine
Piroxicam	Trimeprazine
Polythiazide	Trimethadione
Porfimer	Trioxsalen
Procarbazine	Tripelennamine
Prochlorperazine	Trovafloxacin
Promazine	Valproic acid
Promethazine	Verteporfin
Protionamide	Vinblastine
Protriptyline	Vitamin A
Psoralens	

SUNBURN

Pharmacology

Symptoms related to sunburn result from the skin damage and irritation secondarily associated with overexposure to sunlight or artificial light. Sunburn is most often classified as a first-degree burn (limited to the top layer of the epidermis), causing erythema, tenderness, pain, and, occasionally, skin damage. Second-degree burns may result in blistering and may be associated with fever and chills. The early erythematous reaction is mediated by prostaglandins, therefore aspirin, ibuprofen, and other nonsteroidal antiinflammatory drugs (NSAIDs) may be preferred for the treatment of sunburn. The antiinflammatory effect of these products should also have a beneficial effect on the sunburn. If patients do not tolerate aspirin or NSAIDs, acetaminophen is an acceptable alternative. The prostaglandin-mediated reaction occurs during the first 24 hours. After this phase, a leukocyte-mediated process causes the inflammation. Analgesics may continue to be required for pain relief. Topical hydrocortisone is useful in treating the leukocyte-mediated inflammatory response after the initial prostaglandin-mediated erythematous response. Hydrocortisone in combination with aspirin or an NSAID may provide the most relief for sunburns. The products used to treat the symptoms of sunburn usually include one or more of the following categories:

- **Analgesics** relieve pain and inflammation (except acetaminophen) associated with sunburn. OTC products include aspirin, ibuprofen, naproxen, ketoprofen, and acetaminophen. Information on these individual products will not be discussed in this chapter. For more information, see Fever and Internal Pain, p. 363.
- **Topical hydrocortisone (steroids)** reduces inflammation, irritation, and itching, but does not relieve pain directly; many OTC products include hydrocortisone.
- **Antihistamines** work by competitively inhibiting histamine receptors associated with itching. These products are available both orally and topically. For more information, see Contact Dermatitis, p. 91 and Allergy, p. 187.
- **Aloe vera** is added to products used to treat burns, sunburns, and itching. It may contain substances with a topical anesthetic effect and antibacterial activity. It may also promote a local increase in microcirculation.
- **Topical anesthetics** relieve pain, itching, discomfort, and irritation by reversibly blocking the transmission of nerve impulses. OTC products commonly used to treat sunburn include dibucaine, tetracaine,

lidocaine, and benzocaine. These ingredients are often the main ingredients on which sunburn products are based.

This chapter focuses on products used directly on the sunburn (e.g., topical products containing local anesthetics). For information on the other agents noted above, refer to the appropriate chapter.

Side Effects

Side effects of topical anesthetics are rare; the most common are local skin irritation, stinging, or burning. Hypersensitivity reactions involving the skin have been reported in 1% of patients receiving topical benzocaine. Though rare, if serum concentrations of lidocaine are high enough, systemic effects such as dizziness, nausea, drowsiness, speech disturbances, perioral numbness, muscle twitching, confusion, vertigo, and tinnitus may occur.

Drug Interactions

No clinically significant drug interactions have been reported with these products when they are used appropriately.

Lifespan Considerations

Geriatric

There is no specific recommendation in the elderly population.

Pediatric

Benzocaine is not recommended for use in infants under the age of 1 year. The safety and efficacy of tetracaine has not been determined in children under the age of 12 years. Dosages should be reduced according to age, weight, and physical condition.

Pregnancy

Benzocaine, dibucaine, and tetracaine are all FDA Pregnancy Category C drugs. Lidocaine is a category B drug. The use of topical local anesthetics is only recommended when the potential benefits clearly outweigh the risks to the fetus.

Nursing Mothers

Some topical anesthetics are excreted in breast milk, therefore nursing mothers should consult with a health care professional before using these agents.

Patient Education

- Patients should avoid prolonged exposure to sunlight/artificial light once it is realized that they have experienced a sunburn. Prolonged exposure may worsen the sunburn and symptoms related to it.
- Analgesics should be taken around the clock for the first 24 hours as recommended on the package instruction. If pain continues, the analgesic can be taken on an "as needed" basis (see Fever and Internal Pain, p. 363 for additional information.)
- Cool compresses (e.g., a towel soaked with cool water) should be applied to the sunburned area or the patient should soak the area in a cool bath.
- Perfumes and dyes contained in some moisturizers may be irritating and should be avoided.
- Applying skin moisturizers to the sunburned area may help with the skin peeling. However, use of perfume-containing moisturizers should be avoided because of possible skin irritation.
- Topical hydrocortisone should be used with caution in severe burns with broken skin because the hydrocortisone may promote infection in the wound.
- Antihistamines may help control itching associated with sunburns. In addition, the sedating effects of antihistamines may also help patients sleep.
- Local anesthetics will provide pain relief for 15 to 45 minutes. Application should be limited to times when the pain is especially bothersome, such as at bedtime, and should not be applied more than 3 to 4 times per day, to decrease the risk of adverse effects.
- Topical agents should not be used on broken, raw, or damaged skin.
- Patients should contact a health care professional or acute care center if they experience sunburn to the genital areas, pain or swelling around or in the eyes, or a severe burn to large areas of the body that includes blistering or swelling.

Product Selection

- Patients who experience benzocaine sensitivity may try either lidocaine or dibucaine as an alternative treatment. Benzocaine is an ester anesthetic, whereas lidocaine and dibucaine are amide anesthetics. Cross-sensitivity between the amide and ester anesthetics is rare. If sensitivity to an amide anesthetic occurs, use of that product should be discontinued immediately.

SUGGESTED READING

Wentzell JM: Sunscreens: the ounce of prevention, *Am Fam Phys* 53:1713-1719, 1996.

Product Information: Topical Anesthetics

Brand Name	Dosage Form	Active Ingredient	Other Ingredients
Americaine	Ointment, aerosol	Benzocaine 6%	
Bactine Antiseptic Anesthetic	Liquid, spray	Lidocaine 2.5%	
Dermoplast	Spray	Benzocaine 20%	Menthol, alcohol, lanolin
	Lotion	Benzocaine 8%	Menthol, aloe, lanolin
Lanacane	Cream	Benzocaine 6%	Alcohol, aloe
Lanacane Maximum Strength	Spray	Benzocaine 20%	Aloe
Nupercainal	Ointment	Dibucaine 1%	Acetone sodium, bisulfite
	Cream	Dibucaine 0.5%	Acetone sodium, bisulfite
Pontocaine	Ointment	Tetracaine 0.5%	Menthol
	Cream	Tetracaine 1%	
Solarcaine	Aerosol	Benzocaine 20%	Alcohol
Solarcaine Aloe Extra Burn Relief	Cream, gel, spray	Lidocaine 0.5%	Aloe, alcohol (spray)
Unguentine Plus	Cream	Lidocaine 2%	Chloroxylenol, phenol

Allergy

Ophthalmic allergies can be caused by many external factors, including pollen, animal dander, and cosmetics. Watery eyes and itching are the most common symptoms associated with ophthalmic allergies. The itching can be the source of considerable discomfort. The best treatment for ophthalmic allergies is removal or avoidance of the cause, if known; however, ophthalmic antihistamines and decongestants can help relieve the symptoms.

OPHTHALMIC ANTIHISTAMINES

ANTAZOLINE

PHENIRAMINE

Pharmacology

Antibodies are formed in response to previous exposure to a specific antigen. When these antigens are again encountered, they combine with the preformed antibodies on the surface of mast cells, leading to breakdown (degranulation) of mast cells and spillage of their contents. Mast cells contain large amounts of histamine, as well as other mediators of the allergic response, such as SRS-A (slow reacting substance of anaphylaxis). Pollen and other allergens trapped in the conjunctival sac and tear ducts react with antibodies, leading to a local allergic reaction and the symptoms of itching and watery eyes.

Antihistamines competitively block histamine receptors (H_1 receptors). When the histamine receptor is blocked, histamine cannot stimulate the receptor and cause the allergic reaction.

Side Effects

Because topical antihistamines are not well absorbed into the systemic circulation, side effects are uncommon. Some users may experience a brief tingling sensation when the drops are applied to the eyes.

Drug Interactions

Because of the low systemic absorption of topical antihistamines, significant drug interactions are unlikely.

Lifespan Considerations

Geriatric

Ophthalmic antihistamines are generally safe for use by geriatric patients, if used as directed.

Pediatric

Eye redness in children can occur concurrently with illnesses requiring medical attention, such as colds and measles. Young children should be evaluated before recommending these products.

Pregnancy

The risk associated with topical antihistamines can be expected to be minimal. However, potential benefit must be balanced against risk to the fetus.

Nursing Mothers

Because systemic absorption is low, risk to a nursing infant can be expected to be minimal. However, there is insufficient data on which to make a recommendation.

OPHTHALMIC DECONGESTANTS

PHENYLEPHRINE
NAPHAZOLINE
TETRAHYDROZOLINE
OXYMETAZOLINE

Pharmacology

Ophthalmic decongestants stimulate α-adrenergic receptors in blood vessels, causing vasoconstriction of the conjunctival blood vessels.

Subsequently, this provides symptomatic relief of redness and minor eye irritations. Ophthalmic decongestants (eye drops) are more potent local vasoconstrictors than oral products because they are applied directly into the eye. In normal doses, these products do not enter the circulation in sufficient quantities to be associated with increased blood pressure, but they can be associated with rebound congestion of the conjunctiva as a result of frequent or extended use.

Side Effects

Prolonged or excessive use may cause rebound congestion of the conjunctiva. Phenylephrine may also dilate the pupil if enough of it penetrates the corneal epithelium, but significant dilation is rare in the OTC strength. Individuals most likely to experience the dilatory effects are those who wear contact lenses and instill the medication immediately after removing their contact lenses. Phenylephrine can also cause temporary blurred or unstable vision.

Patients using naphazoline and who also have lightly pigmented irides (e.g., blue or green eyes), wear contacts, or have corneal abrasions appear to experience more of the mydriatic, or dilating, effects of the drug. Mydriasis may precipitate an attack of acute angle-closure glaucoma in predisposed eyes.

Some patients who use tetrahydrozoline may experience a mild, transient stinging after instillation of the drops.

Oxymetazoline appears to be relatively free of ocular and systemic effects.

Patients should be cautioned that liberal or indiscriminate use of ophthalmic decongestants can increase the likelihood of side effects. If signs and symptoms have not resolved within 72 hours, patients should be instructed to seek professional eye care. Waiting longer than 72 hours may cause eye redness and irritation to become worse, increase side effects, or cause a patient to neglect a potentially serious condition.

Drug Interactions

Because of the low systemic absorption of ophthalmic decongestants, clinically significant drug interactions are uncommon.

Lifespan Considerations

Geriatric

Ophthalmic decongestants are generally safe for use by geriatric patients if used as directed for no more than 72 hours. Patients with glaucoma should use ophthalmic decongestants only under the supervision of a health care professional.

Pediatric

Eye redness in children can occur with illnesses that may require medical attention, such as allergies, fevers, colds, and measles. These illnesses must be ruled out before ophthalmic decongestants are recommended for use in children of any age. The following list addresses pediatric considerations by drug:

- **Naphazoline.** Use of naphazoline by infants and children is not recommended because they are especially sensitive to its effects.
- **Phenylephrine and tetrahydrozoline.** There are no data or specific recommendations for use of these products in the pediatric population.
- **Oxymetazoline.** For children age 6 and older, oxymetazoline can be used safely up to 4 times a day for no more than 72 hours. There are no data or specific recommendations for use of this product in children under the age of 6 years.

Pregnancy

Naphazoline, oxymetazoline, phenylephrine, and tetrahydrozoline are all FDA Pregnancy Category C drugs.

Nursing Mothers

Ophthalmic decongestants may be absorbed systemically and distributed into breast milk. These medications have not been reported to cause problems in nursing babies.

Patient Education

- Patients should put 1 or 2 drops into the conjunctival sac of the affected eye every 3 to 4 hours up to a maximum of 4 times a day.
- Patients should not use ophthalmic decongestants for more than 72 hours without consulting a health care professional.
- Patients should be referred to a health care professional if there is an embedded foreign body in the eye, uveitis, flash burns, chemical exposure by splash injury, tear-duct infections or blockage, corneal ulcers, or corneal abrasions.

- Patients experiencing rebound congestion should be referred to a health care professional for differential diagnosis and management.
- Expiration dates on ophthalmic decongestants should be strictly enforced because loss of pharmacologic activity may occur without visible changes in solution color. Once the sterility safety seal on ophthalmic medications is broken, they should be discarded within 30 days; the manufacturer's expiration date does not apply after the seal is broken.
- Patients with glaucoma should not use ophthalmic decongestants except under the advice and supervision of a health care professional because of the risk of acute angle-closure glaucoma.
- Phenylephrine may cause temporary blurred or unstable vision. Patients should use caution while driving or performing other hazardous tasks.
- With prolonged use of ophthalmic decongestants, some patients may experience epithelial xerosis (abnormal dryness).
- Some ointments, drops, nasal sprays, or other products may contain phenylephrine, naphazoline, tetrahydrozoline, or oxymetazoline. However, patients should not use these products in the eye, but should instead use only those products specifically formulated for ophthalmic use.
- Patients should not use these products if the solution changes color or becomes cloudy.
- To avoid contamination, patients should not touch the tip of the container to any surface.
- Patients should replace the cap of the ophthalmic decongestant container immediately after use.
- Contact lenses should be removed before using ophthalmic decongestants.
- For tips on the proper administration of ophthalmic medications, see Box 4-1.

Product Selection

- Because of the potential for adverse drug reactions, ophthalmic decongestants should not be used as an ocular irrigant.
- Patients with itching and red eyes caused by pollen, animal hair, or other allergies may benefit from taking an ophthalmic decongestant/antihistamine combination.
- Patients experiencing watery eyes may also need to take oral antihistamines. For additional information on oral antihistamines, please see Allergy, p. 187.

Box 4-1   Proper Administration of Ophthalmic Medications

1. Always wash hands before administration of any ophthalmic medications.
2. Tilt head backward.
3. To minimize contamination of the container and risk of infection, do not touch the tip of the medication container and do not let the container tip touch the eye or lid during instillation.
4. With clean hands, form a pouch below the bottom eyelashes by pinching together the skin from the inside corner of the eye to the outer corner.
5. Do not instill more than one drop of medication at a time because the eye pouch is not able to hold more than one drop.
6. Look upward just before instilling the drop of ophthalmic medication, then look downward to evenly distribute the medication over the eye.
7. Close the eye gently to allow even distribution of the medication over the eye.
8. If instilling multiple drops of ophthalmic medication into the eye, wait approximately 5 minutes before adding subsequent drops to prevent flushing away the first drop or to prevent the second drop from being diluted by the first.
9. Immediately after instillation, apply gentle pressure to the lacrimal sac (inner corner of the eye) for 3 to 5 minutes to help avoid systemic absorption.
10. Blot excess solution from around the eye.
11. If the eye drops are to be used with ophthalmic ointment, instill the eye drops at least 10 minutes before instilling the ointment to prevent the ointment from becoming a barrier to tear film or corneal penetration of the drop.

SUGGESTED READINGS

Abelson MB, Yamamoto GK, Allansmith MR: Effects of ocular decongestants, *Arch Ophthalmol* 98:856-858, 1980.
Yarborough P: Diabetic eye disease, *US Pharm* 20(11):48-66, 1995.

Product Information: Ophthalmic Decongestants*

Brand Name	Active Ingredient	Pediatric Dose
AK-Nefrin	Phenylephrine 0.12%	
Allerest Eye Drops	Naphazoline 0.012%	
Bausch & Lomb All Clear AR	Naphazoline 0.03%	
Bausch & Lomb All Clear Drops	Naphazoline 0.012%	
Clear Eyes	Naphazoline 0.012%	
Clear Eyes ACR	Naphazoline 0.012%	
Collyrium Fresh	Tetrahydrozoline 0.05%	
Comfort Eye Drops	Naphazoline 0.03%	
Murine Tears Plus	Tetrahydrozoline 0.05%	
Naphcon	Naphazoline 0.012%	
OcuClear	Oxymetazoline 0.025%	≥ age 6: Instill 1 or 2 drops into eye(s) up to 4 times a day
Prefrin Liquifilm	Phenylephrine 0.12%	
Relief†	Phenylephrine 0.12%	
Tetrasine	Tetrahydrozoline 0.05%	
Tetrasine Extra	Tetrahydrozoline 0.05%	
VasoClear	Naphazoline 0.02%	
Visine	Tetrahydrozoline 0.05%	
Visine AC	Tetrahydrozoline 0.05%	
Visine Advanced Relief	Tetrahydrozoline 0.05%	
Visine L.R.	Oxymetazoline 0.025%	≥ age 6: Instill 1 or 2 drops into eye(s) up to 4 times a day

*Adult dose: Instill 1 or 2 drops into eye(s) up to 4 times a day.
†Unit dose (0.3 ml) is preservative free.

Product Information: Ophthalmic Decongestant/Antihistamine Combinations*

Brand Name	Decongestant	Antihistamine
Naphcon-A Solution	Naphazoline 0.025%	Pheniramine maleate 0.3%
Ocuhist	Naphazoline 0.25%	Pheniramine maleate 0.3%
Vasocon A	Naphazoline 0.5%	Antazoline 0.5%
Opcon-A Solution	Naphazoline 0.027%	Pheniramine maleate 0.315%

*Adult dose: Instill 1 or 2 drops into eye(s) up to 4 times a day.

Dry or Irritated Eyes

Dryness and/or irritation are two of the most common problems associated with the eyes. This condition is caused when the normal flow of tears is interrupted, or when there is an abnormality in any of the three layers of the tear film. This condition is characterized by a sandy, gritty feeling in the eye and may be accompanied by other symptoms such as burning, itching, or redness. Individuals develop dry or irritated eyes from many sources, including allergies, medications, contact lenses, and other environmental conditions.

Nonprescription ophthalmic drugs used to treat dry or irritated eyes include artificial tears and lubricants.

ARTIFICIAL TEARS AND OPHTHALMIC LUBRICANTS

Pharmacology

Dry or irritated eyes are typically caused by a dysfunction in the tear layer of the eye that subsequently causes suboptimal lubrication of the ocular surface. A decrease in the amount of tears eventually occurs, which starts a never-ending cycle. Artificial tear solutions offer tearlike lubrication to supplement tear production. The primary benefit of lubricants is to increase the viscosity of existing tears.

Side Effects

Artificial tear solutions may cause mild stinging or temporary blurred vision. Immediately after instillation of ophthalmic ointments, patients may experience blurred vision.

Drug Interactions

There are no known clinically significant drug interactions with artificial tear solutions or lubricants.

Lifespan Considerations

Geriatric

Dry or irritated eyes are frequently associated with the aging process. Because they do not contain active ingredients, artificial tear solutions and lubricants are very useful in the geriatric population to treat dry or irritated eyes.

Pediatric

There are no data or specific recommendations for using these agents in the pediatric population. However, because of the nature of this product, there should not be a problem using it for less than 72 hours.

Pregnancy

There is no FDA pregnancy classification for artificial tear solutions or ophthalmic lubricants. Because of the low systemic absorption of the ingredients listed, these products should be safe to use during pregnancy.

Nursing Mothers

There are no data for the use of artificial tear solutions or ophthalmic lubricants by nursing mothers. Because of the low systemic absorption of the ingredients listed, these products should be safe to use while nursing.

Patient Education

- Artificial tear solutions: Patients should instill 1 to 2 drops into the eye(s) 3 or 4 times daily, as needed.
- Ophthalmic ointments: To apply, patients should pull down the lower lid of the affected eye(s) and apply a small amount (0.25 inch) of ointment to the inside of the eyelid.
- Ophthalmic ointments should not be used for more than 72 hours without consulting a health care professional.
- If eye pain, vision changes, or continued irritation occurs, or if the condition worsens, the patient should contact a health care professional.
- Patients using nonmedicated ophthalmic ointment should be told that they may have temporary blurred vision because the ointment coats the eye. This can be resolved by decreasing the amount of ophthalmic ointment instilled, or by instilling it at bedtime.
- Ophthalmic lubricants should not be used with contact lenses.
- Expiration dates on artificial tear solutions should be strictly adhered

to because loss of pharmacologic activity may occur without visible changes in solution color. Once the sterility safety seal on ophthalmic medications is broken, they should be discarded within 30 days; the manufacturer's expiration date does not apply once the seal is broken.

- To avoid contamination, patients should avoid touching the tip of the container to any surface and should replace the container cap immediately after instillation. For directions on proper administration of ophthalmic medications, see Box 4-1.
- For instructions on proper administration of ophthalmic lubricants, see Box 4-2.

Product Selection

- Some patients may experience a hypersensitivity reaction after use of ophthalmic lubricants that contain a preservative. This type of reaction can be alleviated by switching to a preservative-free ophthalmic lubricant.
- Preservative-free artificial tear solutions are available for patients sensitive to the preservative(s). However, they are more costly and can become easily contaminated by the patient during use.
- Patients may prefer using artificial tears during the day and reserving ophthalmic ointments for use at bedtime because of the potential for blurred vision while using ointments.

Box 4-2   Proper Administration of Ophthalmic Lubricants

1. Always wash hands before administration of any ophthalmic medications.
2. Tilt head backward.
3. Avoid touching the tip of the medication container and do not let the tip touch the eye or lid as the medication is being applied to the eye. This helps to minimize contamination and the risk of infection.
4. With clean hands, form a pouch below the bottom eyelashes by pinching together the inside of the eye to the outer corner.
5. Place ¼ to ½ inch of ointment onto your clean finger, then transfer into the pouch. Close the eye for 1 to 2 minutes and roll the eye around. If more than one eye ointment is to be applied at or about the same time, allow 10 minutes before instilling the other ophthalmic ointment.
6. When ophthalmic ointment or gel is to be used in addition to eye drops, instill the eye drops first, then wait approximately 10 minutes before instilling the ophthalmic ointment or gel.

- Ophthalmic ointments may be preferred because of their longer duration of activity.

SUGGESTED READINGS

Reddy IK, Toedter NM, Khan MA: Dry eye: causes, symptoms and clinical management, US Pharm 23(1):38-55, 1998.
Wright M: Diagnosis and treatment of dry eyes, Practitioner 241(1573):210-212, 214, 216, 1997.

Product Information: Dry or Irritated Eyes*

Brand Name	Ingredients	Comments
Artificial Tears	0.01 % benzalkonium chloride; may also contain EDTA, NaCl, polyvinyl alcohol, hydroxy-propyl methylcellulose	
Adsorbotear	0.4% hydroxyethylcellulose, 1.67% povidone, water soluble polymers, 0.004% thimerosal, 0.1% EDTA	
Akwa Tears	0.01% benzalkonium chloride, 1.4% polyvinyl alcohol, sodium phosphate, EDTA, NaCl	
AquaSite	0.2% PEG-400, 0.1% dextran 70, polycarbophil, NaCl, ESTA, sodium hydroxide	Preservative free in 0.6-ml and 15-ml solutions
Artificial Tears Plus	1.4% polyvinyl alcohol, 0.6% povidone, 0.5% chlorobutanol, NaCl	
Bion Tears	0.1% dextran 70, 0.3% hydroxy-propyl methylcellulose 2910, NaCl, KCl, sodium bicarbonate	Preservative free in 0.45-ml solution
Cellufresh	0.5% carboxymethylcellulose sodium, NaCl	Preservative free in 0.3-ml solution
Celluvisc	1% carboxymethylcellulose, NaCl, KCl, sodium lactate	Preservative free in 0.3-ml solution
Comfort Tears	Hydroxyethylcellulose, 0.005% benzalkonium chloride, 0.02% EDTA	

*Dose: Instill 1 or 2 drops into eye(s) 3 or 4 times a day, as needed.

Product Information: Dry or Irritated Eyes—cont'd

Brand Name	Ingredients	Comments
Dry Eye Therapy	0.3% glycerin, NaCl, KCl, sodium citrate, sodium phosphate	Preservative free in 0.3-ml solution
Dry Eyes	1.4% polyvinyl alcohol, 0.01% benzalkonium chloride, sodium phosphate, EDTA, NaCl	
Isopto Plain	0.5% hydroxypropyl methyl-cellulose 2910, 0.01% benzal-konium chloride, NaCl, sodium phosphate, sodium citrate	
Moisture Drops	0.5% hydroxypropyl methylcellulose, 0.1% povidone, 0.2% glycerin, 0.01% benzalkonium chloride, EDTA, NaCl, boric acid, KCl, sodium borate	
Murine Tears	0.5% polyvinyl alcohol, 0.6% povidone, benzalkonium chloride, dextrose, EDTA, NaCl, sodium bicarbonate, sodium phosphate	
Refresh	1.4% polyvinyl alcohol, 0.6% povidone, NaCl	
Refresh Plus	0.5% carboxymethylcellulose sodium, KCl, NaCl	
Tears Naturale II	0.1% dextran 70, 0.3% hydroxypropyl methylcel-lulose 2910, 0.001% polyquaternium-1, NaCl, KCl, sodium borate	
Tears Naturale Free	0.3% hydroxypropyl methyl-cellulose 2910, 0.1% dextran 70, NaCl, KCl, sodium borate	Preservative free in 0.6-ml solution
Tears Naturale	0.1% dextran 70, 0.01% benzalkonium chloride, 0.3% hydroxypropyl methylcellulose, NaCl, EDTA, hydrochloric acid, sodium hydroxide, KCl	

Product Information: Ophthalmic Lubricants*

Brand Name	Dosage Form	Ingredients	Comments
Akwa Tears	Ointment	White petrolatum, mineral oil, lanolin	Preservative free
Artificial Tears	Ointment	White petrolatum, anhydrous liquid lanolin, mineral oil	
Dry Eyes	Ointment	White petrolatum, mineral oil, lanolin	Preservative free
Duratears Naturale	Ointment	White petrolatum, anhydrous liquid lanolin, mineral oil	Preservative free
HypoTears	Ointment	White petrolatum, light mineral oil	Preservative free
Lacri-Lube NP	Ointment	55.5% white petrolatum, 42.5% mineral oil, 2% petrolatum/lanolin alcohol	Preservative free
Lacri-Lube S.O.P.	Ointment	56.8% white petrolatum, 42.5% mineral oil, chlorobutanol, lanolin alcohols	
LubriTears	Ointment	White petrolatum, mineral oil, lanolin, 0.5% chlorobutanol	
Refresh PM	Ointment	56.8% white petrolatum, 41.5% mineral oil, lanolin alcohols, sodium chloride	Preservative free
Stye	Ointment	55% white petrolatum, 32% mineral oil, boric acid, stearic acid, wheat germ oil	
Tears Renewed	Ointment	White petrolatum, light mineral oil	Preservative free and lanolin free

*Dose: Instill 3 or 4 times daily, as needed.

Canker and Cold Sores

The terms *canker sore* and *cold sore* are often used interchangeably, yet each refers to a distinct type of mouth sore. Canker sores are noninfectious, ulcerative lesions found inside the mouth; they can appear singly or in groups and are often inflamed. The cause is unknown and may be multifactorial, including genetics, stress, injury, or hypersensitivity. Cold sores, also known as *fever blisters*, are more often found outside of the mouth. These inflammatory lesions are caused by the herpes simplex 1 virus and are quite infectious. The virus is often contracted at an early age and lies dormant until an outbreak is triggered by some event stressful to the body. Both types of sores can be very painful and last a similar length of time, usually about 10 days or so. In both instances, only symptomatic relief can be provided because there is no cure for either type of sore.

Nonprescription drugs used to treat canker sores include local anesthetics and oral rinses.

LOCAL ANESTHETICS

BENZOCAINE
BENZYL ALCOHOL
DYCLONINE
LIDOCAINE
TETRACAINE

Pharmacology

Local anesthetics are applied topically to the sores and form a protective layer in addition to facilitating pain relief. They act by suppressing sensory nerve impulse conduction by altering the permeability of the cell membrane to ionic transfer. Absorption through the skin, normally low, is greatly increased because of the ulcerations present in these conditions.

Side Effects

Adverse reactions are dose-related and should be minimal because the doses involved are small. Allergy to any of the ingredients is cause to avoid using a given product. Allergic reactions can include contact dermatitis, lesions, edema, and possibly anaphylactic reactions. Other side effects occasionally seen with these products include stinging, burning, or tenderness. The stinging or burning sensations may be further enhanced by alcohol-based products.

Drug Interactions

There are no known clinically significant drug interactions.

Lifespan Considerations
Geriatric

The rate of occurrence of both canker sores and cold sores diminishes as people approach middle age; therefore the need for these medications in the elderly is greatly reduced.

Pediatric

Canker sores can occur in children under the age of 10 years. As with the geriatric population, the minimum dose and concentration necessary to afford pain relief should be used.

Pregnancy

Lidocaine is an FDA Pregnancy Category B drug. Because these products are applied topically, potential risk to the fetus should be minimal.

Nursing Mothers

No information is available on the use of these medications while nursing.

Patient Education

- Alcohol-containing products may cause a temporary burning or stinging sensation.

- Lesions should be kept moist and clean to promote healing and reduce the possibility of secondary infections.
- Patients should refrain from touching the blisters or pinching or picking at them. These actions could enhance the possibility of secondary infections or prolong the duration of the sores.
- Topical preparations should be kept away from the eyes.
- Treating cold sores present on the tongue or inside of the mouth with anesthetics could lead to numbness and inadvertent biting of the tongue.

Product Selection

- In treating both canker sores and cold sores, patients should avoid products containing menthol, phenol, or camphor because they can promote irritation and increase inflammation.
- Patients should look for a dosage form that helps form a protective layer over the sore and helps to keep the sore from drying out. Protective ingredients include cocoa butter, allantoin, petrolatum, or benzoin tincture.
- Products with lower concentrations of benzocaine or lidocaine at the lowest effective strength for treatment are preferred.

Product Information: Canker and Cold Sores

Brand Name	Dosage Form	Active Ingredients	Canker Sore	Cold Sore
Campho-phenique Cold Sore	Gel	10.8% camphor, 4.7% phenol		X
Kanka	Liquid/film	20% benzocaine benzoin compound tincture	X	
Numzident	Gel	10% benzocaine		X
Orabase	Gel	15% benzocaine	X	X
Orabase-B	Paste	20% benzocaine	X	
Orajel Mouth-Aid	Gel, liquid	20% benzocaine	X	X
Tanac	Gel	1% dyclonine	X	X
Tanac	Liquid	10% benzocaine	X	X
Tanac	Stick	7.5% benzocaine		X
Tanac Roll-On	Liquid	5% benzocaine		X
Viractin	Cream, gel	2% tetracaine		X
Zilactin	Gel	10% benzyl alcohol	X	X
Zilactin-B	Gel	10% benzocaine	X	
Zilactin-L	Liquid	2.5% lidocaine		X

ORAL RINSES

Carbamide peroxide

Hydrogen peroxide

Pharmacology

Oral rinses cleanse mouth ulcerations by releasing oxygen, which floats the particles out of the wound by a foaming action. This decreases inflammation, relieves pain, controls odor-forming bacteria, and promotes healing. These products are used in treating noninfectious canker sores rather than infectious cold sores.

Side Effects

Side effects are not common or expected with oral rinses; however, if inflammation or irritation occurs or worsens, the patient should contact a health care professional.

Drug Interactions

There are no known clinically significant drug interactions.

Lifespan Considerations

Geriatric

There are no concerns specific to this population group for the use of oral rinses.

Pediatric

Oral rinses should not be used for children under the age of 3 without first consulting a health care professional.

Pregnancy

Because these medications are not systemically absorbed, they should not pose any significant risk during pregnancy.

Nursing Mothers

Because these medications are not systemically absorbed, they should not pose any significant risk while nursing.

Patient Education

- If irritation, inflammation, or pain worsens or persists for more than 1 week, the patient should consult a health care professional.
- The patient should avoid contact of the oral rinse with the eyes.
- Oral rinse solutions should be protected from heat or direct lighting.
- Patients should not use oral rinses for more than 7 days unless directed by a health care professional.

Product Selection

There is little difference between products in this category. Both carbamide peroxide and hydrogen peroxide work in essentially the same way. Product choice should be made on ease of application of a given medication.

SUGGESTED READING

Pray WS: Oral mucosal lesions, US Pharm 15(2):21-22, 24-25, 66, 1990.

Product Information: Oral Rinses

Brand Name	Dosage Form	Active Ingredient
Cankaid	Solution	10% carbamide peroxide
Gly-Oxide Liquid	Solution	10% carbamide peroxide
Orajel Perioseptic	Solution	15% carbamide peroxide
Peroxyl	Gel	1.5% hydrogen peroxide
Peroxyl Dental Rinse	Solution	1.5% hydrogen peroxide

Dry Mouth

Dry mouth (xerostomia) is a condition that occurs when salivary glands do not produce sufficient saliva. Saliva is necessary for the breakdown of food and also helps keep bacterial counts low in the mouth. Dry mouth not only makes digestion more difficult, it can also lead to increased risk for infection or dental caries, hinder a person's sense of taste, and cause halitosis. The problem is more prevalent in the elderly and in women, and may be a symptom of an underlying disease such as diabetes or Sjögren's syndrome. Radiation therapy for head and neck cancers frequently causes xerostomia. Drugs that have anticholinergic side effects, such as antihistamines and some antidepressants, are also a potential cause of dry mouth.

Saliva substitutes are used to treat dry mouth.

SALIVA SUBSTITUTES

SODIUM CARBOXYMETHYLCELLULOSE

HYDROXYETHYL CELLULOSE

Pharmacology

The purpose of saliva substitutes is to remoisten and lubricate the inside of the mouth, thus allowing for resumption of more normal eating, tasting, and swallowing of food. The products in this class contain various electrolytes held in a carboxymethylcellulose base or other similar viscous base. The electrolytes help maintain a natural chemical balance inside the mouth, and the cellulose allows the product to adhere better to the inside of the oral cavity.

Side Effects

There are no known clinically significant side effects associated with the use of these products.

Drug Interactions

There are no known clinically significant drug interactions.

Lifespan Considerations

Geriatric

There are no concerns with these medications specific to this population group.

Pediatric

The problems that can lead to dry mouth are seldom a concern in the pediatric population. There are no unique recommendations with the use of these medications for children.

Pregnancy

There are no risks associated with use of these medications during pregnancy.

Nursing Mothers

There are no risks associated with use of these medications while nursing.

Patient Education

- Product canisters should be protected from direct sunlight and excessive heat.
- Saliva substitutes can generally be used as often as necessary with no ill effects.

Product Selection

There is little difference between products in this category because they all have very similar ingredients that work in essentially the same way. Patients should choose a product based on its ease of use.

SUGGESTED READING

Jordan K: A new treatment may alleviate the effects of dry mouth, J Mass Dent Soc 46(2):22-23, 1997.

Product Information: Saliva Substitutes

Brand Name	Dosage Form	Viscosity Agent (Base)
Entertainer's Secret	Solution	Sodium carboxymethylcellulose
Moi-Stir	Solution	Sodium carboxymethylcellulose
Moi-Stir Swabsticks	Solution	Sodium carboxymethylcellulose
Optimoist	Solution	Hydroxyethyl cellulose
Salivart	Solution	Sodium carboxymethylcellulose
Saliva Substitute	Solution	Sodium carboxymethylcellulose
Stoppers 4	Solution	Hydroxyethyl cellulose

Oral Pain, Toothache, and Sensitive Teeth

There are several types of oral and tooth pain. Babies experience teething pain as new teeth break through the gum surface. Adults experience sensitive teeth because of exposed dentin that results from thinning enamel, receding gums, or periodontal surgery. Adults or children can have painful teeth or gums because of ill-fitting dentures or braces or severely chapped lips caused by sun exposure.

Drugs used to treat oral pain/toothache include local anesthetics and preparations for sensitive teeth.

LOCAL ANESTHETICS AND COUNTERIRRITANTS

Local Anesthetics

BENZOCAINE
DYCLONINE

Counterirritants

CAMPHOR
PHENOL
MENTHOL
SALICYLIC ACID

Pharmacology

Local anesthetics are topically applied to the painful site and often provide a protective layer in addition to facilitating pain relief. They act by suppressing sensory nerve impulse conduction by altering the permeability of the cell membrane to ionic transfer. Absorption through the skin, which is normally low, is greatly increased because the skin's surface is often compromised in these conditions. Menthol, camphor, phenol, and salicylic acid are counterirritants and may actually stimulate nerve endings, causing a tingling sensation.

Side Effects

Adverse reactions are dose-related and uncommon. Allergy to any of the ingredients is cause to avoid using a given product. Allergic reactions can include contact dermatitis, lesions, edema, and possibly anaphylactic reactions. The other major side effects with some products is stinging, burning, or tenderness. The stinging or burning sensations may be further enhanced by alcohol-based products. If inflammation is present, it would be best to avoid products containing these ingredients because inflammation or irritation may worsen.

Drug Interactions

There are no known clinically significant drug interactions.

Lifespan Considerations
Geriatric

Because these medications may be necessary to treat denture pain or other minor problems in the mouth, the lowest effective dose and concentration for maintenance of analgesia should be recommended.

Pediatric

There are products formulated specifically for use with teething pain in infants. These products should be used preferentially over similar products because they generally have smaller quantities of the active ingredient and thus less risk of side effects.

Pregnancy

Lidocaine is an FDA Pregnancy Category B drug. Although these medications are not being taken internally, there may still be some risk because of systemic absorption.

Nursing Mothers

There is no information available on the use of these medications while nursing.

Patient Education

- Products with alcohol as an ingredient may cause a temporary burning or stinging sensation on open sores.
- Open lacerations or abrasions should be kept moist and clean to help promote healing and prevent the possibility of secondary infections.

- Patients should refrain from touching sore areas or pinching or picking at them. These actions could enhance the possibility of secondary infections or prolong the duration of the sores.
- Treating lacerations present on the tongue or inside of the mouth with anesthetics could lead to numbness and increase the possibility of trauma when the patient bites the area and does not realize it.
- Because these products can cause numbness, care should be taken to avoid biting one's tongue.

Product Selection

- Patients should use a dosage form that helps form a protective layer over the sore and keeps the sore from drying out. Protective ingredients include cocoa butter, allantoin, petrolatum, or benzoin tincture.
- Patients should try products with lower concentrations of benzocaine or lidocaine and use the lowest effective strength for treatment.

Product Information: Teething Pain

Brand Name	Dosage Form	Active Ingredient
Babee Teething	Lotion	2.5% benzocaine
Baby Anbesol	Gel	7.5% benzocaine
Baby Orajel	Gel	7.5% benzocaine
Baby Orajel Nighttime	Gel	10% benzocaine
Numzit Teething	Gel	7.5% benzocaine
Numzit Teething	Lotion	0.2% benzocaine
Orabase Baby	Gel	7.5% benzocaine

Product Information: Miscellaneous Oral/Tooth Pain

Brand Name	Dosage Form	Active Ingredients	Uses
Anbesol	Gel	6.3% benzocaine, camphor, phenol	Denture irritation, toothache, sore gums
	Liquid	6.3% benzocaine, camphor, menthol, phenol	
Anbesol Maximum Strength	Gel, liquid	20% benzocaine	Denture irritation, toothache, sore gums
Benzodent	Ointment, cream	20% benzocaine	Denture pain
Blistex	Lip balm	Camphor, phenol	Dry, chapped, or sunburned lips
Blistex Lip Medex	Lip balm	Camphor, phenol	Dry, chapped, or sunburned lips
Carmex Lip Balm	Lip balm	Camphor, menthol, phenol, salicylic acid	Dry, chapped, or sunburned lips
Chapstick Medicated Lip Balm	Stick	Camphor, menthol, phenol	Dry, chapped, or sunburned lips
Dent's Double-Action Kit	Liquid, tablets	20% benzocaine, 325 mg acetaminophen	Toothache
Dent's Extra Strength Toothache Gum	Gum	20% benzocaine	Toothache
Dent's Maximum Strength Toothache Drops	Liquid	20% benzocaine	Toothache
Hurricaine	Gel, liquid, or spray	20% benzocaine	Oral pain
Numzident Adult Strength	Gel	10% benzocaine	Denture and braces irritation, toothache, sore gums
Orabase-B	Paste	20% benzocaine	Denture sores, mouth and gum irritation

Orabase Lip	Cream	5% benzocaine, camphor, menthol, phenol	Denture sores, mouth and gum irritation
Orajel	Gel	10% benzocaine	Toothache
Orajel Brace-Aid	Gel	20% benzocaine	Pain, soreness, and irritation caused by orthodontic appliances
Orajel Denture	Gel	10% benzocaine	Denture pain
Orajel, Maximum Strength	Gel, liquid	20% benzocaine	Toothache
Orajel Mouth-Aid	Gel, liquid	20% benzocaine	Chapped lips, sun blisters, mouth and gum sores
Orajel PM, Maximum Strength	Gel	20% benzocaine	Toothache
Orasol	Liquid	6.3% benzocaine, phenol, povidone-iodine	Oral pain
Tanac	Gel	1% dyclonine	Mouth sores
Tanac	Liquid	10% benzocaine	Mouth sores
Tanac	Stick	7.5% benzocaine	Dry, chapped, or sunburned lips
Tanac Roll-On	Liquid	5% benzocaine	Dry, chapped, or sunburned lips
Vaseline Lip Therapy	Ointment	Camphor, menthol, phenol	Dry, chapped, or sunburned lips
Zilactin-B	Gel	10% benzocaine	Mouth sores, cheek bites, gum sores from dental appliances

PREPARATIONS FOR SENSITIVE TEETH

POTASSIUM NITRATE
STRONTIUM CHLORIDE
FLUORIDES

Pharmacology

Potassium nitrate is believed to block transmission of pain along neural pathways, thereby reducing hypersensitivity to hot and cold or other painful stimuli. Fluorides help protect teeth against cavities by forming a protective coating over the enamel.

Side Effects

There are no known clinically significant side effects.

Drug Interactions

There are no known clinically significant drug interactions.

Lifespan Considerations

Geriatric

There are no considerations specific to the geriatric population. As aging occurs, tooth pain is more likely to be indicative of a serious problem caused by natural tooth erosion.

Pediatric

These products should not be used on children under the age of 12 years without consulting a health care professional.

Pregnancy

Pregnant patients should consult a health care professional before using sensitive tooth preparations. Because these medications are topical in nature and should be expectorated rather than swallowed, there is probably little risk associated with their use; however, any systemic absorption may be potentially hazardous.

Nursing Mothers

Nursing mothers should consult a health care professional before using these products. Because they are topical in nature and should be expectorated rather than swallowed, there is probably little risk associated with their use; however, any systemic absorption may be potentially hazardous.

Patient Education

- It may take 2 weeks for significant therapeutic response to become evident.
- Patients should not use these products for longer than 4 weeks without the recommendation of a health care professional.
- Patients should apply at least a 1-inch strip of sensitive tooth preparations to a soft-bristled toothbrush and brush for at least 1 minute twice a day.
- Patients should be sure to brush all sensitive areas of the teeth.

Product Selection

These products are all very similar in nature and content and all come in the form of a toothpaste.

SUGGESTED READINGS

Gossel TA: Hypersensitive teeth: OTCs take the pain away, US Pharm 16(5):23-32, 1991.

Kanapka JA: Over-the-counter dentifrices in the treatment of tooth hypersensitivity, Dent Clin North Am 34(3):545-560, 1990.

Product Information: Sensitive Teeth

Brand Name	Active Ingredients
Aquafresh Sensitive	5% potassium nitrate, sodium fluoride
Crest Sensitivity Protection	5% potassium nitrate, sodium fluoride
Denquel Sensitive Teeth	5% potassium nitrate
Orajel Gold	5% potassium nitrate, sodium monofluorophosphate
Promise Sensitive Teeth	5% potassium nitrate, sodium monofluorophosphate
Baking Soda Sensodyne	5% potassium nitrate, sodium fluoride
Cool Gel Sensodyne	5% potassium nitrate, sodium fluoride
Original Flavor Sensodyne	5% potassium nitrate, sodium monofluorophosphate
Fresh Mint Sensodyne	5% potassium nitrate, sodium monofluorophosphate
Tartar Control Sensodyne	5% potassium nitrate, sodium fluoride
Sensodyne-SC	10% strontium chloride hexahydrate

Allergy

From skin test surveys, it is estimated that 40 to 50 million people in the United States are affected by allergies. Allergic rhinitis, or hay fever, affects nearly 9.3% of Americans, not including those with asthma. According to the National Council on Asthma and Allergy, allergic rhinitis caused 7.6 million physician office visits in 1992. The estimated direct and indirect costs of hay fever in the United States in 1990 totaled $1.8 billion. Patients frequently purchase OTC medications for treatment of allergy symptoms because the condition is so prevalent, and effective medications are available without prescription.

Drugs used to treat allergy include antihistamines, decongestants, and mast cell stabilizers.

ANTIHISTAMINES

BROMPHENIRAMINE
CHLORPHENIRAMINE
CLEMASTINE
DIPHENHYDRAMINE
TRIPOLIDINE

Pharmacology

Antihistamines are used in both the prevention and treatment of allergies. Antibodies are formed in response to previous exposure to a specific antigen. When these antigens are again encountered, they combine with preformed antibodies on the surface of mast cells, leading to breakdown (degranulation) of mast cells and spillage of their contents. Mast cells contain large amounts of histamine, as well as other mediators of the allergic response such as SRS-A (slow reacting substance of anaphylaxis). These mediators (particularly histamine) cause the signs and symptoms of allergy. Major symptoms include rhinorrhea (a clear, watery nasal discharge), nasal congestion secondary to swelling of nasal membranes, watery and itchy eyes caused by trapped pollen in the conjunctival sac and tear ducts, and sneezing.

Taken prophylactically, antihistamines competitively block histamine receptors (H_1 receptors). When the histamine receptor is blocked, histamine cannot stimulate the receptor and cause the allergic reaction. Antihistamines are best utilized prophylactically, but they can also be used to help control the symptoms of allergy once they have already started. Antihistamines decrease mucous secretion because of their anticholinergic side effects, relieving rhinorrhea. Taken after the fact, antihistamines will antagonize new histamine-receptor interactions but do not mitigate the effects of the previously released histamine.

Side Effects

Side effects are caused by the antagonistic effect of antihistamines on the neurotransmitter acetylcholine. Drowsiness, dry mouth, blurred vision, constipation, and urinary retention can occur and are referred to as *anticholinergic side effects*. Antihistamines aggravate glaucoma, particularly acute angle-closure glaucoma, by decreasing outflow of aqueous humor. Nonprescription antihistamines differ in their likelihood to cause these side effects and exhibit large interpatient variability in their effects.

Drug Interactions

Drugs that may interact with antihistamines, and the resulting side effect, include the following:

- CNS depressants such as narcotics and benzodiazepines (Librium, Valium, Ativan, Versed) when used with antihistamines may cause increased drowsiness.
- The following tricyclic antidepressants may increase anticholinergic side effects: amitriptyline (Elavil), nortriptyline (Aventyl, Pamelor), imipramine (Tofranil), doxepin (Sinequan), trimipramine (Surmontil), amoxapine (Asendin), desipramine (Norpramin), protriptyline (Vivactil), and clomipramine (Anafranil).
- The following antispasmodics may also increase anticholinergic side effects: hyoscyamine (Levsin, Anaspaz), glycopyrrolate (Robinul), mepenzolate (Cantil), and dicyclomine (Bentyl).
- Antihistamines may antagonize the pharmacologic effects of the prokinetic agents metoclopramide (Reglan) and cisapride (Propulsid).

- Urinary antispasmodics such as flavoxate (Urispas) and oxybutynin (Ditropan) may increase anticholinergic side effects.

Lifespan Considerations
Geriatric
Antihistamines are problematic in geriatric patients, who are more sensitive to the side effects of these agents. Because antihistamines antagonize the effects of acetylcholine in the CNS and the periphery, acute confusion and disorientation can occur. Excessive drowsiness can lead to falls. Urinary retention and constipation, already a problem for many elderly patients, can be exacerbated by antihistamines. Blurred vision also occurs more commonly in the older population.

Pediatric
In addition to drowsiness, paradoxical excitement can occur in young children. Nonprescription antihistamines are not labeled for use in children under the age of 6 years but are safe and effective when used under the guidance of a health care professional.

Pregnancy
Brompheniramine, clemastine, and triprolidine are FDA Pregnancy Category C drugs. Chlorpheniramine and diphenhydramine are category B drugs. Epidemiologic studies (Schatz Mizeiger, 1997) have demonstrated that diphenhydramine and chlorpheniramine do *not* increase the risk of birth defects if taken during pregnancy. However, indiscriminate use of drugs should be avoided in all pregnant patients. Benefit must be weighed against risk. Data are not available for other antihistamines.

Nursing Mothers
Antihistamines can depress lactation secondary to their anticholinergic effects. The American Academy of Pediatrics generally considers antihistamines to be safe to use while nursing. Caution is recommended in the case of clemastine (Tavist) based on a single case report suggesting the occurrence of anticholinergic side effects in an infant whose mother was taking clemastine (Kok, 1982).

Patient Education
- The beneficial effects of antihistamines must be balanced against the side effects that they can cause.
- Antihistamines work best when taken prophylactically.

- Caution must be exercised when driving or operating machinery while taking antihistamines.
- If patients take antihistamines regularly, they should tell their health care provider because antihistamines can interact with a number of other medications.

Product Selection

- Prophylactic antihistamine therapy may be required during the entire allergy season. Treatment with nonsedating prescription antihistamines might be the preferred option in some allergic patients. This is particularly the case for persons who must maintain a high level of alertness in their work setting, or for geriatric patients.
- Antihistamines must be used cautiously in older patients. If these drugs are required to prevent allergy, the lowest effective dose should be recommended, or nonsedating prescription antihistamines should be prescribed.
- Antihistamines vary in their propensity to cause drowsiness.
- Timed-release antihistamines are more convenient to use and cause fewer side effects because they are slowly released into the circulation, avoiding the higher peak blood levels associated with immediate-release products.
- In patients with allergy and stuffy nose, combination antihistamine/ decongestant products *may* cause less drowsiness. The stimulating effects of decongestants *might* partially offset the drowsiness caused by antihistamines.

REFERENCES

Kok TH et al: Drowsiness due to clemastine transmitted in breast milk, *Lancet* 1(8277):914-915, Apr 17, 1982.

Schatz Mizeiger RS et al: The safety of allergy and asthma medications during pregnancy, *J Allergy Clin Immunol* 100(3):301-306, 1997.

DECONGESTANTS

Oral

PSEUDOEPHEDRINE

PHENYLEPHRINE

PHENYLPROPANOLAMINE

Nasal Sprays

PHENYLEPHRINE
OXYMETAZOLINE
NAPHAZOLINE
XYLOMETAZOLINE

Pharmacology

Decongestants stimulate α-adrenergic receptors in blood vessels, causing vasoconstriction. Vasoconstriction results in shrinkage of the mucous membranes and decreased swelling of the nasal passages and sinuses, improved drainage of the sinuses with resultant decreased sinus pressure, and easier breathing through the nose. Because arteries also contain α receptors, their constriction can exacerbate hypertension. Oral decongestants are less potent vasoconstrictors than topical products but can raise blood pressure in patients predisposed to hypertension. Topical decongestants (nasal sprays) are more potent local vasoconstrictors than oral products because they are applied directly to the nasal membranes. Topical products do not tend to increase blood pressure because systemic absorption is minimal.

Side Effects

Side effects of oral decongestants can include the following: cardiac stimulation (tachycardia), elevated blood pressure, nervousness or sleeplessness, and headache. An association has recently been reported between oral decongestants and increased stroke risk. In one reported case, an oral decongestant caused sufficient cerebral vasoconstriction to cause symptoms of stroke. Although this is only a case report, it does demonstrate that some individuals are extremely sensitive to the vasoconstrictive effects of these drugs. Decongestant nasal sprays do not normally cause systemic side effects, but overuse can cause rebound congestion (rhinitis medicamentosa). In this condition, the nasal membranes become even more congested and swollen as the vasoconstrictive effect starts to wear off. As the nasal spray is used more and more to get relief, the congestion gets progressively worse, and a vicious cycle ensues. Local ischemia, secondary to vasoconstriction, and local irritation are thought to be the mechanisms behind rhinitis medicamentosa. This is the reason that decongestant nasal sprays should not be used continuously for more than 3 to 4 days. When rhinitis medicamentosa occurs, decongestant nasal sprays should be discontinued in favor of oral decongestants or saline nasal spray or drops. Occasionally, intranasal steroids are required to treat rhinitis medicamentosa.

Drug Interactions

- Hypertensive crisis may result when oral decongestants are taken by patients who are also taking monoamine oxidase inhibitors such as phenylzine (Nardil) and tranylcypromine (Parnate).
- Phenylpropanolamine in some OTC diet products may result in additive CSN stimulation and hypertensive effect.

Lifespan Considerations

Geriatric

Older patients are more likely to experience side effects from decongestants. Therefore nasal sprays might be preferred for use in this group, assuming that they are used for less than 3 to 4 days continuously. When oral products are indicated, patients should start with smaller doses and gradually increase as tolerated. Oral decongestants, by virtue of their α-adrenergic activity, can aggravate dysuria secondary to prostatic hypertrophy. Insomnia secondary to oral decongestants also occurs more frequently in older patients. In addition, hypertensive patients should be monitored closely.

Pediatric

Pseudoephedrine is the oral decongestant most commonly used in children. It is available in drops, syrup, and tablets. Phenylpropanolamine is found in combination products. Young children sometimes experience significant CNS stimulation and may appear restless when taking either of these products.

Pregnancy

Studies indicate that pseudoephedrine does not cause an increased risk of birth defects. It is unlikely that phenylephrine or phenylpropanolamine cause an increased birth-defect rate, but studies are inconsistent.

Nursing Mothers

The American Academy of Pediatrics considers pseudoephedrine to be safe for use while nursing. Data regarding phenylephrine and phenylpropanolamine are insufficient to determine safety during nursing. Nasal sprays are safe for both pregnant and nursing women because of their lack of systemic distribution.

Patient Education

- Oral decongestants can increase blood pressure in some patients. If patients have high blood pressure, they should consult a health care professional before taking these medicines.
- Patients should avoid continuous use of topical products for more than 4 days.

Product Selection

- Oral decongestants should be administered with caution in patients with hypertension, hyperthyroidism, diabetes mellitus, cardiovascular disease, coronary artery disease, ischemic heart disease, glaucoma, and prostatic hypertrophy. These are not absolute contraindications; benefit must be weighed against risk. Pseudoephedrine is the preferred agent in hypertensive patients because it causes less systemic vasoconstriction than does phenylephrine or phenylpropanolamine.
- Timed-release products might be less likely to cause side effects because peak blood levels are lower than those with immediate-release products.

MAST CELL STABILIZERS

CROMOLYN SODIUM

Pharmacology

Cromolyn is not an antihistamine or decongestant. Cromolyn nasal spray inhibits the breakdown (degranulation) of sensitized mast cells that occurs after exposure to antigens, blocking the release of histamine and SRS-A (slow-reacting substance of anaphylaxis). It is therefore effective for prevention and treatment of nasal allergy symptoms.

Side Effects

Sneezing, nasal stinging, nasal burning, and nasal irritation are the most commonly reported side effects of cromolyn nasal spray.

Drug Interactions

There are no reported clinically significant drug interactions.

Lifespan Considerations

Geriatric

Because antihistamines are problematic in the older patient and they interact with numerous other drugs, cromolyn nasal spray is a good choice for use in patients exhibiting predominantly nasal symptoms.

Pediatric

Safety and effectiveness in children under the age of 6 years has not been established. From a practical standpoint, young children may not be capable of using a nasal spray correctly.

Pregnancy

Because systemic absorption is very low, risk to a developing fetus is unlikely. However, the data are not sufficient to state that there is no risk.

Nursing Mothers

Because systemic absorption is very low, the amount of cromolyn in breast milk would be expected to be very low. However, information is not available concerning the distribution of cromolyn in breast milk.

Patient Education

Cromolyn works best when used regularly to prevent nasal allergy.

Product Selection

Cromolyn nasal spray is effective in the prevention and treatment of allergic rhinitis. Because it is applied as a nasal spray, it is relatively safe and is not associated with significant side effects compared with anti-histamines and decongestants.

SUGGESTED READINGS

Badhwar AK, Druce HM: Allergic rhinitis, Med Clin North Am 76(4):789-803, 1992.

Ferguson BJ: Allergic rhinitis: recognizing signs, symptoms, and triggering allergens, Postgrad Med 101(5):110-116, 1997.

Ferguson BJ: Cost-effective pharmacotherapy for allergic rhinitis, Otolaryngol Clin North Am 31(1):91-110, 1998.

Wood SF: Review of hay fever. 1. Historical background and mechanisms, Fam Pract 3(1):54-63, 1986.

Product Information: Allergy (Oral Products)

Brand Name	Ingredient Type	Ingredient	Adult Dose	Pediatric Dose	Comments
A.R.M.	Antihistamine	Chlorpheniramine 4 mg	1 tablet every 4-6 hrs		
	Decongestant	Phenylpropanolamine 25 mg			
Actifed	Antihistamine	Tripolidine 2.5 mg	1 tablet every 4-6 hrs	6-12 years: ½ tablet 3-4 times daily	
	Decongestant	Pseudoephedrine 60 mg			
Actifed syrup	Antihistamine	Tripolidine 1.25 mg/5 ml		4 months–2 years: 1.25 ml 3-4 times daily	
	Decongestant	Pseudoephedrine 30 mg/5 ml		2-4 years: 2.5 ml 3-4 times daily	
				4-6 years: 3.75 ml 3-4 times daily	
				6-12 years: 5 ml 3-4 times daily	
Advil Cold & Sinus	Decongestant	Pseudoephedrine 30 mg	1 tablet every 4-6 hrs		
	Analgesic	Ibuprofen 200 mg			
Alka-Seltzer Plus Maximum Strength Sinus Medicine	Antihistamine	Brompheniramine 2 mg	2 tablets every 4 hrs		Effervescent tablet contains 506 mg sodium/tablet
	Decongestant	Phenylpropanolamine 24 mg			
	Analgesic	Aspirin 500 mg			

Continued

Product Information: Allergy (Oral Products)—cont'd

Brand Name	Ingredient Type	Ingredient	Adult Dose	Pediatric Dose	Comments
Allerest 12-Hour Maximum Strength	Antihistamine Decongestant	Chlorpheniramine 12 mg Phenylpropanolamine 75 mg	1 tablet every 12 hrs		Timed-release
Allerest Maximum Strength	Antihistamine Decongestant	Chlorpheniramine 2 mg Pseudoephedrine 30 mg	1 tablet every 4-6 hrs		
Bayer Select Allergy Sinus	Antihistamine Decongestant Analgesic	Chlorpheniramine 2 mg Pseudoephedrine 30 mg Acetaminophen 500 mg	1 tablet every 4-6 hrs		
Benadryl	Antihistamine	Diphenhydramine 25 mg	1-2 tablets every 4-6 hrs		Available as tablets, chewable tablets, capsules
Benadryl Allergy Decongestant Syrup	Antihistamine Decongestant	Diphenhydramine 12.5 mg/5 ml Pseudoephedrine 30 mg/5 ml	2 tsp every 4-6 hrs	*6-12 years:* 1 tsp every 4-6 hrs	
Benadryl Allergy Sinus Headache Formula	Antihistamine Decongestant Analgesic	Diphenhydramine 12.5 mg Pseudoephedrine 30 mg Acetaminophen 500 mg	2 tablets every 6 hrs		

Drug	Category	Ingredients	Adult dose	Pediatric/other dose	Notes
Benadryl elixir	Antihistamine	Diphenhydramine 12.5 mg/5 ml		5 mg/kg/day in divided doses every 4-6 hrs, not to exceed 300 mg/day	
Chlor-Trimeton 12-Hour Allergy	Antihistamine	Chlorpheniramine 12 mg	1 tablet every 12 hrs		Timed-release
Chlor-Trimeton 12-Hour Allergy Decongestant Formula	Antihistamine Decongestant	Chlorpheniramine 12 mg Pseudoephedrine 120 mg	1 tablet every 12 hrs		Timed-release
Chlor-Trimeton 4-Hour Allergy	Antihistamine	Chlorpheniramine 4 mg	1 tablet every 4 hrs		
Chlor-Trimeton 4-Hour Allergy Decongestant	Antihistamine	Chlorpheniramine 4 mg Pseudoephedrine 60 mg	1 tablet every 4 hrs		
Chlor-Trimeton 8-Hour Allergy	Antihistamine	Chlorpheniramine 8 mg	1 tablet every 8 hrs		
Chlor-Trimeton Allergy Sinus Headache	Antihistamine Decongestant Analgesic	Chlorpheniramine 2 mg Phenylpropanolamine 12.5 mg Acetaminophen 500 mg	1 tablet every 4-6 hrs		
Chlor-Trimeton Allergy Syrup	Antihistamine	Chlorpheniramine 2 mg/5 ml		*2-6 years:* 1 mg every 4-6 hrs; *6-12 years:* 2 mg every 4-6 hrs	

Continued

Product Information: Allergy (Oral Products)—cont'd

Brand Name	Ingredient Type	Ingredient	Adult Dose	Pediatric Dose	Comments
Chlor-Trimeton Non-Drowsy 4-Hour	Decongestant	Pseudoephedrine 60 mg	1 tablet every 4-6 hrs		Contains *no* antihistamine
Comtrex Allergy Sinus	Antihistamine Decongestant	Chlorpheniramine 2 mg Pseudoephedrine 30 mg	2 tablets every 6 hrs		
Contac 12-Hour Allergy	Antihistamine	Clemastine 1 mg	1 tablet every 12 hrs		12-hour duration of action
Contac Maximum Strength 12-Hour	Antihistamine Decongestant	Chlorpheniramine 8 mg Phenylpropanolamine 75 mg	1 tablet every 12 hrs		Timed-release
Coricidin D	Antihistamine Decongestant Analgesic	Chlorpheniramine 2 mg Phenylpropanolamine 12.5 mg Acetaminophen 325 mg	2 tablets every 4 hrs	*6-12 years:* 1 tablet every 4 hrs	
Coricidin D Maximum Strength	Antihistamine Decongestant Analgesic	Chlorpheniramine 2 mg Phenylpropanolamine 12.5 mg Acetaminophen 500 mg	2 tablets every 4 hrs		
Coricidin HBP	Antihistamine Analgesic	Chlorpheniramine 2 mg Acetaminophen 325 mg	2 tablets every 4-6 hrs	*6-12 years:* 1 tablet every 4-6 hrs	

Product	Type	Ingredients	Dose	Pediatric Dose	Comments
Coricidin HBP Nighttime Liquid	Antihistamine Analgesic	Diphenhydramine 12.5 mg/15 ml Acetaminophen 325 mg/15 ml	30 ml every 4 hrs	*6-11 years:* 15 ml every 4 hrs	Diphenhydramine promoted as sleep aid in addition to antihistamine activity
Dimetane Elixir	Antihistamine	Brompheniramine 2 mg/5 ml		*<6 years:* 0.125 mg/kg/dose every 6 hrs; maximum 6-8 mg/day *6-12 years:* 2-4 mg every 6-8 hrs; maximum 12-16 mg/day	
Dimetapp Allergy	Antihistamine	Brompheniramine 4 mg	1 tablet every 4 hrs		Available as tablets, gelcaps
Dimetapp Allergy Extentabs	Antihistamine	Brompheniramine 8 mg	1 tablet every 12 hrs		Timed-release
Dimetapp Allergy/ Sinus	Antihistamine Decongestant	Brompheniramine 2 mg Phenylpropanolamine 12.5 mg	2 tablets every 12 hrs		
Dimetapp Cold & Allergy Chewable	Analgesic Antihistamine Decongestant	Acetaminophen 500 mg Brompheniramine 1 mg Phenylpropanolamine 6.25 mg		*6-12 years:* 2 tablets every 4 hrs	

Continued

Product Information: Allergy (Oral Products)—cont'd

Brand Name	Ingredient Type	Ingredient	Adult Dose	Pediatric Dose	Comments
Dimetapp Decongestant Non-Drowsy	Decongestant	Pseudoephedrine 30 mg	2 tablets every 4-6 hrs		Contains *no* antihistamine
Dimetapp Decongestant Pediatric Drops	Decongestant	Pseudoephedrine 7.5 mg/0.8 ml		*<2 years:* 1 mg/kg every 6 hrs *2-5 years:* 15 mg every 6 hrs; maximum 60 mg/24 hrs *6-12 years:* 30 mg every 6 hrs; maximum 120 mg/24 hrs	Orals drops
Dimetapp Elixir	Antihistamine	Brompheniramine 2 mg/5 ml	5-10 ml 3-4 times daily	*1-6 months:* 1.25 ml 3-4 times daily *7-24 months:* 2.5 ml 3-4 times daily *2-4 years:* 3.75 ml 3-4 times daily *4-12 years:* 5 ml 3-4 times daily	
	Decongestant	Phenylpropanolamine 12.5 mg/5 ml			

Name	Category	Ingredients	Dosage	Notes
Dimetapp Maximum Strength 12-Hour Extentabs	Antihistamine Decongestant	Brompheniramine 12 mg Phenylpropanolamine 75 mg	1 tablet every 12 hrs	Timed-release
Dimetapp Maximum Strength 4-Hour	Antihistamine Decongestant	Brompheniramine 4 mg Phenylpropanolamine 25 mg	1 tablet every 4 hrs	
Dimetapp Sinus	Decongestant Analgesic	Pseudoephedrine 30 mg Ibuprofen 200 mg	1 tablet every 4-6 hrs	
Dristan Allergy	Antihistamine Decongestant	Brompheniramine 4 mg Pseudoephedrine 60 mg	1 tablet every 4 hrs	
Dristan Sinus	Decongestant Analgesic	Pseudoephedrine 30 mg Ibuprofen 200 mg	1 tablet every 4-6 hrs	
Drixoral Allergy Sinus Extended Release	Antihistamine Decongestant Analgesic	Dexbrompheniramine 3 mg Pseudoephedrine 60 mg Acetaminophen 500 mg	2 tablets every 12 hrs	Timed-release
Drixoral Non-Drowsy Formula Extended Release	Decongestant	Pseudoephedrine 120 mg	1 tablet every 12 hrs	Timed-release
Efidac/24 Extended Release	Decongestant	Pseudoephedrine 240 mg	1 tablet every 24 hrs	24-hour timed-release

Continued

Product Information: Allergy (Oral Products)—cont'd

Brand Name	Ingredient Type	Ingredient	Adult Dose	Pediatric Dose	Comments
Excedrin Sinus	Decongestant Analgesic	Pseudoephedrine 30 mg Acetaminophen 500 mg	2 tablets every 6 hrs		
Motrin IB Sinus	Decongestant Analgesic	Pseudoephedrine 30 mg Ibuprofen 200 mg	1 tablet every 4-6 hrs		
Novahistine Elixir	Antihistamine Decongestant	Chlorpheniramine 2 mg/5 ml Phenylephrine 5 mg/5 ml	2 tsp every 4 hrs	*6-12 years:* 1 tsp every 4 hrs	
PediaCare Cold- Allergy for Ages 6-12	Antihistamine Decongestant	Chlorpheniramine 1 mg Pseudoephedrine 15 mg		*2-3 years:* 1 tablet every 4-6 hrs *4-5 years:* 1.5 tablets every 4-6 hrs *6-8 years:* 2 tablets every 4-6 hrs *9-10 years:* 2.5 tablets every 4-6 hrs *11 years:* 3 tablets every 4-6 hrs	Chewable tablet

Product	Type	Ingredients	Dosage	Comments
PediaCare Infants Decongestant Drops	Decongestant	Pseudoephedrine 7.5 mg/0.8 ml	*<2 years:* 1 mg/kg every 6 hrs; *2-5 years:* 15 mg every 6 hrs; maximum 60 mg/24 hrs; *6-12 years:* 30 mg every 6 hrs; maximum 120 mg/24 hrs	
Sine-Aid IB	Decongestant, Analgesic	Pseudoephedrine 30 mg, Ibuprofen 200 mg	1 tablet every 4-6 hrs	Available as tablets and gelcaps
Sine-Aid Maximum Strength	Decongestant, Analgesic	Pseudoephedrine 30 mg, Acetaminophen 500 mg	2 tablets every 4-6 hrs	
Sine-Off Maximum Strength Allergy/Sinus	Decongestant, Antihistamine, Decongestant, Analgesic	Chlorpheniramine 2 mg, Pseudoephedrine 30 mg, Acetaminophen 500 mg	2 tablets every 6 hrs	
Sine-Off Maximum Strength No Drowsiness Formula	Decongestant, Analgesic	Pseudoephedrine 30 mg, Acetaminophen 500 mg	2 tablets every 6 hrs	
Sinutab	Decongestant, Analgesic	Pseudoephedrine 30 mg, Acetaminophen 325 mg	2 tablets every 6 hrs	

Continued

Product Information: Allergy (Oral Products)—cont'd

Brand Name	Ingredient Type	Ingredient	Adult Dose	Pediatric Dose	Comments
Sinutab Allergy Sinus Medication Maximum Strength	Antihistamine Decongestant Analgesic	Chlorpheniramine 2 mg Pseudoephedrine 30 mg Acetaminophen 500 mg	2 tablets every 6 hrs		
Sinutab Maximum Strength No Drowsiness	Decongestant Analgesic	Pseudoephedrine 30 mg Acetaminophen 500 mg	2 tablets every 6 hrs		
Sinutab Non-Drying Maximum Strength	Expectorant	Guaifenesin 200 mg	2 tablets every 4 hrs		
Sudafed 12-Hour Extended Release	Decongestant	Pseudoephedrine 120 mg	1 tablet every 12 hrs		Timed release
Sudafed 30 mg	Decongestant	Pseudoephedrine 30 mg	2 tablets every 4-6 hrs	6-12 years: 1 tablet every 4-6 hrs	
Sudafed 60 mg	Decongestant	Pseudoephedrine 60 mg	1 tablet every 4-6 hrs		

Sudafed Children's Liquid	Decongestant	Pseudoephedrine 30 mg/5 ml		*<2 years:* 1 mg/kg every 6 hrs *2-5 years:* 15 mg every 6 hrs; maximum 60 mg/24 hrs *6-12 years:* 30 mg every 6 hrs; maximum 120 mg/24 hrs
Sudafed Maximum Strength Cold & Sinus	Antihistamine Decongestant	Chlorpheniramine 4 mg Pseudoephedrine 60 mg	1 tablet every 4-6 hrs	*6-12 years:* ½ tablet every 4-6 hrs
Sudafed Plus Syrup	Antihistamine Decongestant	Chlorpheniramine 2 mg/5 ml Pseudoephedrine 30 mg/5 ml	2 tsp every 4-6 hrs	*6-12 years:* 1 tsp every 4-6 hrs
Sudafed Sinus	Decongestant Analgesic	Pseudoephedrine 30 mg Acetaminophen 500 mg	2 tablets every 6 hrs	
Tavist-1	Antihistamine	Clemastine 1 mg	1 tablet every 12 hrs	*6-12 years:* ½ tablet every 12 hrs; maximum 3 tablets/day

Continued

Product Information: Allergy (Oral Products)—cont'd

Brand Name	Ingredient Type	Ingredient	Adult Dose	Pediatric Dose	Comments
Tavist-D	Antihistamine Decongestant	Clemastine 1 mg Phenylpropanolamine 75 mg	1 tablet every 12 hrs		Timed release
Teldrin	Antihistamine	Chlorpheniramine 12 mg	1 tablet every 12 hrs		Timed release
Triaminic Allergy	Antihistamine Decongestant	Chlorpheniramine 4 mg Phenylpropanolamine 25 mg	1 tablet every 4 hrs	*6-12 years:* ½ tablet every 4 hrs	
Triaminic Syrup	Antihistamine Decongestant	Chlorpheniramine 2 mg/10 ml Phenylpropanolamine 12.5 mg/10 ml	4 tsp every 4 hrs	*3-12 months:* 1.25 ml every 4 hrs *12-24 months:* 2.5 ml every 4 hrs *2-6 years:* 5 ml every 4 hrs *6-12 years:* 10 ml every 4 hrs	

Product	Class	Ingredients	Dosage	Notes
Triaminic-12	Antihistamine Decongestant	Chlorpheniramine 12 mg Phenylpropanolamine 75 mg	1 tablet every 12 hrs	Timed release
Triaminicin	Antihistamine Decongestant	Chlorpheniramine 4 mg Phenylpropanolamine 25 mg	1 tablet every 4 hrs	
Tylenol Allergy Sinus Maximum Strength	Analgesic Antihistamine Decongestant Analgesic	Acetaminophen 650 mg Chlorpheniramine 2 mg Pseudoephedrine 30 mg Acetaminophen 500 mg	2 tablets every 6 hrs	Available as caplets and gelcaps
Tylenol Severe Allergy	Antihistamine	Diphenhydramine 12.5 mg	2 tablets every 4-6 hrs	
Tylenol Sinus Maximum Strength	Analgesic Decongestant Analgesic	Acetaminophen 500 mg Pseudoephedrine 30 mg Acetaminophen 500 mg	2 tablets every 4-6 hrs	Available as tablets, caplets, and gelcaps

Product Information: Topical Decongestants

Brand Name	Active Ingredient	Adult Dose	Pediatric Dose	Comments
Afrin 4-Hour	Phenylephrine 0.5%	1-2 sprays in each nostril every 4 hrs		
Afrin 12-Hour	Oxymetazoline 0.05%	2-3 sprays/drops in each nostril every 10-12 hrs		Available as spray, pump spray, drops; do not use for more than 3-5 days
Afrin 12-Hour Childrens	Oxymetazoline 0.025%		2-3 sprays/drops in each nostril every 10-12 hrs	Available as spray, drops; do not use for more than 3-5 days
Benzedrex 12	Oxymetazoline 0.05%	2-3 sprays/drops in each nostril every 10-12 hours		Do not use for more than 3-5 days
Dristan	Phenylephrine 0.5%	1-2 sprays in each nostril every 4 hrs		Do not use for more than 3-5 days
Dristan 12-Hour	Oxymetazoline 0.05%	2-3 sprays in each nostril every 10-12 hrs		Do not use for more than 3-5 days
Duration	Oxymetazoline 0.05%	2-3 sprays in each nostril every 10-12 hrs		Do not use for more than 3-5 days

Neo-Synephrine	Phenylephrine 0.5%	2-3 drops/sprays in each nostril every 4 hrs	Do not use for more than 3-5 days
Neo-Synephrine 12-Hour	Oxymetazoline 0.05%	2-3 sprays in each nostril every 10-12 hrs	Do not use for more than 3-5 days
Neo-Synephrine Extra	Phenylephrine 1%	2-3 drops/sprays in each nostril every 4 hrs	Do not use for more than 3-5 days
Neo-Synephrine Mild	Phenylephrine 0.25%	2-3 sprays in each nostril every 4 hrs	Do not use for more than 3-5 days
Neo-Synephrine Pediatric Drops	Phenylephrine .125%	*6-12 years:* 2-3 sprays in each nostril every 4 hrs *Infants:* 1-2 drops every 4 hrs *1-6 years:* 2-3 drops in each nostril every 4 hrs	Do not use for more than 3-5 days
NTZ Long Acting	Oxymetazoline 0.05%	2-3 sprays/drops in each nostril every 10-12 hrs	Do not use for more than 3-5 days
Otrivin	Xylometazoline 0.1%	2-3 drops/sprays in each nostril every 8-10 hrs	Do not use for more than 3-5 days

Continued

Product Information: Topical Decongestants—cont'd

Brand Name	Active Ingredient	Adult Dose	Pediatric Dose	Comments
Privine	Naphazoline 0.05%	1-2 drops/sprays in each nostril every 6 hrs		Do not use for more than 3-5 days
Vicks Sinex 12-Hour	Oxymetazoline 0.05%	2-3 sprays in each nostril every 10-12 hours		Do not use for more than 3-5 days
Vicks Sinex Nasal Spray	Phenylephrine 0.5%	1-2 sprays in each nostril every 4 hrs		Do not use for more than 3-5 days
4-Way Fast Acting	Phenylephrine 0.5% Pyrilamine 0.2% Naphazoline 0.05%	1-2 sprays in each nostril every 4 hrs		Contains topical antihistamine in addition to decongestants
4-Way Menthol Nasal Spray	Phenylephrine 0.5% Pyrilamine 0.2% Naphazoline 0.05%	1-2 sprays in each nostril every 4 hrs		Contains topical antihistamine in addition to decongestants; also contains menthol

Product Information: Mast Cell Stabilizers

Brand Name	Dose
Nasalcrom cromolyn nasal spray	1 spray each nostril 3-4 times daily

Asthma

The National Asthma Education Program defines asthma as being characterized by a reversible airway obstruction (reversing spontaneously or with treatment in the majority of patients), airway inflammation, and hyperresponsiveness of the airways to a variety of stimuli. Bronchodilators and antiinflammatory drugs are used to treat asthma.

Bronchodilators available without a prescription include epinephrine (metered-dose inhaler) and theophylline. There are **no** antiinflammatory drugs (steroids) available without a prescription.

NOTE: Because control of airway inflammation and hyperresponsiveness is critical to the prevention of asthma, this condition can only be treated effectively with prescription products. In addition, OTC epinephrine inhalers are potentially dangerous. Newer, safer prescription products should be used instead. Nonprescription theophylline-containing products do not contain sufficient theophylline to attain and maintain adequate effective levels. **Asthma should NOT be treated with OTC medications.**

Pharmacology

Epinephrine is a sympathomimetic, stimulating α and β receptors. Stimulation of β_2 receptors in the airways causes bronchiolar muscle relaxation, resulting in bronchodilation, increased ciliary action, and inhibition of histamine release from mast cells. Stimulation of β_1 receptors in the heart causes cardiac stimulation, and stimulation of α receptors increases blood pressure. The ideal sympathomimetic would be β_2-specific. Newer prescription drugs are much more β_2-selective and thus less likely to stimulate the heart and raise blood pressure.

Theophylline produces bronchodilation proportionate to its serum concentration. The mechanism by which bronchodilation occurs is not known, but theophylline has been shown to inhibit release of intracellular calcium, competitively antagonize the bronchoconstriction caused by adenosine, and stimulate endogenous catecholamine release. The clinical usefulness of theophylline is limited by its narrow therapeutic range.

Side Effects

Epinephrine and theophylline can cause cardiac arrhythmias, especially in patients with existing heart disease. Tremor, tachycardia, palpitations, anorexia, insomnia, and hypertension can also occur.

Persons with heart disease, thyroid disease, high blood pressure, diabetes, or difficulty urinating because of an enlarged prostate gland should not use these products.

Drug Interactions

Epinephrine can interfere with some medicines used to treat high blood pressure. It must **not** be used by patients taking monoamine oxidase inhibitors (Nardil, Parnate) for depression because a hypertensive crisis could occur. Common medications such as erythromycin, ciprofloxacin, and cimetidine inhibit the metabolism of theophylline, resulting in elevated theophylline blood levels.

Lifespan Considerations
Geriatric

Elderly patients are more likely to have diseases that would be aggravated by epinephrine or theophylline.

Pediatric

These products are not approved for children less than 4 years old. **Childhood asthma can be serious. Do not attempt to treat asthma in a child with nonprescription products**.

Pregnancy

The frequency of congenital anomalies was not increased in a series of women who received epinephrine or theophylline during pregnancy. Therapeutic doses of epinephrine or theophylline are unlikely to pose substantial teratogenic risk, but the data are insufficient to state that there is no risk. In practice, epinephrine should never be used because safer prescription alternatives are available. When theophylline is used, the benefit must be weighed against the possible but unlikely risk to the fetus.

Nursing Mothers

Epinephrine is known to be excreted in breast milk, but the significance has not been studied. As with pregnant women, epinephrine would not be the drug of choice for nursing mothers. The American Academy of Pediatrics considers theophylline to be safe for use while nursing.

Patient Education

- Asthma can be a serious, life-threatening condition.
- Self-treatment is not advised.
- Patients should avoid large amounts of caffeine-containing products if taking epinephrine or theophylline because caffeine also stimulates the heart and might make side effects worse.

Product Selection

Because of the potential seriousness of asthma, safer prescription products are preferred for treatment of asthma.

SUGGESTED READINGS

Davies RJ et al: New insights into the understanding of asthma, Chest 111 (2 suppl):2S-10S, 1997.

Nadel JA, Busse WW: Asthma, Am J Respir Crit Care Med 157(4[2]):S130-S138, 1998.

Vassallo R, Lipsky JJ: Theophylline: recent advances in the understanding of its mode of action and uses in clinical practice, Mayo Clin Proc 73(4):346-354, 1998.

Product Information: Asthma

Brand Name	Ingredients	
	Epinephrine	**Theophylline**
Bronkaid Dual Formula		X
Bronkaid Mist	X	
Primatene Dual Formula		X
Primatene Mist	X	
Primatene Tablets		X

Common Cold and Flu

Viruses cause the common cold and influenza. Because there is no cure for either of these conditions, nonprescription drug products provide symptomatic relief only. Drug classes found in cold and flu remedies include antihistamines, decongestants, cough suppressants, expectorants, and analgesics.

ANTIHISTAMINES

BROMPHENIRAMINE
CHLORPHENIRAMINE
CLEMASTINE
DEXBROMPHENIRAMINE
DIPHENHYDRAMINE
TRIPOLIDINE

Pharmacology

Antihistamines are used in the symptomatic treatment of rhinorrhea associated with the common cold or flu. In response to one or more cold or influenza viruses, an inflammatory response occurs in the nasal epithelial cells. Inflammation causes hyperemia (increased local blood flow), local edema, and rhinorrhea. Antihistamines relieve rhinorrhea associated with the common cold and flu because one of their side effects is reduction of mucous membrane secretions.

Side Effects

Side effects are caused by the antagonistic effect of antihistamines on the neurotransmitter acetylcholine and are dose-related. Referred to as *anticholinergic side effects*, drowsiness, dry mouth, blurred vision, constipation, and urinary retention can occur. Antihistamines can aggravate glaucoma, particularly acute angle-closure glaucoma, by decreasing outflow of aqueous humor. Nonprescription antihistamines differ in their propensity to cause these side effects and exhibit large interpatient variability in their effects (Table 6-1).

Table 6-1
Side Effects Related to Antihistamine Use

Antihistamine	Sedation	Antihistamine effect	Anticholinergic activity
Brompheniramine	Low	High	Moderate
Chlorpheniramine	Low	Moderate	Moderate
Clemastine	Moderate	Low to moderate	High
Diphenhydramine	High	Low to moderate	High
Tripolidine	Low	Moderate to high	Moderate

Drug Interactions

Drugs that may interact with antihistamines, and the resulting side effects, include the following:

- CNS depressants such as narcotics and benzodiazepines (Librium, Valium, Ativan, Versed), when used with antihistamines, may cause increased drowsiness.
- The following tricyclic antidepressants may increase anticholinergic side effects: amitriptyline (Elavil), nortriptyline (Aventyl, Pamelor), imipramine (Tofranil), doxepin (Sinequan), trimipramine (Surmontil), amoxapine (Asendin), desipramine (Norpramin), protriptyline (Vivactil), and clomipramine (Anafranil).
- The following antispasmodics may also increase anticholinergic side effects: hyoscyamine (Levsin, Anaspaz), glycopyrrolate (Robinul), mepenzolate (Cantil), and dicyclomine (Bentyl).
- Prokinetic agents such as metoclopramide (Reglan) and cisapride (Propulsid) may result in antagonism of the prokinetic effect.
- Urinary antispasmodics such as flavoxate (Urispas) and oxybutynin (Ditropan) may increase anticholinergic side effects.

Lifespan Considerations
Geriatric

Antihistamines can be problematic in the geriatric patient because they are more sensitive to the side effects of these agents. Because antihistamines antagonize the effects of acetylcholine in the CNS, acute confusion and disorientation can occur. Excessive drowsiness can lead to falls. Urinary retention and constipation, already a problem for many elderly patients, can be exacerbated by antihistamines. Blurred vision also occurs more commonly in the older population.

Pediatric

In addition to drowsiness, paradoxical excitement can occur in young children. Nonprescription antihistamines are not labeled for use in children under the age of 6 years, but can be used safely under the supervision of a health care professional.

Pregnancy

Brompheniramine, clemastine, and triprolidine are FDA Pregnancy Category C drugs. Chlorpheniramine and diphenhydramine are category B drugs.

Epidemiologic studies (Schatz Mizeiger, 1997) have demonstrated that diphenhydramine and chlorpheniramine do *not* increase the risk of birth defects if taken during pregnancy. However, indiscriminate use of drugs should be avoided in all pregnant patients. Benefit must be weighed against risk. Data are not available for other antihistamines.

Nursing Mothers

Antihistamines can depress lactation secondary to their anticholinergic effects. The American Academy of Pediatrics generally considers antihistamines to be safe to use while nursing. Caution is recommended in the case of clemastine (Tavist) based on a single case report suggesting the occurrence of anticholinergic side effects in an infant whose mother was taking clemastine (Kok, 1982).

Patient Education

Side effects such as drowsiness, dry mouth, and urinary retention can occur with antihistamines. If drowsiness occurs, care must be exercised when driving or working around machinery. If these side effects are bothersome, patients should contact their health care professional for recommendation of an alternative product. When drowsiness interferes with a patient's ability to function, prescription nonsedating antihistamines may be appropriate.

Product Selection

- Diphenhydramine use should be avoided in older patients; other antihistamines should be used cautiously. The lowest effective dose should be recommended, or nonsedating prescription antihistamines should be prescribed.
- Antihistamines exhibit significant interpatient variability in their

effectiveness and side effects. The patient should be questioned about prior usage of antihistamine products and a product chosen that has provided relief without significant side effects.

- Products containing only the ingredients necessary to treat the symptoms of the patient should be recommended. Use of combination or multisymptom products should be avoided when not clearly indicated. Additional drugs carry with them the possibility of side effects.

- Nonsedating prescription antihistamines might be the preferred option in selected patients. This is particularly the case for persons who must maintain a high level of alertness in their work setting, or for geriatric patients.

- Timed-release antihistamines are more convenient and cause fewer side effects because they are slowly released into the circulation, avoiding the higher peak blood levels associated with immediate-release products.

- In patients with allergy and stuffy nose, combination antihistamine/decongestant products *may* cause less drowsiness. The stimulating effects of decongestants *might* partially offset the drowsiness caused by antihistamines.

REFERENCES

Kok TH et al: Drowsiness due to clemastine transmitted in breast milk, *Lancet* 1(8277):914-915, Apr 17, 1982.

Schatz Mizeiger RS et al: The safety of allergy and asthma medications during pregnancy, *J Allergy Clin Immunol* 100(3):301-306, 1997.

DECONGESTANTS

Oral

PSEUDOEPHEDRINE
PHENYLEPHRINE
PHENYLPROPANOLAMINE

Nasal Sprays

PHENYLEPHRINE
OXYMETAZOLINE
NAPHAZOLINE
XYLOMETAZOLINE

Pharmacology

Decongestants stimulate α-adrenergic receptors in blood vessels, causing vasoconstriction. Vasoconstriction results in shrinkage of the mucous membranes and decreased swelling of the nasal passages and sinuses, improved drainage of the sinuses with resultant decreased sinus pressure, and easier breathing through the nose. Because arteries also contain α receptors, their constriction can lead to hypertension. Oral decongestants are less potent vasoconstrictors than topical products but can raise blood pressure in patients predisposed to hypertension. Topical decongestants (nasal sprays) are more potent local vasoconstrictors than oral products because they are applied directly to the nasal membranes. Because topical products are only minimally absorbed into the systemic circulation, they do not tend to raise blood pressure.

Side Effects

Side effects of oral decongestants can include tachycardia, elevated blood pressure, nervousness or sleeplessness, and headache. An association has recently been reported between oral decongestants and increased stroke risk (Sloan et al, 1991). Although only case reports, it is apparent that some individuals are extremely sensitive to the vasoconstrictive effects of these drugs. Decongestant nasal sprays do not cause systemic side effects, but overuse can cause rebound congestion (rhinitis medicamentosa). In this condition, the nasal membranes become even more congested and swollen as the vasoconstrictive effect starts to wear off. As the nasal spray is used more often to get relief, the congestion progressively worsens, and a vicious cycle ensues. Local ischemia, secondary to vasoconstriction, and local irritation are thought to be the mechanisms behind rhinitis medicamentosa. This is the reason that decongestant nasal sprays should not be used continuously for more than 3 to 4 days. When rhinitis medicamentosa occurs, decongestant nasal sprays should be discontinued and oral decongestants or saline nasal spray or drops substituted. Occasionally, prescription intranasal steroids are required to treat rhinitis medicamentosa.

Drug Interactions

- Hypertensive crisis may result when oral decongestants are taken by patients who are also taking monoamine oxidase inhibitors such as phenylzine (Nardil) and tranylcypromine (Parnate).

- Phenylpropanolamine in some OTC diet products may result in additive CSN stimulation and hypertensive effect.

Lifespan Considerations
Geriatric
Older patients are more likely to experience side effects from decongestants. Nasal sprays might be preferred in this patient group, assuming that the decongestants are used for less than 3 to 4 days continuously. When oral products are indicated, patients should start with smaller doses and gradually increase them as tolerated. Oral decongestants, by virtue of their α-adrenergic activity, can aggravate dysuria secondary to prostatic hypertrophy. Insomnia secondary to oral decongestants also occurs more frequently in older patients.

Pediatric
Pseudoephedrine is the oral decongestant most commonly used in children. It is available in drops, syrup, and tablets. Phenylpropanolamine is found in combination products. Young children sometimes experience significant CNS stimulation and may appear restless.

Pregnancy
Phenylephrine, phenylpropanolamine, and pseudoephedrine are all FDA Pregnancy Category C drugs. Epidemiologic studies indicate that pseudoephedrine does not cause an increased risk of birth defects in the first trimester. However, fetal tachycardia has been reported with maternal use of pseudoephedrine (Anastacio et al, 1992). The indiscriminate use of this drug or other decongestants should be avoided during pregnancy.

Nursing Mothers
The American Academy of Pediatrics considers pseudoephedrine to be safe for use while nursing. Data regarding phenylephrine and phenylpropanolamine is insufficient to determine safety during nursing. Nasal sprays are safe for both pregnant and nursing women because of their lack of systemic distribution.

Patient Education
- Nasal sprays are beneficial in the treatment of nasal congestion, but are not effective in relieving sinus congestion because it is difficult for the spray to gain access to the sinuses. Oral products are preferred for sinus pressure.

- Nasal sprays should not be used for more than 3 to 4 days continuously.
- For best results, patients should blow their noses before using nasal sprays.

Product Selection

- Nasal sprays effectively relieve nasal congestion without causing systemic side effects.
- Because nasal sprays do not reach the sinuses, they are ineffective for relief of sinus congestion and pressure.
- Drugs with a longer duration of action, such as oxymetazoline, require fewer daily doses.
- These products should be administered with caution in patients with hypertension, hyperthyroidism, diabetes mellitus, cardiovascular disease, coronary artery disease, ischemic heart disease, glaucoma, and prostatic hypertrophy. These are not absolute contraindications; benefit must be weighed against risk. Pseudoephedrine is the preferred agent in hypertensive patients because it causes less systemic vasoconstriction than does phenylephrine or phenylpropanolamine.
- Timed-release products might be less likely to cause side effects because peak blood levels are lower than with immediate-release products.

REFERENCES

Anastacio GD et al: Fetal tachycardia associated with maternal use of pseudoephedrine, an over-the-counter oral decongestant, J Am Board Fam Pract 5(5):527-528, 1992.

Sloan MA et al: Occurrence of stroke associated with use/abuse of drugs, Neurology 41(9):1358-1364, 1991.

COUGH SUPPRESSANTS

DEXTROMETHORPHAN

DIPHENHYDRAMINE

Pharmacology

Dextromethorphan acts in the CNS to increase the cough threshold. Its antitussive activity is similar to that of codeine, but, unlike codeine, dextromethorphan does not inhibit ciliary action. Antitussive effects persist for 5 to 6 hours after a dose.

Diphenhydramine is an antihistamine with antitussive properties. Although it works centrally, the exact mechanism of action is unknown.

Side Effects

Dextromethorphan is extremely safe and has few, if any, side effects. Drowsiness or gastrointestinal upset have been occasionally reported. Diphenhydramine frequently causes drowsiness and numerous other anticholinergic side effects, such as urinary retention. When compared with dextromethorphan, diphenhydramine is no more efficacious, but causes significantly more side effects.

Drug Interactions

Dextromethorphan has no clinically significant drug interactions. Diphenhydramine can interact with a number of drugs, including the following:

- CNS depressants such as narcotics and benzodiazepines (Librium, Valium, Ativan, Versed), when used with antihistamines, may cause increased drowsiness.
- The following tricyclic antidepressants may increase anticholinergic side effects: amitriptyline (Elavil), nortriptyline (Aventyl, Pamelor), imipramine (Tofranil), doxepin (Sinequan), trimipramine (Surmontil), amoxapine (Asendin), desipramine (Norpramin), protriptyline (Vivactil), and clomipramine (Anafranil).
- The following antispasmodics may also increase anticholinergic side effects: hyoscyamine (Levsin, Anaspaz), glycopyrrolate (Robinul), mepenzolate (Cantil), and dicyclomine (Bentyl).
- Prokinetic agents such as metoclopramide (Reglan) and cisapride (Propulsid) may be antagonized by diphenhydramine.
- Urinary antispasmodics such as flavoxate (Urispas) and oxybutynin (Ditropan) may increase anticholinergic side effects.

Lifespan Considerations
Geriatric

Dextromethorphan is the cough suppressant of choice for the elderly because of its lack of side effects. Diphenhydramine should be avoided because older patients are more sensitive to anticholinergic side effects. Drowsiness, confusion, and delirium caused by central antagonism of acetylcholine can occur in the elderly.

Pediatric

Dextromethorphan is the safest cough suppressant and the preferred agent for use in children. The FDA does not allow dosing information for children under the age of 2 years to appear on nonprescription products. Instead, purchasers are directed to seek the advice of a physician.

Diphenhydramine is safe for use in children but can cause significant drowsiness. Nonprescription labeling directs purchasers to consult a physician for dosages for children under the age of 6 years. Professional dosing is 5 mg/kg/day in divided doses every 6 to 8 hours.

Pregnancy/Nursing Mothers

Dextromethorphan is an FDA Pregnancy Category C drug. Epidemiologic studies have demonstrated no increase in the frequency of congenital anomalies among women who took dextromethorphan during pregnancy (Aselton P et al, 1988). No information has been published regarding the distribution of dextromethorphan in breast milk.

Diphenhydramine is an FDA Pregnancy Category B drug. Epidemiologic studies (Schatz Mizeiger, 1997) have demonstrated that diphenhydramine does *not* increase the risk of birth defects if taken during pregnancy. However, indiscriminate use of drugs should be avoided in all pregnant patients. Benefit must be weighed against risk. Antihistamines such as diphenhydramine can depress lactation secondary to their anticholinergic effects. The American Academy of Pediatrics generally considers antihistamines such as diphenhydramine to be safe to use while nursing.

Patient Education

- Coughing is the body's way of removing unwanted substances from the throat, windpipe, and lungs.
- Coughs are useful (productive) if they cause phlegm to be coughed up. Productive coughs should not be suppressed unless they interfere with sleep or cause discomfort.
- A chronic cough lasting for more than a week or associated with shortness of breath should be referred to a health care professional.
- If blood is seen in the phlegm, patients should consult a health care professional.

Product Selection

Dextromethorphan is more efficacious and causes fewer side effects than diphenhydramine.

REFERENCES

Aselton P et al: First-trimester drug use and congenital disorders, *Obstet Gynecol* 65:451-455, 1988.
Schatz Mizeiger AS et al: The safety of allergy and asthma medications during pregnancy, J *Allergy Clin Immunol* 100(3):301-306, 1997.

EXPECTORANTS

Expectorants decrease the viscosity of phlegm, making it easier to remove the secretions by coughing. Definitive proof that expectorants effectively decrease phlegm viscosity is lacking. Though a number of drugs claim to have expectorant properties, only guaifenesin is considered by the FDA to be generally safe and effective.

Other ingredients claiming to have expectorant properties include ammonium chloride, beechwood creosote, benzoin, camphor, eucalyptus oil, iodides (prescription only), ipecac syrup, menthol, peppermint oil, pine tar, sodium citrate, terpin hydrate, tolu balsam, and turpentine oil.

Guaifenesin is thought to act by stimulating respiratory-tract secretions, decreasing their viscosity. By decreasing the viscosity of secretions, the normal mucociliary mechanism for removing accumulated upper and lower respiratory-tract secretions is enhanced. The adult dose for guaifenesin is 200 to 400 mg every 4 hours with a maximum dose of 2400 mg/day.

Side Effects

Guaifenesin is remarkably free of significant side effects. Rash could occur in patients allergic to guaifenesin but is uncommon.

Drug Interactions

No clinically significant drug interactions have been reported.

Lifespan Considerations

Geriatric

There are no specific concerns or recommendations for the use of guaifenesin with elderly patients.

Pediatric

Guaifenesin is safe for children of all ages.

Pregnancy

Guaifenesin is an FDA Pregnancy Category C drug. Although teratogenicity studies have not been performed, epidemiologic studies have not demonstrated an increased risk for congenital anomalies in infants of women taking guaifenesin during pregnancy. Given the high therapeutic index and lack of significant side effects, guaifenesin is probably safe for administration to pregnant women.

Nursing Mothers

No studies have been performed to determine distribution of guaifenesin in breast milk. However, given its safety, a high benefit to risk ratio exists.

Patient Education

To increase expectoration of respiratory secretions, patients should be advised to increase fluid intake to 6 to 8 8-oz glasses of water daily (if the patient is not fluid-restricted), and to use a cool-mist humidifier to increase humidity of the inspired air.

Product Selection

- Guaifenesin is found in many products.
- Many name brand and generic products contain guaifenesin.

ANALGESICS

Analgesics are found in some combination products sold for the symptomatic relief of achiness associated with colds and the flu. Analgesics found in these products include acetaminophen and salicylates. Information relative to these products can be found in Part IX, p. 363.

Product Selection

It is best to administer analgesics separately if needed. Multipurpose products make sense only if the patient needs all of the ingredients contained in the product.

SUGGESTED READINGS

Hemila H: Vitamin C supplementation and common cold symptoms: problems with inaccurate views, *Nutrition* 12:804-809, 1996.

Kirkpatrick GL: The common cold, *Prim Care* 23(4):657-675, 1996.

Smith MB, Feldman W: Over-the-counter cold medications: a critical review of clinical trials between 1950 and 1991, JAMA 260(17):2258-2263, 1993.

Turner RB: Epidemiology, pathogenesis, and treatment of the common cold, *Ann Allergy Asthma Immunol* 78(6):531-539, 1997.

Product Information: Cough, Cold, and Flu

Brand Name	Ingredient Type	Ingredient	Adult Dose	Pediatric Dose	Comments
A.R.M.	Antihistamine Decongestant	Chlorpheniramine 4 mg Phenylpropanolamine 25 mg	1 tablet every 4-6 hrs	*6-12 years:* ½ tablet every 4-6 hrs	
Actifed Cold & Allergy	Antihistamine Decongestant	Tripolidine 2.5 mg Pseudoephedrine 60 mg	1 tablet every 4-6 hrs	*6-12 years:* ½ tablet 3-4 times daily	
Actifed syrup	Antihistamine Decongestant	Tripolidine 1.25 mg/5 ml Pseudoephedrine 30 mg/5 ml		*4 months-2 years:* 1.25 ml 3-4 times daily *2-4 years:* 2.5 ml 3-4 times daily *4-6 years:* 3.75 ml 3-4 times daily *6-12 years:* 5 ml 3-4 times daily	
Actifed Maximum Strength Cold & Sinus	Antihistamine Decongestant Analgesic	Tripolidine 1.25 mg Pseudoephedrine 30 mg Acetaminophen 500 mg	2 tablets every 6 hrs		
Advil Cold & Sinus	Decongestant Analgesic	Pseudoephedrine 30 mg Ibuprofen 200 mg	1-2 tablets every 4-6 hrs; maximum 6 tablets/24 hrs		

Continued

Product Information: Cough, Cold, and Flu—cont'd

Brand Name	Ingredient Type	Ingredient	Adult Dose	Pediatric Dose	Comments
Alka-Seltzer Plus Cold & Cough Medicine	Antihistamine	Chlorpheniramine 2 mg	2 tablets every 4 hrs		Effervescent tablet contains 506 mg sodium/tablet
	Decongestant	Phenylpropanolamine 24 mg			
	Cough suppressant	Dextromethorphan 10 mg			
	Analgesic	Aspirin 500 mg			
Alka-Seltzer Plus Cold & Cough Medicine Liqui-Gels	Antihistamine	Chlorpheniramine 2 mg	2 gelcaps every 4 hrs	>6 years: 1 gelcap every 4 hrs; maximum 4/day	
	Decongestant	Pseudoephedrine 30 mg			
	Cough suppressant	Dextromethorphan 10 mg			
	Analgesic	Acetaminophen 250 mg			
Alka-Seltzer Plus Cold Medicine	Antihistamine	Chlorpheniramine 2 mg	2 tablets every 4 hrs		Effervescent tablet contains 506 mg sodium/tablet
	Decongestant	Phenylpropanolamine 24 mg			
	Analgesic	Aspirin 325 mg			
Alka-Seltzer Plus Cold Medicine Liqui-Gels	Antihistamine	Chlorpheniramine 2 mg	2 gelcaps every 4 hrs	>6 years: 1 gelcap every 4 hrs; maximum 4/day	
	Decongestant	Pseudoephedrine 30 mg			
	Analgesic	Acetaminophen 250 mg			
Alka-Seltzer Plus Cold & Flu Liqui-Gels Non-Drowsy	Decongestant	Pseudoephedrine 30 mg	2 gelcaps every 4 hrs	6-12 years: 1 gelcap every 4 hrs; maximum 4/day	
	Cough suppressant	Dextromethorphan 10 mg			
	Analgesic	Acetaminophen 325 mg			

Product		Dosage	Comments
Alka-Seltzer Plus Maximum Strength Sinus Medicine	Antihistamine Decongestant	Brompheniramine 2 mg Phenylpropanolamine 24 mg	2 tablets every 4 hrs	Effervescent tablet contains 506 mg sodium/tablet
Alka-Seltzer Plus Night-Time Cold Medicine	Analgesic Antihistamine Decongestant Cough suppressant	Aspirin 500 mg Brompheniramine 2 mg Phenylpropanolamine 24 mg Dextromethorphan 10 mg	2 tablets every 4 hrs	Effervescent tablet contains 506 mg sodium/tablet
Alka-Seltzer Plus Night-Time Cold Medicine Liqui-Gels	Analgesic Antihistamine Decongestant Cough suppressant Analgesic	Aspirin 500 mg Doxylamine 6.25 mg Pseudoephedrine 30 mg Dextromethorphan 10 mg Acetaminophen 250 mg	2 gelcaps HS	Doxylamine is a sedating antihistamine promoted as a sleep aid; product can be taken every 6-8 hrs but causes too much drowsiness for daytime use unless the patient is in bed
Allerest 12-Hour Maximum Strength	Antihistamine Decongestant	Chlorpheniramine 12 mg Phenylpropanolamine 75 mg	1 tablet every 12 hrs	Timed release

Continued

Product Information: Cough, Cold, and Flu—cont'd

Brand Name	Ingredient Type	Ingredient	Adult Dose	Pediatric Dose	Comments
Allerest Headache Strength	Antihistamine Decongestant Analgesic	Chlorpheniramine 2 mg Pseudephedrine 30 mg Acetaminophen 325 mg	2 tablets every 4-6 hrs	>6 years: 1 tablet every 4-6 hrs	
Allerest No-Drowsiness	Decongestant Analgesic	Pseudephedrine 30 mg Acetaminophen 325 mg	2 tablets every 4-6 hrs	6-12 years: 1 tablet every 4-6 hrs; maximum 4/day	
Allerest Sinus Pain Formula	Antihistamine Decongestant Analgesic	Chlorpheniramine 2 mg Pseudephedrine 30 mg Acetaminophen 500 mg	2 tablets every 6 hrs		
Allerest Maximum Strength	Antihistamine Decongestant	Chlorpheniramine 2 mg Pseudephedrine 30 mg	1 tablet every 4-6 hrs		
Benadryl	Antihistamine	Diphenhydramine 25 mg	1-2 tablets (see comments) every 4-6 hrs	>6 years: 1 tablet (see comments) every 4-6 hrs	Available as tablets, chewable tablets, capsules
Benadryl elixir	Antihistamine	Diphenhydramine 12.5 mg/5 ml	2-4 tsp every 4-6 hrs	5 mg/kg/day in divided doses every 4-6 hrs, not to exceed 300 mg/day	
Benadryl Allergy Sinus Headache Formula	Antihistamine Decongestant Analgesic	Diphenhydramine 25 mg Pseudephedrine 30 mg Acetaminophen 500 mg	2 tablets every 6 hrs		

			Adult dose	Pediatric dose
Benadryl Allergy Decongestant syrup	Antihistamine Decongestant	Diphenhydramine 12.5 mg/5 ml Pseudoephedrine 30 mg/5 ml	2 tsp every 4-6 hrs	*6-12 years:* 1 tsp every 4-6 hrs
Benadryl Cold/Flu	Antihistamine	Diphenhydramine 12.5 mg		
Benadryl D	Decongestant Analgesic Antihistamine Decongestant	Pseudoephedrine 30 mg Acetaminophen 500 mg Diphenhydramine 25 mg Pseudoephedrine 30 mg		
Benylin Adult Cough Formula	Cough suppressant	Dextromethorphan 15 mg/5 ml	2 tsp every 6-8 hrs	*6-12 years:* 1 tsp every 6-8 hrs *2-6 years:* ½ tsp every 6-8 hrs
Benylin Expectorant Cough Formula	Cough suppressant Expectorant	Dextromethorphan 15 mg/5 ml Guaifenesin 100 mg/5 ml	2-4 tsp every 4 hrs	*6-12 years:* 1-2 tsp every 4 hrs *2-6 years:* ½ -1 tsp every 4 hrs
Benylin Multi-Symptom Cough Formula	Cough suppressant Expectorant	Dextromethorphan 5 mg/5 ml Guaifenesin 100 mg/5 ml	4 tsp every 4 hrs	*6-12 years:* 2 tsp every 4 hrs *2-6 years:* 1 tsp every 4 hrs

Continued

Product Information: Cough, Cold, and Flu—cont'd

Brand Name	Ingredient Type	Ingredient	Adult Dose	Pediatric Dose	Comments
Benylin Pediatric Formula	Cough suppressant	Dextromethorphan 7.5 mg/5 ml Sodium citrate 7.5 mg/5 ml	4 tsp every 6-8 hrs	*6-12 years:* 2 tsp every 6-8 hrs *2-6 years:* 1 tsp every 6-8 hrs	
Cepacol Children's Sore Throat Formula	Decongestant Analgesic	Pseudoephedrine 15 mg/5 ml Acetaminophen 160 mg/5 ml		*12 years and older:* 4 tsp every 4-6 hrs *6-11 years:* 2 tsp every 4-6 hrs *2-5 years:* 1 tsp every 4-6 hrs	
Cheracol D	Cough suppressant Expectorant	Dextromethorphan 10 mg/5 ml Guaifenesin 100 mg/5 ml	2 tsp every 4 hrs		
Cheracol Plus	Antihistamine Decongestant Cough suppressant	Chlorpheniramine 4 mg/15 ml Phenylpropanolamine 25 mg/15 ml Dextromethorphan 20 mg/15 ml	1 tbsp (15 ml) every 4 hrs		

Cheracol Sinus	Antihistamine	Dexbrompheniramine 6 mg	1 tablet every 12 hrs	Timed release
	Decongestant	Pseudoephedrine 120 mg		
Chlor-Trimeton 12-Hour Allergy	Antihistamine	Chlorpheniramine 12 mg	1 tablet every 12 hrs	Timed release
Chlor-Trimeton 12-Hour Allergy Decongestant Formula	Antihistamine	Chlorpheniramine 12 mg	1 every 12 hrs	Timed release
	Decongestant	Pseudoephedrine 120 mg		
Chlor-Trimeton 4-Hour Allergy	Antihistamine	Chlorpheniramine 4 mg	1 tablet every 4-6 hrs	*6-12 years:* ½ tablet every 4-6 hrs
Chlor-Trimeton 4-Hour Allergy Decongestant	Antihistamine	Chlorpheniramine 4 mg	1 tablet every 4-6 hrs	*6-12 years:* ½ tablet every 4-6 hrs
	Decongestant	Pseudoephedrine 60 mg		
Chlor-Trimeton 8-Hour Allergy	Antihistamine	Chlorpheniramine 8 mg	1 tablet every 8 hrs	
Chlor-Trimeton Allergy syrup	Antihistamine	Chlorpheniramine 2 mg/5 ml		*2-6 years:* 1 mg every 4-6 hrs *6-12 years:* 2 mg every 4-6 hrs

Continued

Product Information: Cough, Cold, and Flu—cont'd

Brand Name	Ingredient Type	Ingredient	Adult Dose	Pediatric Dose	Comments
Chlor-Trimeton Allergy Sinus Headache	Antihistamine Decongestant	Chlorpheniramine 2 mg Phenylpropanolamine 12.5 mg	2 tablets every 6 hrs		
	Analgesic	Acetaminophen 500 mg			
Chlor-Trimeton Non-Drowsy 4-Hour	Decongestant	Pseudoephedrine 60 mg	1 tablet every 4-6 hrs		Contains NO antihistamine
Comtrex Multi-Symptom	Antihistamine Decongestant Analgesic	Chlorpheniramine 2 mg Pseudoephedrine 30 mg Acetaminophen 500 mg	2 tablets every 6 hrs		
Comtrex Deep Chest Cold & Congestion Relief	Decongestant	Phenylpropanolamine 12.5 mg	2 tablets every 4 hrs		
	Cough suppressant	Dextromethorphan 10 mg			
	Expectorant Analgesic	Guaifenesin 200 mg Acetaminophen 325 mg			
Comtrex Maximum Strength	Antihistamine Decongestant Cough suppressant	Chlorpheniramine 2 mg Pseudoephedrine 30 mg Dextromethorphan 15 mg	2 tablets every 6 hrs		
	Analgesic	Acetaminophen 500 mg			

Product	Category	Ingredient	Dosage
Comtrex Maximum Strength Liqui-Gels	Antihistamine	Chlorpheniramine 2 mg	2 tablets every 6 hrs
	Decongestant	Phenylpropanolamine 12.5 mg	
	Cough suppressant	Dextromethorphan 15 mg	
	Analgesic	Acetaminophen 500 mg	
Comtrex Maximum Strength Liquid	Antihistamine	Chlorpheniramine 4 mg/30 ml	2 tbsp (30 ml) every 6 hrs
	Decongestant	Pseudoephedrine 60 mg/30 ml	
	Cough suppressant	Dextromethorphan 30 mg/30 ml	
	Analgesic	Acetaminophen 1000 mg/30 ml	
Comtrex Maximum Strength Non-Drowsy	Decongestant	Pseudoephedrine 30 mg	2 tablets every 6 hrs
	Cough suppressant	Dextromethorphan 15 mg	
	Analgesic	Acetaminophen 500 mg	
Comtrex Maximum Strength Non-Drowsy Liqui-Gels	Decongestant	Phenylpropanolamine 12.5 mg	2 tablets every 6 hrs
	Cough suppressant	Dextromethorphan 15 mg	
	Analgesic	Acetaminophen 500 mg	

Continued

Product Information: Cough, Cold, and Flu—cont'd

Brand Name	Ingredient Type	Ingredient	Adult Dose	Pediatric Dose	Comments
Congestac	Decongestant Expectorant	Pseudoephedrine 60 mg Guaifenesin 400 mg	1 capsule every 4-6 hrs		
Contac 12-Hour Allergy	Antihistamine	Clemastine 1 mg	1 tablet every 12 hrs		12-hour duration of action
Contac 12-Hour Cold	Antihistamine Decongestant	Chlorpheniramine 8 mg Phenylpropanolamine 75 mg	1 tablet every 12 hrs		Timed release
Contac Maximum Strength 12-Hour	Antihistamine Decongestant	Chlorpheniramine 12 mg Phenylpropanolamine 75 mg	1 tablet every 12 hrs		Timed release
Contac Severe Cold & Flu Nighttime	Antihistamine Decongestant Cough suppressant Analgesic	Chlorpheniramine 4 mg/5 ml Pseudoephedrine 60 mg Dextromethorphan 30 mg Acetaminophen 1000 mg			
Contac Severe Cold & Flu Non-Drowsy	Decongestant Cough suppressant Analgesic	Pseudoephedrine 30 mg Dextromethorphan 15 mg Acetaminophen 325 mg	2 tablets every 6 hrs		

Product	Classification	Ingredients	Adult Dosage	Pediatric Dosage	Notes
Contac Severe Cold & Flu	Antihistamine Decongestant Cough suppressant Analgesic	Chlorpheniramine 2 mg Phenylpropanolamine 12.5 mg Dextromethorphan 15 mg Acetaminophen 500 mg	2 tablets every 6 hrs		
Coricidin	Antihistamine Analgesic	Chlorpheniramine 2 mg Acetaminophen 325 mg	2 tablets every 4-6 hrs	6-12 years: 1 tablet every 4-6 hrs	
Coricidin Cold & Flu	Antihistamine Analgesic	Chlorpheniramine 2 mg Acetaminophen 325 mg	2 tablets every 4-6 hrs	6-12 years: 1 tablet every 4-6 hrs	
Coricidin HBP Cough & Cold	Antihistamine Cough suppressant	Chlorpheniramine 4 mg Dextromethorphan 30 mg	1 tablet every 6 hrs		Promoted for patients with hypertension because it does not contain a decongestant
Coricidin HBP Night Time Cough & Cold Liquid	Antihistamine Analgesic	Diphenhydramine 12.5 mg/5 ml Acetaminophen 325 mg/15 ml	2 tbsp (30 ml) every 4 hrs	6-12 years: 1 tbsp (15 ml) every 4 hrs	Best taken at bedtime or when going to bed because diphenhydramine causes significant drowsiness
Coricidin D	Antihistamine Decongestant Analgesic	Chlorpheniramine 2 mg Phenylpropanolamine 12.5 mg Acetaminophen 325 mg	2 tablets every 4 hrs	6-12 years: 1 tablet every 4 hrs	

Continued

Product Information: Cough, Cold, and Flu—cont'd

Brand Name	Ingredient Type	Ingredient	Adult Dose	Pediatric Dose	Comments
Delsym Extended Release	Cough suppressant	Dextromethorphan 30 mg/5 ml	2 tsp every 12 hrs	*6-12 years:* 1 tsp every 12 hrs *2-6 years:* ½ tsp every 12 hrs	This is the only timed-release cough suppressant liquid; more expensive, but more convenient; SHAKE WELL before administering
Diabetic Tussin DM	Cough suppressant Expectorant	Dextromethorphan 10 mg/5 ml Guaifenesin 100 mg/5 ml	2 tsp every 4 hrs	*6-12 years:* 1 tsp every 4 hrs *2-6 years:* ½ tsp every 4 hrs	Contains no sugar, sodium, alcohol, fructose, sorbitol, or dyes
Dimetane Elixir	Antihistamine	Brompheniramine 2 mg/5 ml		*<6 years:* 0.125 mg/kg/dose every 6 hrs; maximum 6-8 mg/day *6-12 years:* 2-4 mg every 6-8 hrs; maximum 12-16 mg/day	

Product	Type	Ingredients	Adult dose	Pediatric dose	Comments
Dimetapp Elixir	Antihistamine	Brompheniramine 2 mg/5 ml	5-10 ml 3-4 times daily	*1-6 months:* 1.25 ml 3-4 times daily *7-24 months:* 2.5 ml 3-4 times daily *2-4 years:* 3.75 ml 3-4 times daily *4-12 years:* 5 ml 3-4 times daily	
	Decongestant	Phenylpropanolamine 12.5 mg/5 ml			
Dimetapp Allergy	Antihistamine	Brompheniramine 4 mg	1 tablet (see comments) every 4 hrs	*6-12 years:* ½ tablet (see comments) every 4 hrs	Available as tablets and gelcaps; gelcaps cannot be halved
Dimetapp Allergy Extentabs	Antihistamine	Brompheniramine 8 mg	1 tablet every 12 hrs		Timed release
Dimetapp Cold & Allergy Chewable Tablet	Antihistamine	Brompheniramine 1 mg		*6-12 years:* 2 tablets every 4 hrs	Chewable
	Decongestant	Phenylpropanolamine 6.25 mg		*2-6 years:* 1 tablet every 4 hrs	
Dimetapp Cold & Cough Maximum Strength Liqui-Gel	Antihistamine	Brompheniramine 4 mg	1 every 4 hrs		
	Decongestant	Phenylpropanolamine 25 mg			
	Cough suppressant	Dextromethorphan 20 mg			

Continued

Product Information: Cough, Cold, and Flu—cont'd

Brand Name	Ingredient Type	Ingredient	Adult Dose	Pediatric Dose	Comments
Dimetapp Decongestant Non-Drowsy	Decongestant	Pseudoephedrine 30 mg	2 tablets every 4-6 hrs		
Dimetapp Decongestant Pediatric Drops	Decongestant	Pseudoephedrine 7.5 mg/0.8 ml		*<2 years:* 1 mg/kg every 6 hrs *2-5 years:* 15 mg every 6 hrs (2-3 droppersful every 6 hr); maximum 60 mg/24 hrs *6-12 years:* 30 mg every 6 hrs; maximum 120 mg/24 hrs	Oral drops
Dimetapp DM Liquid	Antihistamine	Brompheniramine 2 mg/5 ml	2 tsp every 4 hrs	*6-12 years:* 1 tsp every 4 hrs *2-6 years:* ½ tsp every 4 hrs	
	Decongestant	Phenylpropanolamine 12.5 mg/5 ml			
	Cough suppressant	Dextromethorphan 10 mg/5 ml			

Drug	Type	Ingredients	Dosage	Notes
Dimetapp Maximum Strength 12-Hour Extentabs	Antihistamine Decongestant	Brompheniramine 12 mg Phenylpropanolamine 75 mg	1 tablet every 12 hrs	Timed release
Dimetapp Maximum Strength 4-Hour	Antihistamine Decongestant	Brompheniramine 4 mg Phenylpropanolamine 25 mg	1 tablet every 4 hrs	
Dimetapp Sinus	Decongestant Analgesic	Pseudoephedrine 30 mg Ibuprofen 200 mg	1 tablet every 4-6 hrs	
Dorcol Children's Cough Syrup	Decongestant	Pseudoephedrine 15 mg/5 ml		*12-24 months:* 7 drops (0.2 ml)/kg every 4 hrs
	Cough suppressant	Dextromethorphan 5 mg/5 ml		*3-12 months:* 3 drops/kg every 4 hrs
	Expectorant	Guaifenesin 50 mg/5 ml		*6-12 years (46-85 lbs):* 2 tsp every 4 hrs *2-6 years (25-45 lbs):* 1 tsp every 4 hrs
Dristan Allergy	Antihistamine Decongestant	Brompheniramine 4 mg Pseudoephedrine 60 mg	1 tablet every 4 hrs	

Continued

Product Information: Cough, Cold, and Flu—cont'd

Brand Name	Ingredient Type	Ingredient	Adult Dose	Pediatric Dose	Comments
Dristan Cold Maximum Strength No Drowsiness	Decongestant Analgesic	Pseudoephedrine 30 mg Acetaminophen 500 mg	2 tablets every 6 hrs		
Dristan Cold Multi-Symptom	Antihistamine Decongestant Analgesic	Chlorpheniramine 2 mg Phenylephrine 5 mg Acetaminophen 325 mg	2 every 4 hrs		
Dristan Sinus	Decongestant Analgesic	Pseudoephedrine 30 mg Ibuprofen 200 mg	1-2 tablets every 4-6 hrs; maximum 6/24 hrs		
Drixoral Allergy Sinus Extended Release	Antihistamine Decongestant Analgesic	Dexbrompheniramine 3 mg Pseudoephedrine 60 mg Acetaminophen 500 mg	2 tablets every 12 hrs		Timed release
Drixoral Cold & Allergy Sustained Action	Antihistamine Decongestant	Dexbrompheniramine 6 mg Pseudoephedrine 120 mg	1 tablet every 12 hrs		Timed release
Drixoral Cold & Flu	Antihistamine Decongestant Analgesic	Dexbrompheniramine 3 mg Pseudoephedrine 60 mg Acetaminophen 500 mg	2 tablets every 12 hrs		

Product	Action	Ingredients	Adult Dosage	Child Dosage	Notes
Drixoral Cough & Congestion Liquid Caps	Decongestant Cough suppressant	Pseudoephedrine 60 mg Dextromethorphan 30 mg	1 capsule every 6 hrs		
Drixoral Cough & Sore Throat Liquid Caps	Cough suppressant	Dextromethorphan 15 mg	2 capsules every 6-8 hrs	*6-12 years:* 1 capsule every 6-8 hrs	
Drixoral Cough Liquid Caps	Analgesic Cough suppressant	Acetaminophen 325 mg Dextromethorphan 30 mg	1 capsule every 6-8 hrs		
Drixoral Nasal Decongestant Non-Drowsy	Decongestant	Pseudoephedrine 120 mg	1 tablet every 12 hrs		Timed release
Drixoral Non-Drowsy Formula Extended Release	Decongestant	Pseudoephedrine 120 mg	1 tablet every 12 hrs		Timed release
Efidac/24 Extended Release	Decongestant	Pseudoephedrine 240 mg	1 tablet every 24 hrs		24-hour timed release
Excedrin Sinus	Decongestant Analgesic	Pseudoephedrine 30 mg Acetaminophen 500 mg	2 tablets every 6 hrs		
Humibid Guaifenesin Plus	Decongestant Expectorant	Pseudoephedrine 60 mg Guaifenesin 400 mg	1 tablet every 4-6 hrs		
Motrin IB Sinus	Decongestant Analgesic	Pseudoephedrine 30 mg Ibuprofen 200 mg	1-2 tablets every 4-6 hrs; maximum 6/day	*6-12 years:* ½ tablet every 4-6 hrs	

Continued

Product Information: Cough, Cold, and Flu—cont'd

Brand Name	Ingredient Type	Ingredient	Adult Dose	Pediatric Dose	Comments
Naldecon DX Adult Liquid	Decongestant	Phenylpropanolamine 12.5 mg/5 ml	2 tsp every 4 hrs		
	Cough suppressant	Dextromethorphan 10 mg/5 ml			
	Expectorant	Guaifenesin 200 mg/5 ml			
Naldecon DX Children's Liquid	Decongestant	Phenylpropanolamine 6.25 mg/5 ml		6-12 years: 2 tsp every 4 hrs	
	Cough suppressant	Dextromethorphan 5 mg/5 ml		2-6 years: 1 tsp every 4 hrs	
	Expectorant	Guaifenesin 100 mg/5 ml			
Naldecon DX Pediatric Drops	Decongestant	Phenylpropanolamine 6.25 mg/1 ml		2-6 years: 1 ml every 4 hrs	Much more concentrated than syrup
	Cough suppressant	Dextromethorphan 5 mg/1 ml			
	Expectorant	Guaifenesin 50 mg/1 ml			

Product		Ingredient	Dose	
Naldecon EX Children's Liquid	Decongestant	Phenylpropanolamine 6.25 mg/5 ml		
	Expectorant	Guaifenesin 100 mg/5 ml		
Naldecon EX Pediatric Drops	Decongestant	Phenylpropanolamine 6.25 mg/1 ml	2-6 years: 1 ml every 4 hrs	Much more concentrated than syrup
	Expectorant	Guaifenesin 50 mg/1 ml		
Naldecon Senior DX	Cough suppressant	Dextromethorphan 10 mg/5 ml	2 tsp every 4 hrs	
	Expectorant	Guaifenesin 200 mg/5 ml		
Naldecon Senior EX	Expectorant	Guaifenesin 200 mg/5 ml	2 tsp every 4 hrs	
Novahistine Elixir	Antihistamine	Chlorpheniramine 2 mg/5 ml	2 tsp every 4 hrs	6-12 years: 1 tsp every 4 hrs
	Decongestant	Phenylephrine 5 mg/5 ml		
Novahistine DMX Syrup	Decongestant	Pseudoephedrine 30 mg/5 ml	2 tsp every 4 hrs	6-12 years: 1 tsp every 4 hrs
	Cough suppressant	Dextromethorphan 10 mg/5 ml		
	Expectorant	Guaifenesin 100 mg/5 ml		

Continued

Product Information: Cough, Cold, and Flu—cont'd

Brand Name	Ingredient Type	Ingredient	Adult Dose	Pediatric Dose	Comments
Nyquil Children's Cold/Cough Medicine	Antihistamine	Chlorpheniramine 2 mg/15 ml		6-11 years: 15 ml every 6 hrs	
	Decongestant	Pseudoephedrine 30 mg/15 ml		12 years and older: 30 ml every 6 hrs	
	Cough suppressant	Dextromethorphan 15 mg/15 ml			
Ornex No-Drowsiness Formula	Decongestant	Pseudoephedrine 30 mg	2 tablets every 4-6 hrs	6-12 years: 1 tablet every 4-6 hrs	
	Analgesic	Acetaminophen 25 mg			
PediaCare Cold-Allergy for Ages 6-12	Antihistamine	Chlorpheniramine 1 mg		2-3 years (24-35 lbs): 1 tablet every 4-6 hrs	
	Decongestant	Pseudoephedrine 15 mg		4-5 years (36-47 lbs): 1½ tablets every 4-6 hrs	
				6-8 years (48-59 lbs): 2 tablets every 4-6 hrs	
				9-10 years (60-71 lbs): 2½ tablets every 4-6 hrs	
				11 years (72-95 lbs): 3 tablets every 4-6 hrs	

PediaCare Cough-Cold Formula Liquid		
Antihistamine	Chlorpheniramine	1 mg/5 ml
Decongestant	Pseudoephedrine	15 mg/5 ml
Cough suppressant	Dextromethorphan	5 mg/5 ml

2-3 years (24-35 lbs):
  1 tsp every 4-6 hrs
4-5 years (36-47 lbs):
  1½ tsp every 4-6 hrs
6-8 years (48-59 lbs):
  2 tsp every 4-6 hrs
9-10 years (60-71 lbs):
  2½ tsp every 4-6 hrs
11 years (72-95 lbs):
  3 tsp every 4-6 hrs

PediaCare Cough-Cold for Ages 6-12		
Antihistamine	Chlorpheniramine 1 mg	
Decongestant	Pseudoephedrine 15 mg	
Cough suppressant	Dextromethorphan 5 mg	

2-3 years (24-35 lbs):
  1 tablet every 4-6 hrs
4-5 years (36-47 lbs):
  1½ tablets every 4-6 hrs
6-8 years (48-59 lbs):
  2 tablets every 4-6 hrs
9-10 years (60-71 lbs):
  2½ tablets every 4-6 hrs
11 years (72-95 lbs):
  3 tablets every 4-6 hrs

Continued

Product Information: Cough, Cold, and Flu—cont'd

Brand Name	Ingredient Type	Ingredient	Adult Dose	Pediatric Dose	Comments
PediaCare Night Rest Cough-Cold Formula Liquid	Antihistamine	Chlorpheniramine 1 mg/5 ml		*2-3 years (24-35 lbs):* 1 tsp every 4-6 hrs	
	Decongestant	Pseudoephedrine 15 mg/5 ml		*4-5 years (36-47 lbs):* 1½ tsp every 4-6 hrs	
	Cough suppressant	Dextromethorphan 7.5 mg/5 ml		*6-8 years (48-59 lbs):* 2 tsp every 4-6 hrs	
				9-10 years (60-71 lbs): 2½ tsp every 4-6 hrs	
				11 years (72-95 lbs): 3 tsp every 4-6 hrs	
PediaCare Infants Decongestant Drops	Decongestant	Pseudoephedrine 7.5 mg/0.8 ml		*0-3 months (6-11 lbs):* ½ dropper (0.4 ml)	
				4-11 months (12-17 lbs): 1 dropper (0.8 ml)	
				12-23 months (18-23 lbs): 1½ dropper (1.2 ml)	
				2-3 years (24-35 lbs): 2 droppers (1.6 ml)	

Robitussin syrup	Expectorant	Guaifenesin 100 mg/5 ml	2-4 tsp every 4 hrs	*6-12 years:* 1-2 tsp every 4 hrs *2-6 years:* ½-1 tsp every 4 hrs *<2 years:* 12 mg/kg/day in 6 divided doses
Robitussin CF	Decongestant Cough suppressant Expectorant	Phenylpropanolamine 12.5 mg/5 ml Dextromethorphan 10 mg/5 ml Guaifenesin 100 mg/5 ml	2 tsp every 4 hrs	*6-12 years:* 1 tsp every 4 hrs *2-6 years:* ½ tsp every 4 hrs
Robitussin Cold & Cough Liqui-Gels	Decongestant Cough suppressant Expectorant	Pseudoephedrine 30 mg Dextromethorphan 10 mg Guaifenesin 200 mg	2 gelcaps every 4 hrs	*6-12 years:* 1 gelcap every 4 hrs
Robitussin Cold, Cough, & Flu Liqui-Gels	Decongestant Cough suppressant Expectorant Analgesic	Pseudoephedrine 30 mg Dextromethorphan 10 mg Guaifenesin 100 mg Acetaminophen 250 mg	2 gelcaps every 4 hrs	*6-12 years:* 1 gelcap every 4 hrs

Continued

Product Information: Cough, Cold, and Flu—cont'd

Brand Name	Ingredient Type	Ingredient	Adult Dose	Pediatric Dose	Comments
Robitussin Cold NightTime	Antihistamine Decongestant Cough suppressant	Doxylamine 6.25 mg Pseudoephedrine 30 mg Dextromethorphan 15 mg	2 tablets every 6 hrs		
Robitussin DM	Analgesic Cough suppressant Expectorant	Acetaminophen 325 mg Dextromethorphan 10 mg/5 ml Guaifenesin 100 mg/5 ml	2 tsp every 4 hrs	*6-12 years:* 1 tsp every 4 hrs *2-6 years:* ½ tsp every 4 hrs *<2 years:* 1-2 mg dextromethorphan/ kg/day every 6-8 hrs	
Robitussin Maximum Strength Cough liquid	Cough suppressant	Dextromethorphan 15 mg/5 ml	2 tsp every 6-8 hrs	*6-12 years:* 1 tsp every 6-8 hrs *2-6 years:* ½ tsp every 6-8 hrs	
Robitussin Maximum Strength Cough & Cold liquid	Decongestant Cough suppressant	Pseudoephedrine 30 mg/5 ml Dextromethorphan 15 mg/5 ml	2 tsp every 6 hrs		

Product	Category	Ingredient	Dose	Dosing	Notes
Robitussin Night Relief liquid	Antihistamine Decongestant Cough suppressant Analgesic	Pyrilamine 50 mg/30 ml Pseudoephedrine 60 mg/30 ml Dextromethorphan 30 mg/30 ml Acetaminophen 650 mg/30 ml	30 ml HS		Pyrilamine is a sedating antihistamine promoted as a sleep aid; it is too sedating for daytime use unless the patient is going to bed
Robitussin PE	Decongestant Expectorant	Pseudoephedrine 30 mg/5 ml Guaifenesin 100 mg/5 ml	2 tsp every 4 hrs	*6-12 years:* 1 tsp every 4 hrs	
Robitussin Pediatric Cough Liquid	Cough suppressant	Dextromethorphan 7.5 mg/5 ml		*12 years and older:* 4 tsp every 6 hrs *6-12 years:* 2 tsp every 6 hrs *2-6 years:* 1 tsp every 6 hrs	
Robitussin Pediatric Cough & Cold Liquid	Decongestant Cough suppressant	Pseudoephedrine 15 mg/5 ml Dextromethorphan 7.5 mg/5 ml		*12 years and older:* 4 tsp every 6 hrs *6-12 years:* 2 tsp every 6 hrs *2-6 years:* 1 tsp every 6 hrs	

Continued

Product Information: Cough, Cold, and Flu—cont'd

Brand Name	Ingredient Type	Ingredient	Adult Dose	Pediatric Dose	Comments
Robitussin Pediatric Night Relief	Antihistamine Decongestant Cough suppressant	Chlorpheniramine 1 mg/5 ml Pseudoephedrine 15 mg/5 ml Dextromethorphan 7.5 mg/5 ml		*6-12 years:* 2 tsp every 6 hrs *2-6 years:* 1 tsp every 6 hrs	
Robitussin Severe Congestion Liqui-Gels	Decongestant Expectorant	Pseudoephedrine 30 mg Guaifenesin 200 mg	2 gelcaps every 4 hrs	*6-12 years:* 1 gelcap every 4 hrs	
Safe Tussin 30	Cough suppressant Expectorant	Dextromethorphan 30 mg/10 ml Guaifenesin 200 mg/10 ml	2 tsp every 6 hrs	*6-12 years:* 1 tsp every 6 hrs *2-5 years:* ½ tsp every 6 hrs	Contains no sugar, alcohol, dyes, or sodium
Sine-Aid IB	Decongestant Analgesic	Pseudoephedrine 30 mg Ibuprofen 200 mg	1-2 tablets every 4-6 hrs; maximum 6/day		
Sine-Aid Maximum Strength	Decongestant Analgesic	Pseudoephedrine 30 mg Acetaminophen 500 mg	2 tablets (see comments) every 4-6 hrs		Available as tablets and gelcaps
Sine-Off Maximum Strength Allergy/Sinus	Antihistamine Decongestant Analgesic	Chlorpheniramine 2 mg Pseudoephedrine 30 mg Acetaminophen 500 mg	2 tablets every 6 hrs		

Product	Type	Ingredients	Adult Dose	Pediatric Dose	Comments
Sine-Off Maximum Strength No Drowsiness Formula	Decongestant Analgesic	Pseudoephedrine 30 mg Acetaminophen 500 mg	2 tablets every 6 hrs		
Sinutab	Decongestant Analgesic Antihistamine	Pseudoephedrine 30 mg Acetaminophen 325 mg Chlorpheniramine 2 mg	2 tablets every 6 hrs		
Sinutab Allergy Sinus Medication Maximum Strength	Decongestant Analgesic	Pseudoephedrine 30 mg Acetaminophen 500 mg	2 tablets every 6 hrs		
Sinutab Maximum Strength No Drowsiness	Decongestant Analgesic	Pseudoephedrine 30 mg Acetaminophen 500 mg	2 tablets every 6 hrs		
Sudafed (30 mg)	Decongestant	Pseudoephedrine 30 mg	2 tablets every 4-6 hrs	*6-12 years:* 1 tablet every 4-6 hrs	
Sudafed (60 mg)	Decongestant	Pseudoephedrine 60 mg	1 tablet every 4-6 hrs		
Sudafed 12-Hour Extended Release	Decongestant	Pseudoephedrine 120 mg	1 tablet every 12 hrs		Timed release

Continued

Product Information: Cough, Cold, and Flu—cont'd

Brand Name	Ingredient Type	Ingredient	Adult Dose	Pediatric Dose	Comments
Sudafed Cough & Cold Liquid Caps	Decongestant Cough suppressant	Pseudoephedrine 30 mg Dextromethorphan 10 mg	2 every 4 hrs		
Sudafed Cough Syrup	Decongestant Cough suppressant Expectorant	Pseudoephedrine 15 mg/5 ml Dextromethorphan 5 mg/5 ml Guaifenesin 100 mg/5 ml	4 tsp every 4 hrs	6-12 years: 2 tsp every 4 hrs up to 120 mg/day 2-6 years: 1 tsp every 4 hrs up to 60 mg/day <2 years: 4 mg/kg/day every 6 hrs	
Sudafed Maximum Strength Severe Cold Formula	Decongestant Cough suppressant Analgesic	Pseudoephedrine 30 mg Dextromethorphan 15 mg Acetaminophen 500 mg	2 tablets every 6 hrs		
Sudafed Plus	Antihistamine Decongestant	Chlorpheniramine 4 mg Pseudoephedrine 60 mg	1 tablet every 4-6 hrs	6-12 years: ½ tablet every 4-6 hrs	
Sudafed Plus Syrup	Antihistamine Decongestant	Chlorpheniramine 2 mg/5 ml Pseudoephedrine 30 mg/5 ml	2 tsp every 4-6 hrs	6-12 years: 1 tsp every 4-6 hrs	

Drug	Type	Ingredients	Dosage	Notes
Sudafed Severe Cold Formula	Decongestant Cough suppressant	Pseudoephedrine 30 mg Dextromethorphan 15 mg	2 every 6 hrs	
Sudafed Sinus	Analgesic Decongestant	Acetaminophen 500 mg Pseudoephedrine 30 mg	2 every 6 hrs	
Sudafed Children's Liquid	Analgesic Decongestant	Acetaminophen 500 mg Pseudoephedrine 30 mg/5 ml	*<2 years:* 1 mg/kg every 6 hrs *2-5 years:* 15 mg every 6 hrs; maximum 60 mg/24 hrs *6-12 years:* 30 mg every 6 hrs; maximum 120 mg/24 hrs	
Tavist-1	Antihistamine	Clemastine 1 mg	1 tablet every 12 hrs	
Tavist-D	Antihistamine Decongestant	Clemastine 1 mg Phenylpropanolamine 75 mg	*6-12 years:* ½ tablet every 12 hrs; maximum 3 tablets/day 1 tablet every 12 hrs	Timed release

Continued

Product Information: Cough, Cold, and Flu—cont'd

Brand Name	Ingredient Type	Ingredient	Adult Dose	Pediatric Dose	Comments
Tavist Sinus Maximum Strength	Decongestant Analgesic	Pseudoephedrine 30 mg Acetaminophen 500 mg	2 tablets every 6 hrs		
Teldrin	Antihistamine	Chlorpheniramine 12 mg	1 tablet every 12 hrs		Timed release
TheraFlu Flu & Cold Medicine	Antihistamine Decongestant Analgesic	Chlorpheniramine 4 mg Pseudoephedrine 60 mg Acetaminophen 650 mg	1 packet every 4 hrs; maximum 4/24 hrs		Packet contents are dissolved in hot water
TheraFlu Flu, Cold, & Cough Medicine	Antihistamine Decongestant Cough suppressant	Chlorpheniramine 4 mg Pseudoephedrine 60 mg Dextromethorphan 20 mg	1 packet every 4 hrs; maximum 4/24 hrs		Packet contents are dissolved in hot water
TheraFlu Maximum Strength NightTime	Antihistamine Decongestant Cough suppressant Analgesic	Chlorpheniramine 4 mg Pseudoephedrine 60 mg Dextromethorphan 30 mg Acetaminophen 1000 mg	1 packet every 6 hrs; maximum 4/24 hrs		Packet contents are dissolved in hot water

Product	Class	Ingredients	Adult dose	Pediatric dose
TheraFlu Maximum Strength Non-Drowsy Formula	Decongestant Cough suppressant Analgesic	Pseudoephedrine 60 mg Dextromethorphan 30 mg Acetaminophen 1000 mg	1 packet every 6 hrs	
Triaminic syrup	Antihistamine Decongestant	Chlorpheniramine 2 mg/10 ml Phenylpropanolamine 12.5 mg/10 ml	4 tsp every 4 hrs	*3-12 months (12-17 lbs):* ¼ tsp (1.25 ml) every 4 hrs *12-24 months (18-23 lbs):* ½ tsp (2.5 ml) every 4 hrs *2-6 years (24-47 lbs):* 1 tsp (5 ml) every 4 hrs *6-12 years (48-95 lbs):* 4 tsp (20 ml) every 4 hrs
Triaminic Allergy	Antihistamine Decongestant	Chlorpheniramine 4 mg Phenylpropanolamine 25 mg	1 tablet every 4 hrs	*6-12 years:* ½ tablet every 4 hrs

Continued

Product Information: Cough, Cold, and Flu—cont'd

Brand Name	Ingredient Type	Ingredient	Adult Dose	Pediatric Dose	Comments
Triaminic Cold	Antihistamine Decongestant	Chlorpheniramine 2 mg Phenylpropanolamine 12.5 mg	2 tablets every 4 hrs	*6-12 years:* 1 tablet every 4 hrs	
Triaminic Expectorant liquid	Decongestant Expectorant	Phenylpropanolamine 12.5 mg/10 ml Guaifenesin 100 mg/10 ml	4 tsp every 6 hrs	*3-12 months* *(12-17 lbs):* ¼ tsp (1.25 ml) every 4 hrs *12-24 months* *(18-23 lbs):* ½ tsp (2.5 ml) every 4 hrs *2-6 years (24-47 lbs):* 1 tsp (5 ml) every 4 hrs *6-12 years (48-95 lbs):* 4 tsp (20 ml) every 4 hrs	

Triaminic Nite *Light* liquid	Antihistamine	Chlorpheniramine 1 mg/10 ml	4 tsp every 6 hrs	*3-12 months* *(12-17 lbs)*: ¼ tsp (1.25 ml) every 6 hrs	
	Decongestant	Pseudoephedrine 15 mg/5 ml		*12-24 months* *(18-23 lbs)*: ½ tsp (2.5 ml) every 6 hrs	
	Cough suppressant	Dextromethorphan 7.5 mg/10 ml		*2-6 years (24-47 lbs)*: 1 tsp (5 ml) every 6 hrs	
				6-12 years (48-95 lbs): 4 tsp (20 ml) every 6 hrs	
Triaminic Sore *Throat Formula*	Decongestant	Pseudoephedrine 15 mg/5 ml	4 tsp every 6 hrs	*2-6 years*: 1 tsp every 6 hrs	
	Cough suppressant	Dextromethorphan 7.5 mg/5 ml		*6-12 years*: 2 tsp every 6 hrs	
	Analgesic	Acetaminophen 160 mg/5 ml			
Triaminic-12	Antihistamine	Chlorpheniramine 12 mg	1 tablet every 12 hrs		Timed release
	Decongestant	Phenylpropanolamine 75 mg			

Continued

Product Information: Cough, Cold, and Flu—cont'd

Brand Name	Ingredient Type	Ingredient	Adult Dose	Pediatric Dose	Comments
Triaminic-DM syrup	Decongestant	Phenylpropanolamine 12.5 mg/10 ml	4 tsp every 4 hrs	*3-12 months (12-17 lbs):* ¼ tsp (1.25 ml) every 4 hrs *12-24 months (18-23 lbs):* ½ tsp (2.5 ml) every 4 hrs *2-6 years (24-47 lbs):* 1 tsp (5 ml) every 4 hrs *6-12 years (48-95 lbs):* 4 tsp (20 ml) every 4 hrs	
	Cough suppressant	Dextromethorphan 10 mg/10 ml			
Triaminicin	Antihistamine	Chlorpheniramine 4 mg	1 tablet every 4 hrs		
	Decongestant	Phenylpropanolamine 25 mg			
Triaminicol Multi-Symptom Cold tablet	Analgesic	Acetaminophen 50 mg	2 tablets every 4 hrs	*6-12 years:* 1 every 4 hrs	
	Antihistamine	Chlorpheniramine 2 mg			
	Decongestant	Phenylpropanolamine 12.5 mg			
	Cough suppressant	Dextromethorphan 10 mg			

Drug	Category	Ingredients	Adult dosage	Pediatric dosage	Comments
Triaminicol Multi-Symptom Relief liquid	Antihistamine Decongestant Cough suppressant	Chlorpheniramine 1 mg/5 ml Phenylpropanolamine 6.25 mg/5 ml Dextromethorphan 5 mg/5 ml	4 tsp every 4 hrs	*3-12 months (12-17 lbs):* ¼ tsp (1.25 ml) every 4 hrs *12-24 months (18-23 lbs):* ½ tsp (2.5 ml) every 4 hrs *2-6 years (24-47 lbs):* 1 tsp (5 ml) every 4 hrs *6-12 years (48-95 lbs):* 4 tsp (20 ml) every 4 hrs	
Tylenol Allergy Sinus Maximum Strength	Antihistamine Decongestant Analgesic	Chlorpheniramine 2 mg Pseudoephedrine 30 mg Acetaminophen 500 mg	2 caplets (see comments) every 6 hrs		Available as caplets and gelcaps
Tylenol Allergy Sinus NightTime Maximum Strength	Antihistamine Decongestant Analgesic	Diphenhydramine 25 mg Pseudoephedrine 30 mg Acetaminophen 500 mg	2 tablets HS		May be taken more often, but excessive drowsiness may limit use to taking before bedtime

Continued

Product Information: Cough, Cold, and Flu—cont'd

Brand Name	Ingredient Type	Ingredient	Adult Dose	Pediatric Dose	Comments
Tylenol Children's Allergy-D liquid	Antihistamine	Diphenhydramine 12.5 mg/5 ml		*6-11 years (48-95 lbs)*: 2 tsp every 4-6 hrs	
	Decongestant	Pseudoephedrine 15 mg/5 ml			
	Analgesic	Acetaminophen 160 mg/5 ml			
Tylenol Children's Cold Multi-Symptom chewable	Antihistamine	Chlorpheniramine 0.5 mg		*6-12 years*: 4 tablets every 4-6 hrs	
	Decongestant	Pseudoephedrine 7.5 mg		*2-5 years*: 2 tablets every 4-6 hrs	
	Analgesic	Acetaminophen 80 mg			
Tylenol Children's Cold Multi-Symptom liquid	Antihistamine	Chlorpheniramine 1 mg/5 ml		*6-12 years*: 2 tsp every 4-6 hrs	
	Decongestant	Pseudoephedrine 15 mg/5 ml		*2-5 years*: 1 tsp every 4-6 hrs	
	Analgesic	Acetaminophen 160 mg/5 ml			

Product	Class	Ingredient	Dosage
Tylenol Children's Cold Multi-Symptom Plus Cough liquid	Antihistamine	Chlorpheniramine 1 mg/5 ml	*6-12 years:* 2 tsp every 4-6 hrs
	Decongestant	Pseudoephedrine 15 mg/5 ml	*2-5 years:* 1 tsp every 4-6 hrs
	Cough suppressant	Dextromethorphan 5 mg/5 ml	
	Analgesic	Acetaminophen 160 mg/5 ml	
Tylenol Children's Cold Plus Cough chewable	Antihistamine	Chlorpheniramine 0.5 mg	*6-12 years:* 2 tablets
	Decongestant	Pseudoephedrine 7.5 mg	
	Cough suppressant	Dextromethorphan 2.5 mg	
	Analgesic	Acetaminophen 80 mg	
Tylenol Children's Flu Formula	Antihistamine	Chlorpheniramine 1 mg/5 ml	*6-11 years:* 2 tsp every 6-8 hrs
	Decongestant	Pseudoephedrine 15 mg/5 ml	
	Cough suppressant	Dextromethorphan 7.5 mg/5 ml	
	Analgesic	Acetaminophen 160 mg/5 ml	

Continued

Product Information: Cough, Cold, and Flu—cont'd

Brand Name	Ingredient Type	Ingredient	Adult Dose	Pediatric Dose	Comments
Tylenol Children's Sinus liquid	Decongestant	Pseudoephedrine 15 mg/5 ml		*6-11 years:* 2 tsp every 4-6 hrs	
	Analgesic	Acetaminophen 160 mg/5 ml		*2-5 years:* 1 tsp every 4-6 hrs	
Tylenol Cold Multi-symptom No Drowsiness Formula	Decongestant	Pseudoephedrine 30 mg	2 tablets every 6 hrs	*6-11 years:* 1 tablet every 6 hrs	
	Cough suppressant	Dextromethorphan 15 mg			
	Analgesic	Acetaminophen 325 mg			
Tylenol Cold Infant drops	Decongestant	Pseudoephedrine 7.5 mg/0.8 ml		*2-3 years (24-35 lbs):* 2 droppersful (1.6 ml) every 4-6 hrs	
	Analgesic	Acetaminophen 80 mg/0.8 ml			
Tylenol Cough liquid	Cough suppressant	Dextromethorphan 30 mg/15 ml	15 ml every 6-8 hrs	*6-11 years:* 7.5 ml every 6-8 hrs	
	Analgesic	Acetaminophen 650 mg/15 ml			

Product	Type	Ingredient	Dose	Notes
Tylenol Cough with Decongestant liquid	Decongestant Cough suppressant Analgesic	Pseudoephedrine 60 mg/15 ml Dextromethorphan 30 mg/15 ml Acetaminophen 650 mg/15 ml	15 ml every 6-8 hrs	
Tylenol Flu	Decongestant Cough suppressant Analgesic	Pseudoephedrine 30 mg Dextromethorphan 15 mg Acetaminophen 500 mg	2 tablets every 6 hrs	
Tylenol Flu NightTime Maximum Strength	Antihistamine Decongestant Analgesic	Diphenhydramine 25 mg Pseudoephedrine 30 mg Acetaminophen 500 mg	2 tablets HS	May be taken more often, but drowsiness may limit use to bedtime
Tylenol Multi-Symptom Cold Medication	Antihistamine Decongestant Cough suppressant Analgesic	Chlorpheniramine 2 mg Pseudoephedrine 30 mg Dextromethorphan 15 mg Acetaminophen 325 mg	2 tablets every 6 hrs	*6-11 years:* 1 tablet every 6 hrs

Continued

Product Information: Cough, Cold, and Flu—cont'd

Brand Name	Ingredient Type	Ingredient	Adult Dose	Pediatric Dose	Comments
Tylenol Multi-Symptom Cough liquid	Cough suppressant Analgesic	Dextromethorphan 30 mg/15 ml Acetaminophen 650 mg/15 ml	15 ml every 6-8 hrs	6-11 years: 7.5 ml every 6-8 hrs	
Tylenol Multi-Symptom Cough with Decongestant	Decongestant Cough suppressant Analgesic	Pseudoephedrine 60 mg/15 ml Dextromethorphan 30 mg/15 ml Acetaminophen 650 mg/15 ml	15 ml every 6-8 hrs	6-11 years: 7.5 ml every 6-8 hrs	
Tylenol Sinus Maximum Strength	Decongestant Analgesic	Pseudoephedrine 30 mg Acetaminophen 500 mg	2 tablets (see comments) every 4-6 hrs		Available as tablets, caplets, and gelcaps
Vicks 44 Cough, Cold & Flu Relief Liquicaps	Antihistamine Decongestant Cough suppressant	Chlorpheniramine 2 mg Pseudoephedrine 30 mg Dextromethorphan 10 mg	2 gelcaps every 4 hrs	6-12 years: 1 gelcap every 4 hrs	
Vicks 44 Dry Hacking Cough	Analgesic Cough suppressant	Acetaminophen 250 mg Dextromethorphan 15 mg/5 ml	2 tsp every 6-8 hrs		

Vicks 44 Dry Hacking Cough & Head Congestion	Decongestant	Pseudoephedrine 20 mg/5 ml	3 tsp every 6 hrs
	Cough suppressant	Dextromethorphan 10 mg/5 ml	
Vicks 44 Non-Drowsy Cough & Cold Relief Liquicaps	Decongestant	Pseudoephedrine 60 mg	1 gelcap every 6 hrs
	Cough suppressant	Dextromethorphan 30 mg	
Vicks 44E Chest Cold & Chest Congestion	Cough suppressant	Dextromethorphan 20 mg/15 ml	3 tsp every 4 hrs
	Expectorant	Guaifenesin 200 mg/15 ml	
Vicks 44M Cough, Cold & Flu Relief	Antihistamine	Chlorpheniramine 1 mg/5 ml	4 tsp every 6 hrs
	Decongestant	Pseudoephedrine 15 mg/5 ml	
	Cough suppressant	Dextromethorphan 7.5 mg/5 ml	
	Analgesic	Acetaminophen 162 mg/5 ml	

Continued

Product Information: Cough, Cold, and Flu—cont'd

Brand Name	Ingredient Type	Ingredient	Adult Dose	Pediatric Dose	Comments
Vicks 44d Pediatric Dry Hacking Cough & Head Congestion	Decongestant	Pseudoephedrine 30 mg/15 ml		*12 years and older:* 30 ml every 6 hrs	
	Cough suppressant	Dextromethorphan 15 mg/15 ml		*6-11 years:* 15 ml every 6 hrs	
				2-5 years: 7.5 ml every 6 hrs	
Vicks 44e Pediatric Chest Cold & Chest Congestion	Cough suppressant	Dextromethorphan 10 mg/15 ml		*12 years and older:* 30 ml every 4 hrs	
	Expectorant	Guaifenesin 100 mg/15 ml		*6-11 years:* 15 ml every 4 hrs	
				2-5 years: 7.5 ml every 4 hrs	
				12-23 months: 6.25 ml every 4 hrs	
				6-11 months: 5 ml every 4 hrs	

Product	Category	Ingredient	Dosage
Vicks 44m *Pediatric Cough & Cold Relief*	Antihistamine	Chlorpheniramine 2 mg/15 ml	*12 years and older:* 30 ml every 4 hrs
	Decongestant	Pseudoephedrine 30 mg/15 ml	*6-11 years:* 15 ml every 4 hrs
	Cough suppressant	Dextromethorphan 15 mg/15 ml	*2-5 years:* 7.5 ml every 4 hrs
			12-23 months: 6.25 ml every 4 hrs
			6-11 months: 5 ml every 4 hrs
Vicks DayQuil *Multi-Symptom Cold/Flu Relief*	Decongestant	Pseudoephedrine 60 mg/30 ml	*6-11 years:* 15 ml every 4 hrs
	Cough suppressant	Dextromethorphan 20 mg/30 ml	30 ml every 4 hrs
	Expectorant	Guaifenesin 200 mg/30 ml	
	Analgesic	Acetaminophen 650 mg/30 ml	
Vicks DayQuil *Multi-Symptom Cold/Flu Relief Liquicaps*	Decongestant	Pseudoephedrine 30 mg	*6-11 years:* 1 gelcap every 4 hrs
	Cough suppressant	Dextromethorphan 10 mg	2 gelcaps every 4 hrs
	Expectorant	Guaifenesin 100 mg	
	Analgesic	Acetaminophen 250 mg	

Continued

Product Information: Cough, Cold, and Flu—cont'd

Brand Name	Ingredient Type	Ingredient	Adult Dose	Pediatric Dose	Comments
Vicks Nyquil Hot Therapy	Antihistamine Decongestant Cough suppressant Analgesic	Doxylamine 12.5 mg Pseudoephedrine 60 mg Dextromethorphan 30 mg Acetaminophen 1000 mg	1 packet HS		May be taken more often, but drowsiness limits use to bedtime
Vicks Nyquil Multi-Symptom Cold/Flu Relief Liquicaps	Antihistamine Decongestant Cough suppressant Analgesic	Doxylamine 6.25 mg Pseudoephedrine 30 mg Dextromethorphan 10 mg Acetaminophen 250 mg	2 gelcaps every 4 hrs		
Vicks Nyquil Multi-Symptom Cold/Flu Relief liquid	Antihistamine Decongestant Cough suppressant Analgesic	Doxylamine 12.5 mg/30 ml Pseudoephedrine 60 mg/30 ml Dextromethorphan 30 mg/30 ml Acetaminophen 1000 mg/30 ml	30 ml HS		May be taken more often, but drowsiness limits use to bedtime

Vaginal Yeast Infections

Vaginal infections are commonly caused by bacteria, trichomonads, and yeast. Of these culprits, only yeast infections have treatments that are available over the counter. *Candida albicans* and other *Candida* species cause the majority of yeast infections in women. *Candida* sp. are part of the normal flora in the vagina; symptoms evolve when there is an overgrowth of yeast caused by alteration in the vaginal flora (e.g., individuals taking broad-spectrum antibiotics) or a change in the vaginal pH. In addition, a warm, moist environment with an abundance of glucose allows for the proliferation of yeast, a situation often seen in diabetics and women wearing tight clothing or undergarments/pantyhose made of synthetic materials. Symptoms of yeast infection include pruritus, external burning, burning with urination, and vaginal discharge (normally thick and white).

Antifungal products are used to treat vaginal yeast infection.

ANTIFUNGAL PRODUCTS

CLOTRIMAZOLE

MICONAZOLE

BUTOCONAZOLE

TIOCONAZOLE

Pharmacology

All of the agents listed above are fungicidal against *C. albicans*. These agents exert their effect by altering cell membranes, resulting in increased membrane permeability, secondary metabolic effects, and growth inhibition. Clotrimazole is also fungistatic.

273

Side Effects

The incidence of side effects with antifungal products is rare. Side effects that may occur are irritation, sensitization, vulvovaginal burning, skin rash, vaginal soreness, headache, allergic contact dermatitis, swelling, itching, burning, dysuria, and dysmenorrhea. These side effects are more likely to occur with the initial application of the vaginal preparation. Although these side effects have been reported as being caused by antifungal products, many of these symptoms are experienced by women with candidal infections with or without treatment.

Lifespan Considerations

Geriatric

There are no unique recommendations for the geriatric population.

Pediatric

Vaginal products should not be used in girls under the age of 12 years unless directed by a health care professional. The safety and efficacy of these products in children have not been established.

Pregnancy

No adverse effects or complications are reported in infants born to women treated with antifungal agents. During pregnancy, manual insertion of a suppository is recommended over the use of an applicator. Vaginal antifungal products should only be used under the direction of a health care professional. Small amounts of these drugs may be absorbed through the vagina and should be used during the first trimester only when absolutely necessary.

Nursing Mothers

It is not known whether these drugs are excreted in breast milk. Patients should temporarily discontinue nursing during the course of administration.

Patient Education

- Pregnant women should not use any vaginal products without first consulting their health care professional.
- To prevent contamination, patients should open applicators just before administration of the product. Nondisposable applicators should be cleaned with warm, soapy water and rinsed thoroughly after each use.

- Medication should be inserted high into vagina (except during pregnancy).
- Patients should complete a full course of therapy, even if symptoms disappear or menstruation begins.
- If burning or irritation develop, the patient should notify a health care professional.
- Patients should not have sexual intercourse during the treatment period.
- Patients should use a sanitary napkin or minipad to prevent staining of clothing, but should not use a tampon.
- Ingredients in these preparations may weaken latex prophylactics such as condoms and diaphragms, which should not be used within 72 hours of treatment.
- If symptoms recur within 2 months, the patient should be referred to a health care professional.

Product Selection

- Vaginal antifungal products come in package sizes specific for the duration of therapy, which may be 1, 3, or 7 days. All therapies are clinically equivalent in efficacy.
- The 1-day or 3-day therapies may be preferred because of increased patient compliance.

Product Information: Vaginal Yeast Infections

Brand Name	Ingredient	Dosage Forms	Directions for Use
Femcare	Clotrimazole	7 100-mg suppositories with 1 applicator or 45-g tube of 1% cream with 1 reusable or 7 disposable applicators	Apply daily for 7 days
Femstat 3	Butoconazole	2% cream with 3 measured-dose disposable applicators or 3 prefilled applicators	Apply daily for 3 days
Gyne-Lotrimin 3	Clotrimazole	3 vaginal inserts	Apply daily for 3 days
Gyne-Lotrimin 7	Clotrimazole	7 100-mg suppositories with 1 applicator or 45-g tube of 1% cream with 1 reusable or 7 disposable applicators	Apply daily for 7 days
Gyne-Lotrimin Combination Pack	Clotrimazole	7 500-mg suppositories with 1 applicator and a 7-g tube of 1% cream for external use	Apply daily for 7 days
Monistat 1	Tioconazole	4.6-g tube of 6.5% ointment in a single prefilled, disposable applicator	Apply once
Monistat 3	Miconazole	3 200-mg suppositories with 1 applicator or 3 prefilled applicators	Apply daily for 3 days
Monistat 3	Miconazole	3 vaginal suppositories with reusable applicator or 3 disposable applicators and 7-g tube of 1% cream for external use	Apply daily for 3 days
Monistat 7	Miconazole	7 100-mg suppositories with 1 applicator or 45-gram tube of 1% cream with 1 reusable or 7 disposable applicators	Apply daily for 7 days
Monistat 7 Combination Pack	Miconazole	7 100-mg suppositories with 1 applicator and a 9-g tube of 2% cream for external use	Apply daily for 7 days
Mycelex-3	Butoconazole	28-g tube of 2% cream with 3 disposable applicators or 3 prefilled applicators	Apply daily for 3 days
Mycelex Twin Pack	Clotrimazole	7 500-mg suppositories with 1 applicator and a 7-g tube of 1% cream for external use	Apply daily for 7 days
Mycelex-7	Clotrimazole	7 100-mg suppositories with 1 applicator or 45-g tube of 1% cream with 1 reusable or 7 disposable applicators	Apply daily for 7 days
Vagistat-1	Tioconazole	4.6-g tube of 6.5% ointment in a single prefilled, disposable applicator	Apply once

Vaginal Irritation/Dryness

Vaginal irritation or dryness may be caused by a number of culprits, including menopause, infection, and sexual intercourse. Products used to treat vaginal irritation and/or dryness utilize a combination of ingredients to lessen the discomfort.

VAGINAL IRRITATION

POVIDONE-IODINE

TRIPELENNAMINE

BENZOCAINE

RESORCINOL

Pharmacology

The ingredients most commonly found are povidone-iodine, tripelennamine, benzocaine, and resorcinol. Povidone-iodine is thought to have antiseptic or germicidal activity and also relieves minor irritation. Tripelennamine relieves external irritation. Benzocaine is a topical and local anesthetic used to temporarily relieve minor pain, itching, and irritation. Resorcinol is a counterirritant used for its anesthetic or antipruritic properties.

Side Effects

The incidence of side effects with these products is rare. Because povidone-iodine can be absorbed from the vagina, its use should be avoided in pregnant patients and those with a thyroid abnormality.

Lifespan Considerations
Geriatric
Vaginal atrophy associated with aging is a common cause of dryness.

Pediatric
Vaginal products should not be used in girls under the age of 12 years unless under the direction of a health care professional. The safety and efficacy of these products in children have not been established.

277

Pregnancy

With the exception of povidone-iodine, these products are designed for external use and are safe for use during pregnancy if used properly. Use of povidone-iodine in pregnant women should be avoided because of the potential for absorption of iodine through the vagina.

Nursing Mothers

It is not known whether these drugs are excreted in breast milk. Patients should temporarily discontinue nursing during the course of administration.

Patient Education

- Pregnant women should not use any vaginal products without first consulting their health care professional.
- Patients should not insert medication high into vagina if pregnant.
- Patients should notify a health care professional if burning or irritation develop.
- Patients should use a sanitary napkin or minipad to prevent staining of clothing, but should not use a tampon.
- Ingredients in these preparations may weaken latex prophylactics such as condoms and diaphragms, which should not be used within 72 hours of treatment.

Product Selection

These products are equally effective.

Product Information: Vaginal Irritation

Brand Name	Ingredient	Dosage Forms	Directions for Use
Betadine	Povidone-iodine	10% gel or solution in various sizes or 7 10% suppositories with 1 reusable applicator	For duration of symptoms or 7 days
Gynecort Maximum Strength	Hydrocortisone 1%	30-g tube of cream	Apply 3-4 times daily; for external use for duration of symptoms
Vagi-Gard	Benzocaine 5%, benzalkonium chloride 0.13%	30-g tube of cream	For duration of symptoms or 7 days
Vagi-Gard Maximum Strength	Benzocaine 20%, benzalkonium chloride 0.13%	30-g tube of cream	For duration of symptoms or 7 days
Vaginex Hydrocortisone Formula	Hydrocortisone 1%	30-g tube of cream	Apply 3-4 times daily; for external use for duration of symptoms; scented and unscented formulas
Vagisil	Benzocaine and resorcinol	5% benzocaine and 2% resorcinol in a 30-g tube of cream	Apply 3-4 times daily; for external use for duration of symptoms
Vagisil Maximum Strength Formula	Benzocaine 20%	30-g tube of cream	Apply 3-4 times daily; for external use for duration of symptoms
Yeast Guard Maximum Strength	Benzocaine and resorcinol	20% benzocaine and 3% resorcinol in a 30-g tube of cream	Apply 3-4 times daily; for external use for duration of symptoms

VAGINAL DRYNESS

CAPRYLIC/CAPRIC TRIGLYCERIDE, GLYCERIN, AND LAURETH-23

BLEND OF POLYETHYLENE GLYCOLS, A SURFACTANT, AND A GLYCERIDE

GLUCONO DELTA LACTATE, SODIUM HYDROXIDE, GLYCERIN, CHLORHEXIDINE GLUCONATE, AND HYDROXYMETHYLCELLULOSE

GLYCERIN, PROPYLENE GLYCOL AND SODIUM CARBOXYMETHYLCELLULOSE, SODIUM ALGINATE, AND SORBIC ACID

Pharmacology

These products consist of moisturizers, emollients, and surfactants to lessen the discomfort associated with a dry vaginal canal.

Side Effects

The incidence of side effects with these products is rare. Some discomfort in the form of burning or irritation may be associated with their use initially because of the severity of the dryness being treated, much like hand lotion may burn slightly when applied to very dry skin. After the products have been used sufficiently to begin to cure the problem, this initial burning or irritation will subside.

Lifespan Considerations
Pediatric
Vaginal products should not be used in girls under the age of 12 years unless under the direction of a health care professional. The safety and efficacy of these products in children have not been established.

Pregnancy
No adverse effects or complications are reported in infants born to women treated with these agents. During pregnancy, manual insertion is recommended over the use of an applicator. These products should be used only under the direction of a health care professional.

Nursing Mothers
These drugs are not known to be absorbed systemically and present no known risk to babies when used by nursing mothers.

Patient Education

- Pregnant women should not use any vaginal products without first consulting their health care professional.
- Patients should clean the applicator with warm, soapy water and rinse thoroughly after each use.
- Patients should notify a health care professional if burning or irritation develop.
- A health care professional should also be notified if vaginal dryness persists or is not aided by use of these products.

SUGGESTED READINGS

Deutchmann ME, Leaman DJ, Thomason JL: Vaginitis: diagnosis is the key, *Patient Care* 28:39-61, 1994.

Ferris DG, Dekle C, Litaker MS: Women's use of over-the-counter antifungal medications for gynecologic symptoms, J *Fam Pract* 42:595-600, 1996.

McCombs J: When to treat vaginal yeast infections with nonprescription products, *Pharmacy Times* 61:20-24, 1995.

Product Information: Vaginal Dryness*

Brand Name	Ingredients
CondomMate	Polyethylene glycols, a surfactant, and a glyceride
K-Y	Glucono delta lactate, sodium hydroxide, glycerin, chlorhexidine gluconate, and hydroxymethylcellulose
Lubrin	Caprylic/capric triglyceride, glycerin, and laureth-23
Personal Lubricant	Glycerin, propylene glycol and sodium carboxymethylcellulose, sodium alginate, and sorbic acid
Replens Vaginal Moisturizer	Glycerin, mineral oil, polycarbophil, carbomer 934P
Vaginex Moisture Replenishing Therapy	Glycerin, aloe vera, carbomer, glycol
Vagisil Intimate Moisturizer	Water, glycerin, propylene glycol

*Directions for use: Apply as needed.

Nutritional Supplements

ORAL NUTRITIONAL SUPPLEMENTS

Many persons are unable to meet their nutritional needs through diet alone. This may be particularly true of patients with chronic disease, multiple consecutive illnesses, unintentional weight loss, or physical impairment of chewing or swallowing ability. Elderly patients often fall into one or more of these categories. Box 8-1 lists some of the reasons why patients may not be able to meet their nutritional needs through a normal diet.

It is important to identify the reasons for inadequate nutritional intake. It may be possible to correct the problem without dependence on oral nutritional supplements. Financial problems and physical disabilities can make it difficult to purchase and prepare meals. Providing supplements without correction of the underlying cause can perpetuate the problem and frustrate the health care professional and the patient.

When patients require additional nutrients to complement food intake, the diet can be enhanced with high-calorie and high-protein foods such as nonfat dry milk, cream, butter/margarine, salad dressings, cheese, gravies, etc. Other patients will need partial or complete replacement of meals with oral nutritional supplements. When oral supplements are the sole source of nutrition, problems such as taste fatigue and noncompliance can arise. Patients requiring long-term oral nutritional replacement therapy may benefit from placement of an enteral feeding access. It is preferable for patients to receive nutrition via the gastrointestinal tract because it is more physiologic, less expensive, and safer than parenteral nutritional support. The focus of this chapter will be on oral nutritional products. Information regarding tube feeding is beyond the scope of this book.

Formula Selection

There are more than 100 commercially available enteral formulas. These formulas are categorized according to nutrient composition

Box 8-1 Hindrances to Adequate Oral Intake	
Depression	Nausea and vomiting
Fluid and electrolyte abnormalities	Pain
Impaired functional status	Poor dentition
Impaired mental status	Shortness of breath
Inability to purchase food or	Swallowing difficulties
prepare meals	Unpalatable food
Medications	Vitamin and mineral deficiencies

(standard and disease specific) and digestion required (polymeric and elemental). Pertinent information about enteral formulas includes the following:

- Standard formulas are polymeric, meaning that they require digestion.
- Elemental formulas are "predigested" and require absorption only. Elemental formulas are comprised of partially or completely hydrolyzed nutrients.
- Disease-specific formulas can be polymeric or elemental. These formulas vary in nutrient content based on particular disease-state requirements. Some formulas have nutrients added, limited, or omitted to meet the nutritional needs of specific patient populations.
- Products prepared with milk contain lactose, which may not be tolerated by patients with some gastrointestinal disorders.
- Product selection should be based on patient preference for taste, accessibility, and cost. It is possible to exchange comparable formulas without detriment to the patient.

Healthcare facilities choose the enteral nutrition products that they stock based on vendor service contracts. Patients are often discharged from a health care facility on the "house formula." It is important to evaluate the efficacy and cost of a particular formula in the outpatient setting. Generic oral nutritional supplements can significantly reduce costs while providing quality nutrition. Categorizing nutritional supplements by content and not by brand name provides the health care professional more flexibility to substitute an equivalent product for a more costly one. The oral nutritional supplement product information table at the end of this chapter organizes formulas according to nutrient content and similar characteristics. This information can be used to compare products. Some products are widely available at pharmacies, grocery stores, or discount stores. Other, less widely used products, might need to be ordered for the patient.

Table 8-1
Choosing a Disease-Specific Formula

Formula type	Composition	Indications
Diabetic	Reduced carbohydrate levels, higher percentage of fat and fiber	Brittle diabetes, poor glycemic control with standard fiber formula
Fat malabsorption	Reduced long-chain fats, higher percentage of medium-chain triglycerides	Steatorrhea, inflammatory bowel disease, surgical resection of the terminal ileum, chylothorax
Hepatic	Enriched with branched-chain amino acids, reduced aromatic amino-acid content	Hepatic encephalopathy
Renal	Reduced protein content, concentrated urine volume, restricted electrolyte content	*Predialysis:* Minimal protein to reduce need for dialysis *Chronic renal replacement therapy:* Moderate protein content
Pulmonary	Reduced carbohydrate content, increased fat content	Carbon dioxide retention, COPD

Given the large number of available products, how does one choose the appropriate supplement for a patient? Questions for the health care professional to consider include the following:

- What is the reason for recommending an oral nutritional supplement to the patient? Does the patient have a physical impairment, particular disease process, physiologic hindrance, or functional incapacity? Information on choosing a disease-specific formula can be found in Table 8-1.
- If there is no organ dysfunction, a standard polymeric formula is preferred.
- Polymeric formulas are less expensive and can be more palatable because they are available in a variety of flavors.
- Oral nutritional supplements include liquids, soups, puddings, and food bars.
- Certain formulas are designed for feeding-tube infusion and are less palatable.

- Patients undergoing chemotherapy prefer formulas that are less sweet tasting. These patients sometimes have a heightened sensitivity for sweetness, which can contribute to nausea.
- Specialty formulas should be used only in patients who meet the criteria, because these formulas are more expensive and can be difficult to obtain.
- Specialty formulas can be unpalatable because of added nutrients.
- Elemental formulas are bitter because of the amino acid content. These formulas are not well suited for oral consumption.

Flavoring Oral Nutrition Supplements

Oral nutritional products can be flavored with items such as syrups, spices, and extracts, or with commercial flavoring packets. The possibilities are limited only by the patient's imagination and ability to tolerate the additive. Suggested flavorings for nutritional supplements can be found in Box 8-2.

Box 8-2   Suggestions for Flavoring Nutritional Supplements

Flavored syrups	Commercial flavor packets
Chocolate	**Nestle**
Maple	Apricot
Strawberry	Blue raspberry
Caramel	Bubble gum
Flavored extracts	Cappuccino
Vanilla	Cherry
Butterscotch	Chocolate
Maple	Chocolate dream
Almond	Citrus sunrise
Coffee (regular or flavored)	French vanilla
Ice cream or flavored yogurt	Grape
Whipped cream/whipped	Strawberry-banana
topping	Vanilla
Fresh, frozen, or canned	**Ross**
fruit	Cherry
Peanut butter	Lemon
Spices	Orange
Cinnamon	Pecan
Nutmeg	Strawberry

When recommending oral nutritional supplements, health care professionals should start the patient with 1 to 2 supplements per day if the supplement is to be taken in conjunction with an oral diet. Patients can feel overwhelmed if told to consume supplements more often. Taste fatigue is the reason that many patients stop consuming an oral nutritional supplement. The less variety of flavors or the more unpalatable the formula, the more quickly the patient will experience taste fatigue. If oral nutrition supplements are the sole source of nutritional support, use of a feeding tube may be preferred to consistently meet the patient's nutritional requirements.

Patients should be encouraged to use nutritional supplements to augment caloric intake when possible and to purchase the vanilla-flavored products by the case to save money. Use of flavorings to provide taste variety should also be encouraged. The addition of vitamins and minerals to oral nutrition supplements affects the flavor. Patients who do not tolerate this taste may need to enhance their diet with high-calorie and high-protein food items instead.

Determining Calorie and Protein Goals

Estimation of calorie and protein needs can be accomplished using established formulas. There are more than 200 mathematical formulas available for estimating caloric needs. Some of the calculations are designed for use in specific patient populations, such as those with burns, cystic fibrosis, or head trauma. Although there are caveats to using standardized formulas to estimate nutritional requirements, the following simple calculation can be used to estimate a patient's caloric and protein target for nutritional repletion or maintenance:

Calories (use actual body weight)

20 kcal/kg for weight loss

30 kcal/kg for weight maintenance

40 kcal/kg for weight gain

NOTE: 1 lb = 2.2 kg

Protein (use ideal body weight)

0.6-0.8 g/kg for patients with renal failure (no dialysis) and hepatic encephalopathy

0.8-1.0 g/kg for normal nutrition

1.0-1.25 g/kg for patients who are moderately malnourished

1.25-1.5 g/kg for patients who are severely malnourished

Ideal body weight calculation

Men: 50 kg + 2.3 (inches height over 60)

Women: 45 kg + 2.3 (inches height over 60)

Monitoring

After determination of a caloric goal and initiation of oral nutritional supplementation, the patient's weight and laboratory values should be monitored to determine the efficacy of the regimen. Based on objective and subjective data, the feeding regimen should be adjusted to obtain the desired outcome. Items to be monitored include the following:

- Weight change over time (compare with usual body weight)
- Gastrointestinal tolerance (nausea, diarrhea, distension)
- Hydration status (monitor intake/output, pulse rate)
- Wound healing
- Changes in functional status (ability to perform activities of daily living)
- Laboratory values

	Normal value
Serum albumin	3.5-5.0 g/dL
Serum prealbumin	17-40 mg/dL
Total cholesterol	<200 mg/dL

All levels should be monitored as needed.

Patient Education

- Identify the etiology of inadequate oral intake.
- Initiate nutritional intervention with encouragement of increased intake of calories and protein.
- Remind patients that adequate nutrition is an integral part of their medical therapy and recovery.
- Consult a registered dietitian for assistance with counseling patients on food selection and preparation and with selection of the appropriate oral nutrition supplement.

ORAL REHYDRATION SOLUTIONS AND SPORTS DRINKS

The adult human body is composed of 55% to 75% water (10 to 12 gallons). To meet fluid requirements, adults should drink 8 to 12 cups of fluid per day or 30 to 35 ml/kg/day. Fluid intake is stimulated by thirst. Elderly, aphasic, and mentally incompetent patients are at risk of receiving inadequate fluid and developing dehydration. Water is often called the *forgotten nutrient*. It is the ideal fluid to meet hydration requirements because it is absorbed quickly, is naturally low in sodium, and contains no fat or caffeine.

Oral Rehydration Solutions

Oral rehydration solutions (ORS) have been used since 1986 to combat severe dehydration from diarrheal disease. Infant mortality from dehydration significantly dropped when mothers were taught to prepare a rehydration solution to give to their children with diarrhea.

The World Health Organization developed an oral rehydration solution to combat dehydration associated with cholera. The solution utilizes the sodium-glucose transport mechanism in the intestinal brush border to facilitate absorption of sodium and water. This solution contains 90 mmol/L sodium, which compensates for the sodium losses associated with cholera. However, this amount of sodium may contribute to hypernatremia in patients with less severe sodium losses.

Patient populations likely to benefit from ORS include those with high fluid and electrolyte loss from the gastrointestinal tract, such as patients with fistulas, enteric drains, wounds, diarrhea, and emesis. Oral rehydration solutions should be consumed as long as the patient experiences symptoms of dehydration.

Sports Drinks

ORS should not be confused with sports drinks (Table 8-2). ORS are designed to replace salts and water in proportions needed by ill patients. Sports beverages are designed to provide an energy source and salt replacement in healthy athletes. Sports drinks should not be recommended as fluid replacement for gastrointestinal losses and dehydration. When sports drinks are consumed by patients with diarrhea and dehydration, water reabsorption in the intestine can be reduced, diarrhea and vomiting aggravated, and electrolytes inadequately replaced.

Sports drinks have become popular with athletes for replacement of fluids and electrolytes after a workout. Sports drinks are promoted to

Table 8-2
Comparison of ORS and Sports Drinks

Ingredients	Rehydration solutions	Sports drinks
Sodium	45-90 mEq/L	7-20 mEq/L
Potassium	20-25 mEq/L	3-8 mEq/L
Chloride	35-80 mEq/L	4-27 mEq/L
Carbohydrate	20-40 gm/L	25-84 gm/L

replace fluid and electrolytes (sodium and potassium) lost in perspiration. Sports drinks also contain carbohydrate as an energy source.

Patient Education

- Sports drinks are indicated only when an athlete participates in strenuous exercise for 60 minutes or longer.
- Encourage athletes to drink water for hydration during a workout. The only beverage required for most athletes or sports enthusiasts is water.
- Selection of a sports beverage should be based on fluid and electrolyte requirements, palatability, glycemic control, allergies, and cost.
- ORS or sports drinks should not be consumed by persons who are salt sensitive, such as those with hypertension, congestive heart failure, renal insufficiency, or liver failure.
- Rehydration solutions tend to contain more electrolytes and less carbohydrate than sports drinks.
- ORS are recommended for patients with large gastrointestinal losses and dehydration.

SUGGESTED READINGS

A.S.P.E.N. Board of Directors: Guidelines for the use of parenteral and enteral nutrition in adults and pediatric patients, JPEN 17(4 suppl):1SA-52SA, 1993.

Gottschlich MM, Shronta EP, Hutchins AM: Defined formula diets. In Rombeau JL, Rol Andeli RH, editors: *Clinical nutritional enteral and tube feeding*, Philadelphia, 1997, WB Saunders.

Lipschitz DA: Approaches to the nutritional support of the older patient, *Clin Geriatr Med* 11(4):715-724, 1995.

Matarese LE: Rationale and efficacy of specialized enteral nutrition, *Nutr Clin Prac* 9:58-64, 1994.

Ryan M: Sports drinks: research asks for reevaluation of current recommendations, *J Am Diet Assoc* 97:S197-S198, 1997.

Product Information: Oral Nutritional Supplements

Type of Supplement	Calories/Can or Packet	Grams Protein/ Can or Packet	Cans Required for 100% RDA
Polymeric, Isotonic, No Fiber	237-250	9-15	5-8
Ensure			
Ensure HN			
NuBasics			
NuBasics VHP*			
Resource			
Sustacal Basic			
Sustacal Liquid			
Polymeric, Isotonic, with Fiber	250-260	9-11	4-8
Ensure with Fiber			
NuBasics with Fiber			
Sustacal with Fiber			
Calorically Dense, No Fiber	355-375	13-15	3-6
Ensure Plus			
Ensure Plus HN			
NuBasics Plus			
Resource Plus			
Sustacal Plus			
Milk-Based			
Carnation Instant Breakfast	160-250	10-12	4
Sustacal Powder	200-290	13-21	4
Age-Specific Formulas			
Pediatric	237-250	7-8	4
Kindercal			
Nutren Jr. With Fiber			
Nutren Jr. Without Fiber			
Pediasure			

RDA, Recommended Daily Allowances.
*High protein (>55 g/L).
†Higher nitrogen for patients on chronic dialysis.

Continued

Product Information: Oral Nutritional Supplements—cont'd

Type of Supplement	Calories/Can or Packet	Grams Protein/ Can or Packet	Cans Required for 100% RDA
Age-Specific Formulas—cont'd			
Geriatric			
ProBalance	300	13.5	4
Disease-Specific Formulas			
Diabetes	237-250	10-12	4-6
Choice DM			
Diabetisource			
Glucerna			
Glytrol			
Fat malabsorption	320	14	5
Lipisorb			
Travasorb MCT			
Hepatic	375-400	10-15	4
Hepatic Aid II (negligible electrolytes)			
NutriHep			
Pulmonary	355-375	15-18	4-6
NutriVent			
Pulmocare			
Respalor			
Renal	475-500	7-17	4
Amin-Aid (minimal electrolytes)			
Magnacal Renal†			
Nephro†			
Novasource Renal†			
RenalCal (no electrolytes or fat-soluble vitamins)			
Suplena			

Continued

Product Information: Oral Nutritional Supplements—cont'd

Type of Supplement	Calories/Can or Packet	Grams Protein/ Can or Packet	Cans Required for 100% RDA
Other Supplements			
Liquid supplements	160-165	8-10	
Citrotein			
Nubasics Coffee drink			
Nutrition bars	120-145/bar	4-6	
Choice DM			
Ensure			
Nubasics			
Puddings	240-250	7	
Ensure			
Sustacal			
Unsure			
Soups	250	9	
NuBasics			

Product Information: Oral Rehydration Solutions and Sports Drinks

	Sodium (mEq/L)	Potassium (mEq/L)	Carbohydrates (g/L)
Oral Rehydration Solutions			
Cera Lyte	70	20	40
Infalyte	50	25	30
Pedialyte	45	20	25
Rehydrate	75	20	25
WHO solution	90	20	20
Sports Drinks			
10-K	10	3	60
AllSport	10	5	84
Gatorade	20	3	50
Gatorade Light	15	3	25
Hy 5	7	8	55
Powerade	10	3	80

Vitamins and Minerals

Vitamins and minerals are essential to health. Because the body is incapable of synthesizing most of these compounds, they must be obtained in the diet. Most experts agree that the best source of vitamins and minerals is the diet and that supplements should not be required if the diet is well balanced. Whether one consumes a well-balanced diet determines the need for supplementation. The Recommended Daily Allowance (RDA) is the minimum daily requirement for vitamins and minerals as established by the U.S. government. In most cases, a balanced diet is capable of providing the RDA of the essential vitamins and minerals.

Examples of situations when vitamin/mineral supplements might be appropriate include the following:

- Patients with diseases associated with vitamin/mineral deficiency, such as alcoholism, drug-induced vitamin deficiency (antitubercular medications), osteoporosis, and pernicious anemia.
- Anything that interferes with the consumption of a balanced diet, such as "fad" or vegetarian diets, malnutrition, loss of appetite (whether idiopathic or the result of disease [e.g., depression, cancer]), or physical inability to take food by mouth (physical blockade or dysfunction of the GI tract).
- Patients receiving total parenteral nutrition (TPN), peripheral parenteral nutrition (PPN), or enteral nutrition (tube feedings).

It must be acknowledged that many individuals take large doses of vitamins, minerals, and nutritional supplements in the hope of preventing or treating disease or enhancing performance. The "natural product" or "food supplement" industry has grown exponentially in recent years to create and fulfill demand for these products. Many therapeutic claims for these products are made, with most being scientifically unsubstantiated. Anecdotal evidence, extrapolation from animal data, in vitro experiments, or known effects of deficiency (no matter how rare or regardless of whether is it possible to create the same deficiency in humans) forms the basis for most claims. There is no Food and Drug Administration (FDA) oversight of these products because they are classified as food supplements, not vitamins or drugs. Although the FDA does recommend daily intakes for vitamins and minerals (Table 8-3), it does not evaluate therapeutic claims as it is required to do for prescription medications. This means that as long as

Table 8-3
1989 National Research Council* Recommended Dietary Allowances†

Age (years) or condition	Weight‡		Height		Protein (g)	Fat-soluble vitamins				Water-soluble vitamins							Minerals					
	kg	lb	cm	in		Vitamin A (RE)§	Vitamin D (µg)‖	Vitamin E (mg α-TE)¶	Vitamin K (µg)	Vitamin C (mg)	Thiamin (mg)	Riboflavin (mg)	Niacin (mg NE)#	Vitamin B$_6$ (mg)	Folate (µg)	Vitamin B$_{12}$ (µg)	Calcium (mg)	Phosphorus (mg)	Magnesium (mg)	Iron (mg)	Zinc (mg)	Iodine (µg)
Infants																						
0.0-0.5	6	13	60	24	13	375	7.5	3	5	30	0.3	0.4	5	0.3	25	0.3	400	300	40	6	5	40
0.5-1.0	9	20	71	28	14	375	10	4	10	35	0.4	0.5	6	0.6	35	0.5	600	500	60	10	5	50
Children																						
1-3	13	29	90	35	16	400	10	6	15	40	0.7	0.8	9	1.0	50	0.7	800	800	80	10	10	70
4-6	20	44	112	44	24	500	10	7	20	45	0.9	1.1	12	1.1	75	1.0	800	800	120	10	10	90
7-10	28	62	132	52	28	700	10	7	30	45	1.0	1.2	13	1.4	100	1.4	800	800	170	10	10	120
Men																						
11-14	45	99	157	62	45	1000	10	10	45	50	1.3	1.5	17	1.7	150	2.0	1200	1200	270	12	15	150
15-18	66	145	176	69	59	1000	10	10	65	60	1.5	1.8	20	2.0	200	2.0	1200	1200	400	12	15	150
19-24	72	160	177	70	58	1000	10	10	70	60	1.5	1.7	19	2.0	200	2.0	1200	1200	350	10	15	150
25-50	79	174	176	70	63	1000	5	10	80	60	1.5	1.7	19	2.0	200	2.0	800	800	350	10	15	150
51+	77	170	173	68	63	1000	5	10	80	60	1.2	1.4	15	2.0	200	2.0	800	800	350	10	15	150

Women

Age																					
11-14	46	101	157	62	46	800	10	8	45	50	1.1	1.3	15	1.4	150	2.0	1200	1200	280	15	12	150
15-18	55	120	163	64	44	800	10	8	55	60	1.1	1.3	15	1.5	180	2.0	1200	1200	300	15	12	150
19-24	58	128	164	65	46	800	10	8	60	60	1.1	1.3	15	1.6	180	2.0	1200	1200	280	15	12	150
25-50	63	138	163	64	50	800	5	8	65	60	1.1	1.3	15	1.6	180	2.0	800	800	280	15	12	150
51+	65	143	160	63	50	800	5	8	65	60	1.0	1.2	13	1.6	180	2.0	800	800	280	10	12	150
Pregnant					60	800	10	10	65	70	1.5	1.6	17	2.2	400	2.2	1200	1200	320	30	15	175
Lactating																						
1st 6 months					65	1300	10	12	65	95	1.6	1.8	20	2.1	280	2.6	1200	1200	355	15	19	200
2nd 6 months					62	1200	10	11	65	90	1.6	1.7	20	2.1	260	2.6	1200	1200	340	15	16	200

*Food and Nutrition Board, National Academy of Sciences.

†The allowances, expressed as average daily intakes over time, are intended to provide for individual variations among most normal persons as they live in the United States under usual environmental stresses. Diets should be based on a variety of common foods to provide other nutrients for which human requirements have been less well defined. See the RDA publication for detailed discussion of allowances and of nutrients not tabulated.

‡Weights and heights of Reference Adults are actual medians for the U.S. population of the designated age, as reported by NHANES II. The use of these figures does not imply that the height-to-weight ratios are ideal.

§Retinol equivalents. 1 retinol equivalent = 1 μg retinol or 6 μg β-carotene.

‖As cholecalciferol. 10 μg cholecalciferol = 400 IU of vitamin D.

¶α-Tocopherol equivalents. 1 mg d-α tocopherol = 1 α-TE.

#1 ne (niacin equivalent) is equal to 1 mg of niacin or 60 mg of dietary tryptophan.

a product is not considered "harmful," various claims can be made for its benefit. However, not all claims are false; some of these products have been appropriately studied and found to be beneficial. The fact that large quantities of these products have been and continue to be sold, however, does not guarantee efficacy or safety.

This chapter will cover four categories of vitamins and minerals: fat-soluble vitamins, water-soluble vitamins, minerals, and selected natural and herbal products.

FAT-SOLUBLE VITAMINS

Fat-soluble vitamins are vitamins A, D, E, and K. They are stored in the liver. The liver stores are utilized by the body whenever dietary intake is inadequate, making deficiencies of these vitamins uncommon in well-nourished individuals.

Vitamin A

The term *vitamin* A encompasses a number of compounds referred to as *retinoids* and *carotenoids*. Most retinoids and carotenoids are converted in the body to substances having vitamin A activity. The RDA is expressed in International Units (IU). One IU is equal to 0.3 mcg retinol or 0.6 mcg beta carotene.

Functions

Vitamin A is necessary for formation of rhodopsin (required for night vision), integrity of epithelial tissues, lysosome stability, and glycoprotein synthesis.

Sources

Preformed vitamin A is found in fish, liver, egg yolk, butter, cream, and vitamin A–fortified margarines. Carotenoids are found in dark green, leafy vegetables and yellow-orange vegetables.

Effects of Deficiency and Toxicity

A vitamin-A deficiency can result in night blindness, increased susceptibility to infection, drying and hyperkeratinization of the skin, loss of appetite, impaired taste and smell, and impaired equilibrium. Toxicity may cause headache, peeling of skin, hepatosplenomegaly, and bone thickening.

Therapeutic Uses

Vitamin A analogs, such as Retin-A and Accutane (available by prescription), are useful in treatment of acne and other skin conditions and might be useful in the prevention of certain types of skin cancers. Beta-carotene might reduce the risk of lung cancer and certain oral cancers.

Patient Education

- Supplementation of the fat-soluble vitamins may be necessary in patients with malabsorption syndromes.
- Large doses of vitamin A may increase the hypoprothrombinemic effect of warfarin.
- Prolonged use of cholestyramine (Questran) or mineral oil may reduce absorption of vitamin A and lead to deficiency.
- Vitamin A supplementation should be avoided in patients taking isotretinoin (Accutane) because it is a vitamin-A analog and vitamin A toxicity could occur.

Vitamin D

Vitamin D is a generic term that includes a number of structurally similar chemicals and their metabolites.

Functions

Vitamin D is necessary for proper formation of the skeleton (mineralization of bones), calcium, and phosphorus homeostasis.

Sources

Cholecalciferol (vitamin D_3) is the natural form of vitamin D that is formed in the skin when exposed to sunlight. Vitamin D is also found in fortified milk, fish liver oils, butter, egg yolk, and liver. The liver and kidneys are required for conversion of vitamin D to its active form. 25-Hydroxycholecalciferol is formed in the liver and then further hydroxylated in the kidneys to the most active form: 1,25-dihydroxycholecalciferol.

Effects of Deficiency and Toxicity

A deficiency can result in rickets and osteomalacia, whereas toxicity can lead to anorexia, renal failure, and metastatic calcification.

Therapeutic Uses

Vitamin D is used as an adjunct with calcium for the treatment and prevention of osteoporosis.

Patient Education

- Causes of vitamin-D deficiency include dietary deficiency, gastrointestinal disorders (such as hepatobiliary disease, malabsorption, or chronic pancreatitis), chronic renal failure, phosphate depletion, renal tubular disease, or prolonged parenteral nutrition without proper vitamin-D supplementation.
- The elderly may be at special risk for development of vitamin-D deficiency because of inadequate exposure to sunlight (especially in the winter months). Vitamin-D supplementation may be appropriate.
- Chronic cholestyramine (Questran) or mineral oil use may cause decreased absorption of vitamin D and lead to deficiencies.
- Patients with renal disease may require 25-hydroxy or 1,25-dihydroxycholecalciferol (available by prescription only) because they may not be able to convert vitamin D into its active forms.

Vitamin E

The term *vitamin* E describes a number of naturally occurring plant compounds (tocopherols and tocotrienols). These compounds possess varying degrees of vitamin-E activity. For this reason, the potency of vitamin-E products is standardized in IUs.

Functions

Vitamin E functions as an antioxidant (protects cell membranes from oxidative damage or destruction) and a free-radical scavenger. It may be involved in heme biosynthesis, steroid metabolism, and collagen formation.

Sources

Vitamin E is found in vegetable oil, wheat germ, leafy vegetables, egg yolk, margarine, beans, and lentils.

Effects of Deficiency and Toxicity

Vitamin E deficiency may lead to red blood cell (RBC) hemolysis, neurologic damage, creatinuria, and ceroid (age pigment) deposition. The effects of toxicity are not known.

Therapeutic Uses and Claims

Therapeutic uses include treatment of claudication and fibrocystic breast disease. Many claims have been made regarding the benefits of vitamin E. It *may* be helpful in preventing certain cancers because of its antioxidant and free-radical scavenging effects. Studies have demonstrated possible benefits in prevention of atherosclerosis and Alzheimer's disease. Vitamin E may help to prevent heart disease caused by coronary thrombosis and scarring. In addition, it may help to slow down the aging process, reduce skin wrinkles, repair varicose veins, and treat hot flashes. It may also help to regulate menstrual flow. *Conclusive evidence of efficacy is lacking for some of these claims.*

Patient Education

- Vitamin E appears to be safe because patients tolerate large doses without side effects. Benefit of daily doses exceeding 1000 IUs is doubtful.
- The average daily diet contains 3 mg to 15 mg of vitamin E. Benefits of larger doses are unproven.
- High-dose vitamin E may potentiate the anticoagulant effect of warfarin (Coumadin).
- Supplementation of the fat-soluble vitamins may be necessary in patients with malabsorption syndromes.

Vitamin K

Functions

Vitamin K is necessary for the formation of prothrombin and other clotting factors. It is thus required for normal blood coagulation.

Sources

Vitamin K_1 (phytonadione) is present in pork liver, vegetable oils, and many vegetables, such as spinach, kale, cabbage, and cauliflower. Vitamin K_2 (menaquinone) is synthesized by bacteria in the colon.

Effects of Deficiency and Toxicity

Deficiencies of vitamin K are rare because the combination of diet and bacterial synthesis normally meets the daily requirement; however, a deficiency can cause hemorrhage. Toxicity may lead to kernicterus.

Therapeutic Uses

Vitamin K is used therapeutically to reverse the effects of warfarin and to prevent hemorrhage in newborns.

Patient Education

- Therapeutic doses of vitamin K are sold by prescription only. A few multiple-vitamin products contain small amounts of vitamin K.
- Confusion exists regarding whether the vitamin-K content of foods affects patients taking warfarin. It is not necessary for these patients to stop eating foods containing vitamin K; instead they should continue to eat a balanced diet. Patients taking warfarin should be instructed not to abruptly change their diet. The warfarin dose is adjusted to the target INR based on the dietary factors present.
- Vitamin-K deficiency can be caused by breastfeeding, severe liver disease, malabsorption syndromes, biliary obstruction, ulcerative colitis, and chronic use of broad-spectrum antibiotics, which kill off intestinal bacteria that synthesize Vitamin K.

WATER-SOLUBLE VITAMINS

The water-soluble vitamins include the B vitamins, vitamin C, and folic acid (folate). They are not stored by the body, thus the RDA must be consumed either through diet or supplements. A balanced diet should provide the RDA. Generally speaking, toxicity is rare because these vitamins are not stored.

Vitamin B$_1$ (Thiamine)

Functions

Thiamine is important in carbohydrate metabolism, central and peripheral nerve cell function, and myocardial function.

Sources

Thiamine is found in dried yeast, whole grains, meat, enriched cereal products, nuts, beans, and potatoes.

Effects of Deficiency and Toxicity

A thiamine deficiency can result in beriberi, both infantile and adult types. Principal effects for adults include peripheral neuropathy, cardiac failure, and Wernicke-Korsakoff syndrome. Principle causes of thiamine deficiency include alcoholism, malabsorption syndromes, prolonged diarrhea, and pregnancy. No toxic effects have been noted.

Therapeutic Uses

Thiamine is used in the treatment of thiamine-responsive inborn errors of metabolism and treatment of thiamine deficiency.

Vitamin B$_2$ (Riboflavin)

Functions

Riboflavin is essential for cell growth, energy, and protein metabolism. It also helps to maintain the health of mucous membranes and is involved in the cytochrome P-450 enzyme system that metabolizes many drugs.

Sources

Riboflavin is found primarily in milk, cheese, liver, eggs, and enriched cereal products. Most plants contain trace amounts.

Effects of Deficiency and Toxicity

Pure riboflavin deficiency probably does not occur alone but could occur along with other vitamin deficiencies in malnourished patients or vegetarians. A deficiency can cause cheilosis, angular stomatitis, corneal vascularization, amblyopia, and sebaceous dermatitis. The effects of toxicity are unknown.

Therapeutic Uses

There are no known therapeutic uses for riboflavin.

Vitamin B$_3$ (Niacin, Nicotinic Acid)

Functions

Niacin is necessary for the oxidative-reductive reactions of cellular respiration and for carbohydrate metabolism.

Sources

Niacin is found in dried yeast, meats, fish, liver, whole grains, enriched cereal products, green vegetables, and beans.

Effects of Deficiency and Toxicity

A severe deficiency of niacin results in pellagra (dermatitis, diarrhea, dementia, neuropathy, glossitis, stomatitis, proctitis). A less severe deficiency may cause weakness, anorexia, and indigestion. Pellagra is rare, occurring most often in alcoholics and malnourished patients. Toxicity can cause nausea, vomiting, diarrhea, hepatotoxicity, skin lesions, tachycardia, hypertension, and flushing.

Therapeutic Uses

In high doses, niacin lowers LDL cholesterol and triglycerides. It is also used to treat pellagra.

Patient Education

- Niacin therapy for hyperlipidemia should be done only under medical supervision. Results of laboratory studies should be monitored for indications of hepatotoxicity.
- The large doses used to treat hyperlipidemias (1 g to 2 g three times daily) are associated with flushing and the sensation of warmth. This side effect can be minimized by taking a 325-mg aspirin tablet or 200 mg of ibuprofen 30 minutes before taking niacin.
- Stomach upset caused by high-dose niacin therapy can be minimized by taking the dose with meals.
- Niacinamide is not associated with stomach upset but neither does it lower lipids.

Vitamin B$_6$ (Pyridoxine)

Functions

Pyridoxine serves as a cofactor for more than 60 enzymes, including decarboxylases, synthetases, transaminases, and hydroxylases. It is important in heme production and linoleic acid metabolism.

Sources

Pyridoxine is found in dried yeast, liver, organ meats, whole-grain cereals, fish, and beans.

Effects of Deficiency and Toxicity

Pyridoxine deficiency may cause convulsions, peripheral neuropathy, and sideroblastic anemia. Toxicity can lead to severe sensory neuropathy.

Therapeutic Uses and Claims

Pyridoxine is used therapeutically in the treatment of deficiency states and to prevent drug-induced peripheral neuropathy secondary to pyridoxine deficiency. Unsubstantiated claims have been made that pyridoxine relieves or treats nervousness.

Patient Education

- The tuberculosis drugs isoniazid (INH) and cycloserine can cause peripheral neuropathy by antagonizing pyridoxine. Daily pyridoxine supplementation (usually 50 mg) is recommended while patients take these drugs.
- Patients taking levodopa for Parkinson's disease should avoid supplemental pyridoxine. Levodopa is taken in large doses to gain entry into the brain, where it is converted by decarboxylases to dopamine, which improves the symptoms of the disease. Supplemental pyridoxine enhances the peripheral conversion of levodopa into dopamine, which cannot cross the blood-brain barrier. Persons taking Sinemet can take supplements containing pyridoxine because Sinemet contains a peripheral decarboxylase inhibitor that blocks peripheral dopamine formation.
- Because deficiency of pyridoxine causes peripheral neuropathy, vitamin B_6 is promoted for prevention and treatment of "nervousness." This is a spurious claim.

Vitamin B_{12} (Cyanocobalamin)

Functions
Vitamin B_{12} is important in the formation and development of red blood cells; deoxyribonucleic acid (DNA) synthesis; fat, protein, and carbohydrate metabolism; and formation of myelin (important to neural function). It is also involved in choline, methionine, and folate metabolism.

Sources
Vitamin B_{12} is found in liver, meats, eggs, milk, and milk products.

Effects of Deficiency and Toxicity
The effects of deficiency are pernicious anemia, glossitis, atrophic gastritis, achlorhydria, neurologic degeneration, and dementia. True B_{12}-deficiency is uncommon except in strict vegetarians and persons unable to absorb vitamin B_{12} because of lack of intrinsic factor (those with pernicious anemia). The effects of toxicity are unknown.

Therapeutic Uses and Claims

Some claim that vitamin B_{12} increases energy. This claim is unsubstantiated and is grounded in the fact that energy loss is a symptom of anemia that can be caused by deficiency of this vitamin. Correction of the underlying anemia with vitamin supplementation is associated with increased energy.

Patient Education

- Anemias must be evaluated by means of laboratory tests to determine their cause. Laboratory studies should include B_{12}, folate, iron, and iron-binding studies. If B_{12} is found to be deficient, the level of intrinsic factor should be measured to determine if the cause of B_{12}-deficiency is dietary or caused by lack of absorption.
- Drugs inhibiting gastric-acid production, such as H_2 receptor antagonists (ranitidine, cimetidine, and nizatidine) and proton pump inhibitors (omeprazole and lansoprazole), may decrease the absorption of vitamin B_{12}.
- Dietary deficiency can be treated with oral supplementation. Pernicious anemia must be treated with Vitamin B_{12} injections (either intramuscular or subcutaneous) for the lifetime of the patient.

Folic Acid (Folate)

Functions

Folic acid is important in red blood cell development and the synthesis of purines, pyrimidines, and DNA. It is critical to neural-tube development in the fetus.

Sources

Sources of folic acid include liver, lean beef, yeast, leafy vegetables, beans, some fruits, eggs, and whole-grain cereals.

Effects of Deficiency and Toxicity

A deficiency of folic acid can lead to megaloblastic anemia, sore mouth, diarrhea, CNS symptoms (irritability, forgetfulness), and neural-tube defects in the fetus. Toxic effects are unknown.

Therapeutic Uses

Folic acid is used in the treatment of anemia caused by folic acid deficiency, and in the prevention of neural-tube defects in the developing fetus.

Patient Education

- The patient's diet should include some uncooked sources of folic acid. Dietary folates are destroyed by heat.
- Because folic acid can mask the signs of pernicious anemia, it should not be started until an anemia workup is completed.
- Folic-acid requirements are higher in infancy, pregnancy, and in lactating women; during blood loss; and in hypermetabolic states such as hyperthyroidism.
- **It is currently recommended that pregnant women take a daily prenatal vitamin containing folic acid.** Folic acid deficiency is associated with fetal neural-tube defects.

Vitamin C (Ascorbic Acid)

Functions

Vitamin C is an antioxidant, necessary for formation of collagen and connective tissue, osteoid, and dentin. It assists in iron absorption and in maintaining integrity of the capillaries.

Sources

Vitamin C is found in green and red peppers, broccoli, spinach, tomatoes, potatoes, strawberries, oranges, and other citrus fruits. Meat, fish, poultry, eggs, and dairy products contain some vitamin C.

Effects of Deficiency and Toxicity

Deficiencies are rare but effects include malaise; weakness; capillary hemorrhages and petechiae; swollen, hemorrhagic gums; bone changes; and scurvy. Toxicity may cause increased oxalate excretion, causing nephrolithiasis or hemolysis in patients with glucose 6-phosphate dehydrogenase deficiency.

Therapeutic Uses and Claims

Vitamin C enhances iron absorption and aids in wound healing. Claims have been made that vitamin C builds resistance to infection, prevents and treats the common cold, and prevents cancer.

Patient Education

- Vitamin-C deficiency is rare because this substance is found in many foods. The typical American diet should provide many times the RDA.
- Lower-than-normal levels of vitamin C have been reported in women

taking oral contraceptives, in smokers, and in some institutionalized elderly patients.
- Vitamin C may aid in wound healing. A double-blind placebo controlled study demonstrated that vitamin C may be helpful in minimizing pressure ulcers (Thomas, 1997).
- A trial of vitamin C might be reasonable in patients who bruise easily, because vitamin-C deficiency leads to increased capillary friability.
- Studies have shown that vitamin C reduces the formation of colon polyps, which some consider to be precancerous lesions. Further studies are needed to determine whether this will translate into fewer cases of colon cancer (Watson, 1986).
- Reasonable doses of vitamin C are apparently safe and well tolerated.

Biotin

Functions
Biotin is necessary for at least nine enzymes involved in fat, amino acid, and carbohydrate metabolism. No RDA has been established.

Sources
Biotin is found in liver, egg yolk, cauliflower, salmon, carrots, bananas, and yeast.

Effects of Deficiency and Toxicity
Because biotin is available in a variety of foods, deficiencies are rare; however, a deficiency may lead to glossitis or dermatitis. A severe deficiency can cause nausea, vomiting, lassitude, muscle pain, anorexia, and depression. Toxic effects are unknown.

Therapeutic Uses and Claims
Claims have been made that biotin helps to promote healthy hair and skin, but these claims are unsubstantiated.

Pantothenic Acid

Functions
Pantothenic acid is important in cholesterol, steroid, and fatty-acid synthesis; carbohydrate metabolism; and synthesis of acetylcholine. No RDA has been established for pantothenic acid, but 4 mg to 7 mg daily is thought to be safe and adequate.

Sources
Pantothenic acid is found in meat, liver, milk, eggs, vegetables, beans, and whole-grain cereals.

Effects of Deficiency and Toxicity
Deficiencies of pantothenic acid are rare but can cause somnolence, fatigue, headache, paresthesia of the hands or feet, and gastrointestinal complaints. Toxic effects are unknown.

Therapeutic Uses
Pantothenic acid is used to treat burning-feet syndrome.

Carnitine
Functions
Carnitine is involved in fatty-acid utilization/regulation.

Sources
Carnitine is found in dairy products and meat, especially red meats. It is also synthesized in the body from lysine and methionine.

Effects of Deficiency and Toxicity
No specific deficiency or toxicity symptoms have been noted in humans.

Therapeutic Uses and Claims
No therapeutic uses are known, and there is no recommended daily allowance. Claims have been made that carnitine protects against cardiovascular disease and memory loss, prevents some diseases of the nervous system (such as Alzheimer's disease and tardive dyskinesia), can be used to treat Alzheimer's disease, treats liver damage caused by alcoholism, and lowers cholesterol levels in human serum. These claims are unsubstantiated.

Choline
Functions
Choline is involved in the production of acetylcholine and platelet aggregating factor (PAF). It also affects the mobilization of fat from the liver.

Sources

Choline's major source is lecithin, which is used as a thickener in several foods, including mayonnaise, margarine, and ice cream.

Effects of Deficiency and Toxicity

Effects of choline deficiency and toxicity are unknown. No RDA has been established.

Therapeutic Uses and Claims

No therapeutic uses are known for choline. Claims have been made that choline helps with proper function of the nervous system, including mood, behavior, orientation, personality traits, and judgment. These claims are unsubstantiated.

Inositol

Functions

Inositol is a component of phospholipids.

Sources

Inositol is found in beans, calves' liver, cantaloupe, most citrus fruit, lecithin granules, lentils, nuts, oats, pork, rice, veal, wheat germ, and whole-grain products.

Effects of Deficiency and Toxicity

Effects of inositol deficiency and toxicity are unknown. No RDA has been established, and deficiencies do not exist in humans.

Therapeutic Uses and Claims

No therapeutic uses are known. Claims have been made that inositol protects against cardiovascular disease, peripheral neuritis associated with diabetes, and hair loss; helps maintain healthy hair; functions as a mild antianxiety agent; helps control blood-cholesterol levels; promotes the body's production of lecithin; and treats constipation with its stimulating effect on muscular action of the colon. These claims are unproved.

Para-aminobenzoic Acid

Functions

Para-aminobenzoic acid (PABA) is part of the coenzyme tetrahydrofolic acid. It aids in the metabolism and utilization of amino acids and is also supportive of blood cells, particularly the RBCs. PABA supports folic-acid production by the intestinal bacteria. PABA is important to skin, hair pigment, and intestinal health. Used as a sunscreen, it also can protect against the development of sunburn and skin cancer from excess ultraviolet light exposure.

Sources
PABA is found in bran, brown rice, kidney, liver, molasses, sunflower seeds, wheat germ, and whole-grain products.

Effects of Deficiency and Toxicity
Problems related to PABA deficiency are rare. No RDA has been established. Toxic effects are unknown.

Therapeutic Uses and Claims
No therapeutic uses are known. Claims have been made that PABA rejuvenates the skin, treats arthritis, stops hair loss, restores color to graying or white hair, and treats anemia, constipation, headaches, and skin disorders. These claims are unsubstantiated.

Pangamic Acid (Vitamin B_{15})
Functions
There are no known functions for vitamin B_{15}.

Sources
Vitamin B_{15} is found in brewers yeast, whole brown rice, sesame seeds, and pumpkin seeds.

Effects of Deficiency and Toxicity
Effects of deficiency and toxicity of vitamin B_{15} are unknown.

Therapeutic Uses and Claims
No therapeutic uses are known. Claims have been made that vitamin B_{15} protects against cancers, stimulates the immune system, lowers cholesterol, and helps to treat drug addiction, diabetes, heart disease, and alcoholism. These claims are unsubstantiated.

Patient Education
- Vitamin B_{15} is not a vitamin because pangamic acid is **not** a necessary nutrient.

- There is some concern regarding the safety of pangamic acid. Until this issue is resolved, it should not be recommended.

MINERALS

Calcium

Functions

Calcium is required for development and maintenance of bones and teeth. It is involved in a number of enzyme systems, biosynthesis of a number of critical substances, regulation of muscle contraction and relaxation, and clotting of blood, and is necessary for function of cardiovascular and neuromuscular cells.

Sources

Calcium is found in dairy products, meat, fish, eggs, cereal products, beans, fruits, and vegetables.

Effects of Deficiency and Toxicity

Because calcium is critical to physiologic function, the body will "borrow" calcium from the bones when there is insufficient dietary intake. A deficiency can cause osteoporosis, muscle spasms and cramps, tooth decay, convulsions, personality disorders, mental retardation, and growth retardation. Toxicity can lead to hypercalcemia, loss of gastrointestinal tone, renal failure, and psychosis.

Therapeutic Uses

Calcium is used in the prevention and treatment of osteoporosis, correction of calcium deficiencies, and prevention and treatment of hyperphosphatemia (renal patients).

Patient Education

- Dairy products are sufficient to provide the RDA of calcium for most adults.
- RDAs are expressed in milligrams of elemental calcium. The various salt forms contain different percentages of elemental calcium (Table 8-4).
- Postmenopausal women (especially those not taking hormone replacement therapy) should consume 1500 mg of elemental calcium/day.

Table 8-4
Calcium Salts

Calcium salt	Percentage elemental calcium	Conversion to elemental calcium
Calcium acetate	25	500 mg = 125 mg elemental
Calcium lactate	13	500 mg = 65 mg elemental
Calcium glucobionate	6.5	1.8 g = 115 mg elemental
Calcium gluconate	9	500 mg = 45 mg elemental
Calcium citrate	21	950 mg = 200 mg elemental
Calcium carbonate	40	650 mg = 250 mg elemental
Tricalcium phosphate	39	500 mg = 195 mg elemental

- Calcium carbonate and calcium phosphate are insoluble and should be taken with meals because low pH is required for absorption. Patients taking H_2 antagonists (ranitidine, cimetidine, nizatidine) or proton pump inhibitors (omeprazole or lansoprazole) should take a soluble calcium salt such as calcium citrate, calcium lactate, or calcium gluconate.
- Vitamin D is required for optimum absorption of calcium. Calcium products with vitamin D might be beneficial for patients who are homebound or who do not receive adequate sunlight.
- Calcium binds with several medications, including quinolone antibiotics, tetracyclines, and alendronate. If concurrent administration is required, doses should be staggered.

Phosphorus
Functions
Phosphorus is an integral component of bones and teeth, acid-base balance, and nucleic acids. It is also involved in energy production.

Sources
Phosphorus is present in most foods, especially protein-rich foods and grains.

Effects of Deficiency and Toxicity
Phosphorus deficiency may cause irritability, weakness, blood disorders, and gastrointestinal and renal dysfunction. Toxicity may lead to renal

failure. Because phosphorus is contained in many foods, deficiency is usually secondary to other factors, such as binding of phosphorus by aluminum-containing antacids or calcium, or diabetic ketoacidosis.

Therapeutic Uses
Phosphorus is used to correct hypophosphatemia.

Magnesium
Functions
Magnesium is important in the formation of bones and teeth, nerve conduction, and muscle contraction. It is also involved in enzyme systems.

Sources
Magnesium is contained in most unprocessed foods, especially vegetables, nuts, legumes and unmilled grains, and seafoods.

Effects of Deficiency and Toxicity
Magnesium deficiency may cause neuromuscular irritability, apathy, and depression. Toxicity may lead to hypotension, respiratory failure, or cardiac arrhythmias. Dietary deficiency is rare and is usually due to alcoholism, diabetes, chronic diarrhea, renal dysfunction, or renal wasting caused by some drugs (platinum derivatives).

Therapeutic Uses
Magnesium is used to correct hypomagnesemia.

Patient Education
Magnesium binds with several medications, including quinolone antibiotics, tetracyclines, and alendronate. If concurrent administration is required, doses should be staggered.

Iron
Functions
Iron is required for hemoglobin and myoglobin formation. It is also involved in enzyme function.

Sources
With the exception of dairy products, iron is present in most foods.

Effects of Deficiency and Toxicity
Iron deficiency can lead to anemia, exhaustion, koilonychia, sore tongue, angular stomatitis, and decreased work performance. Toxicity can lead to hemochromatosis, cirrhosis, and skin pigmentation.

Therapeutic Uses
Iron is used therapeutically to correct iron-deficiency anemia.

Patient Education
- Though iron is present in most foods, absorption is poor. It is estimated that only 5% to 20% is absorbed.
- Approximately 60% to 70% of iron is found as hemoglobin in RBCs. The remainder is stored in the liver and other sites.
- Anemia secondary to low dietary intake may take years to develop.
- Infants who are fed cow's milk may develop iron-deficiency anemia because cow's milk contains little iron.
- Menstruation and pregnancy can cause iron-deficiency anemia.
- Anemia can occur secondary to blood loss as seen in peptic ulcer disease, esophageal varices, diverticulitis, ulcerative colitis, and colon cancer. These secondary causes of iron-deficiency anemia should be investigated.
- RDAs are expressed as elemental iron. Various salt forms contain different percentages of elemental iron (Table 8-5).
- Providing the RDA will correct iron-deficiency anemia, but larger amounts are necessary to rebuild the normal stores. In treating iron-deficiency anemia, it is recommended that patients take 3 to 4 tablets daily for 3 months. Assuming the patient's diet is

Table 8-5
Elemental Iron Salts

Iron salt	Percentage elemental iron	Dose conversion
Ferrous sulfate	20	300 mg = 60 mg elemental
Ferrous gluconate	11.6	300 mg = 35 mg elemental
Ferrous fumarate	33	200 mg = 66 mg elemental

adequate, iron supplementation could cease at that point. Patients with inadequate dietary iron intake can generally receive the RDA if they take 1 325-mg ferrous sulfate tablet (or equivalent) daily.

- Food is capable of decreasing iron absorption by as much as 50%. However, some patients cannot tolerate the gastrointestinal irritation caused by iron preparations, so they must take iron with meals. Ferrous gluconate *may* cause less gastrointestinal irritation than ferrous sulfate. Timed-release iron products also minimize gastrointestinal upset, but absorption is decreased because less iron is absorbed distally to the duodenum.
- Constipation can occur when iron supplements are taken. Attention must be paid to adequate fiber and fluid intake. Stool softeners may help alleviate the constipation.
- Iron products must be kept out of the reach of children. The brightly colored tablets can be mistaken for candy and ingested. As few as 15 325-mg ferrous sulfate tablets can be fatal to a child. Rapid medical treatment prevents serious outcomes.
- Iron binds to several medications, including quinolone antibiotics, tetracyclines, and alendronate. If concurrent administration is required, doses should be staggered.

Zinc

Functions
Zinc is an integral part of at least 70 enzymes. It is important to insulin function, reproduction, skin integrity, wound healing, and growth.

Sources
Zinc is found in animal products, oysters, liver, legumes, peanuts, and whole-grain cereals.

Effects of Deficiency and Toxicity
A zinc deficiency can cause growth retardation, loss of appetite, skin changes, altered immune function, hypogonadism, alopecia, impaired taste and smell, and poor wound healing. A zinc deficiency is uncommon and is usually secondary to gastrointestinal losses or parenteral nutrition without trace mineral supplementation. Toxic effects are unknown.

Therapeutic Uses
Zinc is used to correct deficiencies and improve wound healing.

Patient Education

- Zinc gluconate lozenges may decrease the duration of the common cold.
- A trial of zinc might be of benefit in patients with poor wound healing.

Iodine
Functions
Iodine is necessary for formation of thyroid hormones.

Sources
Iodine is found in iodized salt, saltwater fish, and shellfish.

Effects of Deficiency and Toxicity
An iodine deficiency can lead to goiter, cretinism, and impaired fetal growth and brain development. However, since the introduction of iodized salt in the United States, iodine deficiency is rarely seen. One-fourth teaspoonful of iodized salt contains approximately 100 mcg of iodine. Additional iodine supplementation should not be required. Iodine toxicity can lead to myxedema.

Therapeutic Uses
Iodine is used to prevent radiation damage to the thyroid gland.

Selenium
Functions
Selenium is required for the enzyme glutathione peroxidase.

Sources
Selenium is found in meats, seafoods, and some cereal grains.

Effects of Deficiency and Toxicity
Selenium deficiencies can lead to cardiomyopathy, muscle pain, and abnormal nails. Selenium deficiency is rare, but has been reported in patients with cirrhosis, and those receiving long-term parenteral nutrition without trace mineral supplementation. Selenium toxicity can cause loss of hair and nails, and dermatitis.

Therapeutic Uses
Selenium is used therapeutically to correct and prevent selenium deficiencies.

Chromium

Functions

Chromium is required for efficient glucose utilization. It may also be involved in protein synthesis.

Sources

Chromium is found in liver, fish, whole grains, and milk.

Effects of Deficiency and Toxicity

Chromium deficiency may lead to impaired glucose function. Toxic effects are unknown.

Therapeutic Uses

No therapeutic use has been established. Little is known regarding the incidence and role for chromium supplementation.

Copper

Functions

Copper is necessary for copper metalloenzymes involved in iron absorption. It is required for CNS function and bone formation.

Sources

Copper is found in organ meats (especially liver), shellfish, chocolate, whole-grain cereals, and nuts.

Effects of Deficiency and Toxicity

A deficiency of copper may cause impaired iron absorption with resultant anemia. This deficiency is uncommon. Toxicity may cause CNS, kidney, and liver damage (Wilson's disease).

Therapeutic Use

Copper is used for supplementation in patients receiving parenteral nutrition.

Potassium

Functions

Potassium is important for muscle activity, nerve transmission, intracellular acid-base balance, and water homeostasis.

Sources
Potassium is found in milk and dairy products, bananas, prunes, and raisins.

Effects of Deficiency and Toxicity
A potassium deficiency can cause hypokalemia, paralysis, and cardiac disturbances. Toxicity can lead to hyperkalemia, paralysis, and cardiac disturbances.

Therapeutic Uses
Potassium is used to correct and prevent hypokalemia.

Patient Education

- Potent diuretics can cause potassium wasting. Careful attention must be paid to prevent hypokalemia.
- Prescription timed-release potassium products are preferred when supplementation is necessary. Nonprescription potassium tablets should be avoided.
- Significant renal impairment can lead to hyperkalemia. Potassium supplementation can be dangerous to renal patients.

Fluorine

Functions
Fluorine is important for bone and teeth formation.

Sources
Fluorine is found in most municipal water supplies and in plant and animal products.

Effects of Deficiency and Toxicity
A fluorine deficiency can lead to dental caries. Toxicity can lead to fluorosis.

Therapeutic Uses
Fluorine is use to prevent dental caries and osteoporosis.

Patient Education

Fluoride supplements should be administered to children who consume nonfluoridated water (well water).

Manganese

Functions

Manganese is involved in glucose utilization, synthesis of cartilage components, and certain enzyme systems.

Sources

Manganese is found in vegetables, fruits, nuts, and whole-grain cereals.

Effects of Deficiency and Toxicity

A manganese deficiency may cause symptoms involving the hair or nails, nausea, and decreased phospholipids and triglycerides. Toxic effects are unknown.

Therapeutic Uses

There are no known therapeutic uses.

Patient Education

Dietary sources should provide sufficient manganese.

Molybdenum

Functions

Molybdenum is a cofactor for several enzymes, including xanthine oxidase.

Sources

Molybdenum is found in milk, organ meats, beans, breads, and cereals.

Effects of Deficiency and Toxicity

The effects of a deficiency are not known. Toxicity may cause goutlike symptoms.

Therapeutic Uses

There are no known therapeutic uses.

Patient Education

Dietary intake is apparently sufficient.

Silicon, Tin, Vanadium

Silicon, tin, and vanadium are presumed to be involved in cellular function, although deficiency states have not been described. It is apparent that diet supplies adequate amounts of these substances.

Selected Natural/Herbal Products

Many claims are made for the numerous "natural" or "herbal" products available in pharmacies and health-food stores. Although many of these claims are unsubstantiated, some data exists on which we can make rational decisions. "Natural" products have gained wide acceptance in Europe. In response to this widespread use, the German Federal Health Agency established a commission in 1978 charged with the task of reviewing the literature to determine the safety and effectiveness of the many natural products sold in Germany. The commission (Commission E) has published approximately 300 monographs to date. These monographs represent the best information available regarding many of these products. Table 8-6 provides a summary of common herbs and their purported benefits.

Product Selection

Vitamin B and C Complexes

- Vitamin B and C complexes usually contain the common B vitamins (B_1, B_2, B_3, B_6, B_{12}), vitamin C, and/or vitamin E, iron, and biotin.
- These products do not contain fat-soluble vitamins such as vitamins A or D, or minerals other than iron.
- Vitamin B and C complexes are promoted for increasing "energy" and decreasing "stress."
- Generic brands are inexpensive and equally effective.
- If vitamin supplementation is required, consider recommending a complete multivitamin formula.

Multivitamins

- There are many different brands and formulas of multivitamins; some are more complete than others.
- Multivitamins commonly contain both fat-soluble and water-soluble vitamins; some contain minerals.
- Little practical difference exists between brands.

Table 8-6
Selected Herbal Products

Herbal product	Purported benefits
Ginger	Indigestion, motion sickness
Bearberry	Short-term treatment of urinary tract inflammation
Black cohosh	PMS, dysmenorrhea, nervous conditions associated with menopause
Buckthorn bark	Stimulant laxative
Chamomile	Gastrointestinal spasms, gastrointestinal tract inflammation
Chinese ephedra (ma huang)	Asthma bronchoconstriction
Clove oil	Local anesthetic, antiseptic
Cranberry	Prevention of urinary tract infections
Echinacea	Supportive measure in the treatment of recurrent respiratory and urinary tract infections
Garlic	To support dietetic measures for treatment of hyperlipoproteinemia and to prevent age-related changes in blood vessels
Gingko	Effective for treatment of cerebral circulatory disorders, intermittent claudication
Goldenrod	Antispasmodic, diuretic, antiinflammatory
Horehound	Bronchial cough, dyspepsia, loss of appetite
Horse chestnut (topical)	Chronic venous insufficiency, leg pain
Iceland moss, marshmallow root, plantain leaves, slippery elm	Throat irritation, cough
Licorice	Short-term gastrointestinal ulcer therapy
Milk thistle (silymarin)	Chronic inflammation of the liver, cirrhosis
Nettle root	BPH
Parsley, birch leaves, lovage root	Reduce urinary tract inflammation, facilitate passage of kidney stones
Passion flower	Nervous unrest
Sage	Antiseptic, local antiinflammatory (mouthwash)
Saw palmetto	Benign prostatic hypertrophy (BPH)
Senega snakeroot	Expectorant
St. John's wort (hypericin)	Depression
Thyme	Cough, bronchitis
Turmeric, boldo, dandelion	Dyspepsia
Valerian	Sleep aid, minor tranquilizer

- "House" brands or generic brands are less expensive and equally effective.
- One tablet/capsule daily provides many times the minimum daily requirement of common vitamins and minerals.

Women's Formulas

- Women's formula vitamins generally contain additional calcium but not enough to replace the need for additional calcium supplements, especially in postmenopausal women.
- These products generally contain more iron than other products.

Men's Formulas

Men's formula vitamins generally contain additional amounts of antioxidants, such as vitamin E, and sometimes less iron.

Senior Formulas

Senior formulas tend to be similar to multivitamin formulas with additional minerals and antioxidants.

Prenatal Vitamins

- Prenatal vitamins contain fat-soluble vitamins A, D, E, common B vitamins, additional calcium and iron, and sometimes larger amounts of folic acid.
- It is important that pregnant women receive at least 400 mcg daily of folic acid to prevent neural-tube defects.

Vitamins for the Eyes

- Vitamins for the eyes contain antioxidants such as vitamin E and beta carotene.
- These products are promoted as good for vision.

Children's Vitamins

- Children's vitamins are sold in chewable and liquid forms.
- There is little practical difference between brands.
- Products are targeted specifically at children, with brand names such as Bugs Bunny, Sesame Street, and Flintstones.
- Generic brands are equally good and less expensive than brand names.

Calcium Products

- Dosing of calcium products is based on elemental calcium.
- Name brands are expensive compared with store or generic brands.

- Calcium should be given in divided doses because large doses are poorly absorbed.

Iron Products
- Name brands and timed-release iron products are expensive.
- Dosing of iron products is based on elemental iron content.
- Store brands or generic brands are much less expensive.

SUGGESTED READINGS

Halbert SC: Diet and nutrition in primary care: from antioxidants to zinc, *Prim Care* 24(4):825-843, 1997.

Meydani M, Meisler JG: A closer look at vitamin E: can this antioxidant prevent chronic diseases? *Postgrad Med* 102(2):199-201, 1997.

Morrow JD, Kelsey K: Folic acid for prevention of neural tube defects: pediatric anticipatory guidance, *J Pediatr Health Care* 12(2):55-59, 1998.

Mossad SB et al: Zinc gluconate lozenges for treating the common cold: a randomized, double-blind, placebo-controlled study, *Ann Intern Med* 125:81-88, 1996.

Probart CK, Bird PJ, Parker KA: Diet and athletic performance, *Med Clin North Am* 77(4):757-772, 1993.

Watson RR, Leonard TK: Selenium and vitamins A, E, and C: nutrients with cancer prevention properties, *J Am Diet Assoc* 86(4):505-510, 1986.

Williamson BL et al: Structural characterization of contaminants found in commercial preparations of melatonin: similarities to case-related compounds from L-tryptophan associated with eosinophilia-myalgia syndrome, *Chem Res Toxicol* 11(3):234-240, 1998.

Vitamin C Studies
Hemila H: Vitamin C and plasma cholesterol: critical reviews, *Food Science and Nutrition*, 32(1):33-57, 1992.

Jacques PF: Effects of vitamin C on high-density lipoprotein cholesterol and blood pressure, *J Am Col Nutr* 11(2):139-144, 1992.

Thomas DR: The role of nutrition in prevention and healing of pressure ulcers, *Clin Geriatr Med* 13(3):497-511, 1997.

Product Information: Vitamin B Complex*

Vitamin	Geritol Tonic	Stresstabs	Stresstabs With Iron	Stresstabs With Zinc	Surbex-T
C (mg)	—	500	500	500	500
E (IU)	—	30	30	30	—
B_1 (mg)	2.5	10	10	10	15
B_2 (mg)	2.5	10	10	10	10
B_3 (mg)	50	100	100	100	100
B_6 (mg)	0.5	5	5	5	5
Folic acid (mcg)	—	400	400	400	—
B_{12} (mcg)	—	12	12	12	10
Biotin (mcg)	—	45	45	45	—
Pantothenic acid (mg)	2	20	20	20	20
Iron (mg)	18	—	18	—	—
Zinc (mg)	—	—	—	23.9	—
Copper	—	—	—	3	—

*None of these products contain calcium or magnesium.

Product Information: Calcium Supplements

Brand Name	Vitamin D (IU)	Calcium (Elemental) (mg)	Other
Caltrate 600		600	
Caltrate 600 + D	200	600	
Caltrate 600 Plus Chewable	200	600	Magnesium 40 mg Zinc 7.5 mg Copper 1 mg Manganese 1.8 mg Boron 250 mcg
Caltrate Plus	200	600	Magnesium 40 mg Zinc 7.5 mg Copper 1 mg Manganese 1.8 mg Boron 250 mcg
Citracal		200	
Citracal + D	200	315	
Oscal 250 + D	125	250	
Oscal 500		500	
Oscal 500 + D	125	500	
Posture		600	
Posture-D	125	600	
Tums 500 Chewable		500	

Product Information: Iron Supplements

Brand Name	Iron Content (Elemental) (mg)
Feosol caplets	50
Feosol tablets	65
Fergon	27
Fer-In-Sol drops	15 mg/0.6 ml
Ferro-Sequels	50
Slow FE	50
Slow FE plus Folic Acid	50

Product Information: Prenatal Vitamins

Vitamin	Natalins	Stuart Prenatal
A (IU)	4000	4000
C (mg)	70	100
D (IU)	400	400
E (IU)	15	11
B_1 (mg)	1.5	1.84
B_2 (mg)	1.6	1.7
B_3 (mg)	17	18
B_6 (mg)	2.6	2.6
Folic acid (mcg)	500	800
B_{12} (mcg)	2.5	4
Calcium (mg)	200	200
Iron (mg)	27	60
Magnesium (mg)	100	—
Zinc (mg)	15	25
Copper (mg)	1.5	—

Product Information: Children's Formula Vitamins

Vitamin	Bugs Bunny With Extra C	Centrum Jr Plus Extra C	Centrum Jr Plus Extra Calcium	Centrum Jr Plus Iron	Flintstones	Flintstones Complete	Flintstones Plus Iron	Poly-Vi-Sol drops	Poly-Vi-Sol With Iron	Poly-Vi-Sol With Iron drops	Sesame Street Complete	Sesame Street Extra C	Tri-Vi-Sol drops	Tri-Vi-Sol With Iron drops	Vi-Daylin Plus Iron drops
A (IU)	2500	2500	2500	2500	2500	5000	2500	1500	2500	1500	2750	2750	1500	1500	1500
C (mg)	250	150	30	30	60	60	60	35	60	35	40	80	35	35	35
D (IU)	400	200	200	200	400	400	400	400	400	400	200	200	400	400	400
E (IU)	15	15	15	15	15	30	15	5	15	5	10	10	—	—	5
B_1 (mg)	1.05	0.75	0.75	0.75	1.05	1.5	1.05	0.5	1.05	—	0.75	0.75	—	—	0.5
B_2 (mg)	1.2	0.85	0.85	0.85	1.2	1.7	1.2	0.6	1.2	0.6	0.85	0.85	—	—	0.6
B_3 (mg)	13.5	10	10	10	13.5	20	13.5	8	13.5	8	10	10	—	—	8
B_6 (mg)	1.05	1	1	1	1.05	2	1.05	0.4	1.05	0.4	0.7	0.7	—	—	0.4
Folic acid (mcg)	300	200	200	200	300	400	300	—	300	—	200	200	—	—	—

B₁₂ (mcg)	4.5	3	3	3	4.5	6	4.5	2	4.5	—	3	3	—	—	—
Biotin (mcg)	—	22.5	22.5	22.5	—	40	—	—	—	—	15	—	—	—	—
Pantothenic acid (mg)	—	5	5	5	—	10	—	—	—	—	5	5	—	—	—
Calcium (mg)	—	54	80	54	—	100	—	—	—	—	80	—	—	—	—
Iron (mg)	—	9	9	9	—	18	15	—	12	10	10	—	—	10	10
Phosphate (mg)	—	25	25	25	—	100	—	—	—	—	—	—	—	—	—
Iodine (mcg)	—	75	75	75	—	150	—	—	—	—	75	—	—	—	—
Magnesium (mg)	—	20	20	20	—	20	—	—	—	—	20	—	—	—	—
Zinc (mg)	—	7.5	7.5	7.5	—	15	—	—	8	—	8	—	—	—	—
Copper (mg)	—	1	1	1	—	2	—	—	0.8	—	1	—	—	—	—
K (mcg)	—	5	5	5	—	—	—	—	—	—	—	—	—	—	—
Manganese (mg)	—	0.5	—	0.5	—	—	—	—	—	—	—	—	—	—	—
Chromium (mcg)	—	10	—	10	—	—	—	—	—	—	—	—	—	—	—
Molybdenum (mcg)	—	10	—	10	—	—	—	—	—	—	—	—	—	—	—

Product Information: Adult Multivitamins

Vitamin	Centrum	Centrum Liquid	Geritol Complete	Myadec	One A Day Maximum	One A Day Mens	One A Day Womens	Theragran-M	Unicap M
A (IU)	5000	2500	6000	5000	5000	5000	5000	5000	5000
C (mg)	60	60	60	60	60	90	60	90	60
D (IU)	400	400	400	400	400	400	400	400	400
E (IU)	30	30	30	30	30	45	30	30	30
B_1 (mg)	1.5	1.5	1.5	1.7	1.5	2.25	1.5	3	1.5
B_2 (mg)	1.7	1.7	1.7	2	1.7	2.55	1.7	3.4	1.7
B_3 (mg)	20	20	20	20	20	20	20	20	20
B_6 (mg)	2	2	2	3	2	3	2	3	2
Folic acid (mcg)	400	—	400	400	400	400	400	400	—
B_{12} (mcg)	6	6	6	6	6	9	6	9	6
Biotin (mcg)	30	300	45	30	30	—	—	30	—
Pantothenic acid (mg)	10	10	10	10	10	10	10	10	10
Calcium (mg)	162	—	162	162	130	—	450	40	60
Iron (mg)	18	9	18	18	18	—	27	18	—
Phosphate (mg)	109	—	125	125	100	—	—	31	45
Iodine (mcg)	150	150	150	150	150	150	—	150	150

Magnesium (mg)	100	—	100	100	100	100	—	100	—
Zinc (mg)	15	3	15	15	15	15	15	15	15
Copper (mg)	2	—	2	2	2	2	—	2	2
Potassium (mg)	80	—	40	40	37.5	37.5	—	7.5	5
K (mcg)	25	—	25	25	—	—	—	28	—
Selenium (mcg)	20	—	75	25	10	87.5	—	21	1
Manganese (mg)	3.5	—	2.5	2.5	2.5	3.5	—	3.5	—
Chromium (mcg)	65	—	15	25	10	150	—	26	—
Molybdenum (mcg)	160	—	15	25	10	75	—	32	—
Chloride (mg)	72	—	35	—	34	34	—	7.5	—
Nickel (mcg)	5	—	5	5	—	2	—	—	—
Tin (mcg)	10	—	10	10	—	—	—	—	—
Silicon (mg)	2	—	0.08	10	—	—	—	—	—
Venadium (mcg)	10	—	10	10	—	—	—	—	—
Boron (mcg)	150	—	—	150	—	—	—	—	—

Product Information: Senior Formula Vitamins

Vitamin	Centrum Silver	Geritol Extend	One A Day 50 Plus	Unicap Senior
A (IU)	5000	3333	5000	5000
C (mg)	60	60	120	60
D (IU)	400	200	400	200
E (IU)	45	15	60	15
B_1 (mg)	1.5	1.2	4.5	1.2
B_2 (mg)	1.7	1.4	3.4	1.4
B_3 (mg)	20	15	20	16
B_6 (mg)	3	2	6	2.2
Folic acid (mcg)	400	200	400	400
B_{12} (mcg)	25	2	30	—
Biotin (mcg)	30	—	30	—
Pantothenic acid (mg)	10	—	15	10
Calcium (mg)	200	130	120	100
Iron (mg)	4	10	—	10
Phosphate (mg)	48	100	—	77
Iodine (mcg)	150	150	150	150

Magnesium (mg)	100	35	100	30
Zinc (mg)	15	150	22.5	15
Copper (mg)	2	—	2	2
Potassium (mg)	80	—	37.5	5
K (mcg)	10	80	20	—
Selenium (mcg)	20	70	105	—
Manganese (mg)	3.5	2.5	4	—
Chromium (mcg)	130	15	180	—
Molybdenum (mcg)	160	15	93.75	—
Chloride (mg)	72	35	342	—
Nickel (mcg)	5	5	—	—
Tin (mcg)	—	10	—	—
Silicon (mg)	2	0.08	—	—
Venadium (mcg)	10	102	—	—
Boron (mcg)	150	—	—	—

Weight Reduction

Weight reduction is a difficult assignment for patients. The sociologic, emotional, and physiologic effects of food penetrate all aspects of our lives. The etiology of excess body weight can be an energy imbalance, genetic predisposition, and/or sedentary lifestyle.

In this age of instant gratification and "miracle" drugs, weight control continues to require hard work and determination. If a weight-loss method sounds easy and too good to be true, it probably is. If all the products that promised easy weight loss were effective, obesity would not remain the problem it is today. Americans spend more than $30 billion per year on pills, potions, and programs that promise to induce weight loss, many of which do not work. The most effective means of achieving weight loss is a reduction in calorie intake below energy expenditure. In other words, consume fewer calories than you burn. This can be done by reducing calorie intake or increasing physical activity.

The Centers for Disease Control and Prevention (CDC) estimates that one third of all American adults are obese. Obesity is associated with multiple medical problems including heart disease, diabetes, hypertension, hyperlipidemia, stroke, certain cancers, arthritis, and pulmonary dysfunction. Patients do not have to achieve ideal body weight to benefit from a weight-loss and exercise program. A loss of 5% to 10% of body weight can lower the associated health risks of obesity.

Obesity can be identified by using body mass index (BMI) or comparing the patient's current weight to an ideal body weight.

$$\text{Body Mass Index (BMI)} = \frac{\text{Weight (kg)}}{\text{Height (m}^2)}$$

BMI	Interpretation of BMI
19-25	Appropriate for those ages 19-34
21-27	Appropriate for those over the age of 35
>27.5	Obesity
27.5-30	Mild obesity
30-40	Moderate obesity
>40	Severe or morbid obesity

$$\% \text{ Ideal Body Weight} = \frac{\text{Actual body weight}}{\text{Ideal body weight} \times 100}$$

Result	Interpretation of Ideal Body Weight
110% to 120%	Overweight
>130%	Obese
>200%	Morbid obesity

Remember that excess weight is not always excess fat. Weight lifters, for instance, are often above ideal body weight because of muscle development. On the flip side, there are many people who are within ideal body weight range who have a high proportion of body fat. There are tests to determine the percentage of body fat (underwater weighing, skin caliper measurements, and bioelectrical impedance), but they are not generally available. When in doubt, patients can use the "pinch an inch" test:

• Pinch a fold of skin on the back of the mid–upper arm between your thumb and forefinger.
• A fold greater than 1-inch thick suggests excess fat.

Not all patients who want to lose weight are obese. Many patients who complain about their weight are slightly overweight or within ideal body weight but are sedentary. These patients should consider beginning an exercise regimen to improve physical conditioning. In fact, all patients should include exercise with their weight-loss program. Dieting alone can contribute to loss of lean body mass. Exercise promotes retention and improvement in lean body mass while using fat stores for energy needs as long as carbohydrate intake is not increased. Guidelines for effective weight loss can be found in Box 8-3.

Exercise is the most powerful tool for weight loss. Aerobic exercise

---

Box 8-3   Guidelines for Effective Weight Loss

• Focus on a feeling of well-being and not just appearance.
• Identify a realistic weight goal.
• Weight loss is a long-term process; setbacks can occur.
• Periodic indulgences can avoid feelings of deprivation.
• Weight management requires an attitude and behavior change and not a quick-fix diet.
• Exercise and diet modifications should be individualized to meet the patient's lifestyle and preferences.

promotes cardiovascular benefits as well. Exercise should be started gradually and only after approval of the primary care provider. Endurance will improve over time. Any activity is better than none. Ideally, exercise should be 20 to 30 minutes per day and can be divided into 10- to 15-minute periods throughout the day. Benefits of exercise include the following:

- Energy is expended with activity.
- Muscle mass is maintained and fat is used for energy.
- Basal metabolic rate is increased with exercise and remains elevated for 12 hours after the workout is completed.
- Physical exertion is a great stress reliever.
- Firming muscles through exercise improves the appearance.

Health care professionals should remind patients that weight loss occurs proportionally and not just where they notice the fat (i.e., hips, thighs, upper arm, and abdomen).

Health care professionals should stress the following when discussing weight loss with patients:

- A variety of foods should be consumed to provide proper nutrients and prevent taste fatigue.
- Encourage intake of fruits, vegetables, and whole-grain products.
- Portion control is vital.
- Reduce intake of fats by:
  Consuming lean meats, poultry, and fish
  Preparing foods by baking, broiling, or poaching
  Using low-fat or fat-free substitutes (but watch calorie content!)
  Using oils and fats in moderation
  Reading food labels to identify calorie and fat content
- Consume alcohol in moderation (alcohol stimulates the appetite and provides non-nutritional calories).
- Consult a Registered Dietitian for assistance in developing an individualized meal plan.

Estimating the number of calories a patient needs to promote weight loss involves intuition and guesswork. The number depends on the size, age, gender, and activity level of the person involved. A quick and easy method for estimating the number of calories needed for weight loss is to allow 20 calories per kilogram of actual body weight. Typical weight-loss calorie levels are 1200 calories for women and 1800 calories for men. However, the appropriateness of the calorie level chosen needs to be evaluated according to weight loss achieved and patient tolerance. Too restrictive a calorie level can be difficult to follow and discourage long-term adherence needed for effective weight loss.

For any weight-loss program to be successful, the patient and health care professional must set realistic goals. The following guidelines should be considered:

- Weight-loss goals should be set in increments.
- Allow gradual weight loss of one half to 1 lb a week.
- Celebrate achievement of incremental goals.
- Set calorie level within reasonable limits.
- Adjust calorie level to maintain compliance.
- Gradual calorie reduction may improve compliance.
- Moderation, not exclusion, of favorite high-fat foods is the key to compliance.
- Encourage exercise.
- Any activity is better than none.
- Encourage exercise program based on patient's preference and endurance.
- Gradually increase intensity and length of time of exercise.

Support from health care professionals, family members, and friends is critical for weight reduction to be effective. There are many saboteurs who will try to impede weight-loss success. Health care professionals should provide encouragement and positive feedback to their patients who are struggling with this difficult assignment.

Pharmacologic agents discussed in this chapter include phenylpropanolamine and benzocaine, liquid diets, chromium, and other "natural" products.

PHENYLPROPANOLAMINE AND BENZOCAINE

Pharmacology

The brain centers that control appetite are located in the hypothalamus. There appears to be an appetite control center and "satiety center." It is believed that the satiety center normally turns the appetite center off after food is ingested. The ventral noradrenergic bundle is a group of nerve fibers that controls the satiety center. Amphetamines are believed to suppress appetite by stimulating the ventral noradrenergic bundle. Phenylpropanolamine is a chemical cousin to amphetamines and may reduce appetite by the same mechanism. Benzocaine is a local anesthetic. The mechanism by which it causes weight reduction is unknown, however it is not the result of a local anesthetic effect in the oral cavity.

Side Effects

Phenylpropanolamine can stimulate the nervous system, causing nervousness, restlessness, insomnia, dizziness, and anxiety. If taken in excess, increased blood pressure and cardiac stimulation can occur. Phenylpropanolamine may increase blood glucose levels. Intracranial hemorrhage has rarely been associated with excessive doses and/or prolonged use. Patients with diabetes, heart disease, or untreated hyperthyroidism should be evaluated before taking phenylpropanolamine-containing products. Benzocaine is relatively free from side effects, except for the possibility of allergic reactions in patients sensitive to benzocaine or lidocaine.

Drug Interactions

Products containing phenylpropanolamine should **never** be taken by patients concurrently taking MAO inhibitors (Nardil, Parnate) because a hypertensive crisis can occur. Phenylpropanolamine also has additive effects with other sympathomimetics.

Lifespan Considerations

Geriatric

Phenylpropanolamine-containing products should be used cautiously in older patients because they often have diseases that relatively contraindicate their use. Hypertension, heart disease, and diabetes are more common in older patients.

Pediatric

These products are not recommended for use in children.

Pregnancy

Studies have not demonstrated an increased risk of birth defects among babies born to women who took phenylpropanolamine during pregnancy. No animal teratology studies have been published. Phenylpropanolamine is unlikely to pose serious teratogenic risk but the data are insufficient to state that there is no risk. Benzocaine products have not been studied, so their use should be avoided by pregnant women.

Nursing Mothers

There is no information available regarding the distribution of phenylpropanolamine or oral benzocaine products in breast milk. These products should not be used while nursing.

Patient Education

- These products will not magically cause weight loss. Patients should not be swayed by the many testimonials regarding these products. Diet and exercise can affect weight loss independent of weight-loss products.
- Weight loss requires burning more calories than one takes in. Effective weight loss is not easy.

Product Selection

- The efficacy of these products is difficult to assess given the lack of well-controlled scientific studies.
- These products are intended for short-term use (less than 3 months) during which time patients needs to make significant changes in their eating habits and lifestyle.
- These products are sold as a number of formulations, including those with caffeine, vitamin C, and other assorted vitamins. There is insufficient evidence to support the added benefit of these additional ingredients. An appropriate diet should include enough variety of foods to provide essential vitamins and nutrients.

LIQUID DIETS

Pharmacology

Most liquid diets contain protein, carbohydrates, nutrients, and vitamins and are intended to replace food that would contain more calories. A typical liquid diet provides approximately 900 calories daily, which is sufficient to cause weight loss in most individuals. Liquid diets do not contain appetite suppressants.

Side Effects

Short-term use is not associated with significant side effects in most patients. Patients with renal insufficiency should be monitored because of the protein content of the liquid. Diabetic patients may require adjustment of oral medications or insulin if they use these products. Long-term use has been associated with cholecystitis.

Drug Interactions

Little data is available on any possible drug interactions with liquid diets.

Lifespan Considerations

Geriatric

Liquid diets should not be used in older patients until a complete physical assessment has been conducted.

Pediatric

These products should not be used by children unless the benefits clearly outweigh any risks involved.

Pregnancy

Pregnant women require additional nutrients that may not be supplied by these products. Weight maintenance rather than weight reduction is the goal in pregnant patients.

Nursing Mothers

Nursing mothers may require additional nutrients not supplied in sufficient amounts by these products. The desire to lose weight must be balanced with the intake of sufficient nutrients for mother and infant.

Patient Education/Product Selection

- Liquid diets replace food that would otherwise be ingested. A flaw with these products is that they do not encourage long-term changes in eating habits.
- To be effective, these products must replace meals that have a higher number of calories. If they are taken in addition to food, they may actually cause weight gain.
- A reasonable approach to the use of these products might entail replacement of breakfast and lunch with these products, followed by an appropriate dinner meal.

CHROMIUM

Chromium is marketed as a natural product and not as a drug. There are limited data regarding the safety and efficacy of chromium products.

Pharmacology

It is claimed that the lack of chromium in the diet causes inefficient action of insulin, leading to inefficient carbohydrate metabolism, which in turn results in the storage of fat. Chromium-containing products claim to improve insulin activity and decrease fat storage. In addition, it is claimed that chromium deficiency, with the resultant insulin inefficiency, causes reduced glucose levels in the brain. Sensing this, the appetite control center is stimulated, creating a "false hunger." It is known that chromium is involved in insulin function, however its significance in the nondiabetic patient is not known.

Side Effects

Widespread use of chromium has not been associated with significant reported side effects. Patients with renal insufficiency might tend to accumulate chromium.

Drug Interactions

There are probably no significant drug interactions, but available information is insufficient to make a definitive statement.

Lifespan Considerations

Geriatric

Information on the use of chromium in the elderly is insufficient to make a recommendation.

Pediatric

Information on the use of chromium in children is insufficient to make a recommendation.

Patient Education/Product Selection

- More is unknown about chromium than is known. Many claims are made regarding the benefits of this mineral, including benefits in diabetic patients and enhancing of the immune system. At this point, scientific evidence is lacking.
- Many chromium-containing, natural weight-loss products contain other "natural" ingredients. The efficacy of these substances is unproved.

OTHER "NATURAL PRODUCTS"

Many "natural" products are promoted as aids to weight reduction (among their many other claims). Because they are promoted as "natural products" and "food supplements," the FDA has no jurisdiction over such products. Most of the information contained in this section constitutes product claims. Conclusive scientific evidence as to their effectiveness is lacking. Sound scientific data regarding these products are lacking. The following is a list of common "natural" products promoted as aids to weight reduction:

- **Garcinia cambogia:** Said to decrease sugar cravings and to interrupt the Krebs Cycle, an important step in the body's fat-storage process.
- **Guarana:** Contains chemicals similar to caffeine and theophylline. Claimed to raise the metabolic rate, causing more calories to be burned.
- **Ginger root:** Claimed to be a stimulant.
- **Kola nut:** Contains caffeine and other stimulants. Claimed to increase metabolism.
- **Choline, inositol, betaine, l-carnitine:** Claimed to improve fat metabolism or pull fat out of the tissues.
- **Calcium pyruvate:** Claims to increase metabolism, burn fat, and add lean muscle.
- **Ginseng, gotu kola:** Claim to increase metabolism.
- **Chitomax:** A fiber that claims to bind to fat in the stomach, preventing its absorption.
- **Cinnamon bark:** Claimed to raise metabolism.
- **Ma huang:** Contains ephedrine, which is claimed to boost energy, improve blood circulation, and to stimulate the burning of stored fat.
- **Bladderwrack:** Contains natural iodine, claims to raise metabolic rate.

Side Effects

Information is insufficient to be specific. However, stimulating or thermogenic substances may stimulate the heart and raise blood pressure. Insomnia and nervousness may also occur. Ma huang is a natural source of ephedrine, which is a known CNS stimulant. The FDA has banned ephedrine from OTC drug products because of its side effects and abuse potential.

Drug Interactions

Information is insufficient to be specific. However, stimulants such as ma huang (contains ephedrine), guarana, and kola nut (both contain caffeine and theophylline-type chemicals) could be expected to display additive CNS stimulation when taken with other CNS stimulants such as theophylline or albuterol.

Lifespan Considerations

Geriatric
No specific information is available.

Pediatric
No information is available.

Patient Education/Product Selection

- Products containing thermogenic substances or stimulants should not be taken without professional advice.
- Efficacy information is anecdotal. There is no hard science on which to make product selections.

SUGGESTED READINGS

Alger S et al: Effect of phenylpropanolamine on energy expenditure and weight loss in overweight women, Am J Clin Nutr 57(2):120-126, 1993.

Cerulli J et al: Chromium picolinate toxicity, Ann Pharmacother 32(4):428-431, 1998.

Duyff RL, editor: The American Dietetic Association's complete food and nutrition guide, Minneapolis, 1996, Chromimed Publishing.

Gottschlich MM, Matarese LE, Shronts EP, editors: Nutrition support dietetics core curriculum, ed 2, Silver Spring, Md, 1992, American Society for Parenteral and Enteral Nutrition.

Rushing PA et al: Acute administration of phenylpropanolamine fails to affect resting energy expenditure in men of normal weight, Obes Res 5(5):470-473, 1997.

Ryan DH: Medicating the obese patient, Endocrinol Metab Clin North Am 25(4):989-1004, 1996.

Zelaski CJ: Exercise for weight loss: what are the facts? J Am Diet Assoc 95(12):1414-1417, 1995.

Product Information: Weight Loss

Brand Name	Active Ingredients	Other Ingredients	Comments
Acutrim 16 Hour Timed-release	Phenylpropanolamine 75 mg		
Acutrim Late Day Strength Timed-release	Phenylpropanolamine 75 mg		
Acutrim Maximum Strength Timed-Release	Phenylpropanolamine 75 mg		Immediate release
Appedrine	Phenylpropanolamine 75 mg	Vitamins	
Chitosan-C	Chromium	Chitomax	
Chroma-Slim	Chromium	Ginseng, gotu kola, vitamin B_6	
Citrimax	Chromium	Garcinia cambogia	
Dexatrim Caffeine Free Extended Duration	Phenylpropanolamine 75 mg		
Dexatrim Caffeine Free Plus Vitamins	Phenylpropanolamine 75 mg	Vitamins	
Dexatrim Caffeine Free with Vitamin C Timed-Release	Phenylpropanolamine 75 mg	Vitamin C 180 mg	
Diet System 6	Chromium	Kola nut extract, guarana extract, ginger root, choline, inositol, betaine, l-carnitine, vitamins, and minerals	
Fat Burner	Chromium	Kola nut extract, cinnamon bark, mustard seed, grapefruit rind, l-carnitine	
Fat Burner Drink	Chromium	l-Carnitine, inositol, "herbal energy blend," "micronutrient blend"	No calories

Continued

Product Information: Weight Loss—cont'd

Brand Name	Active Ingredients	Other Ingredients	Comments
Fat Burner Bar	Chromium	Garcinia cambogia, kola nut extract, protein, carbohydrates	130 calories/bar
Mini Slims Timed-Release	Phenylpropanolamine 75 mg		
Permathene-12	Phenylpropanolamine 75 mg		
Permathene-12 with Vitamin C	Phenylpropanolamine 75 mg	Vitamin C 180 mg	
Permathen16 Timed Release	Phenylpropanolamine 75 mg		
Protrim	Phenylpropanolamine 37.5 mg		Immediate release
	Benzocaine 9 mg		
Protrim SR	Phenylpropanolamine 75 mg		
Pyruvate-C	Chromium	Calcium pyruvate	
SeQuester	—	"Special" fiber mixture	
SlimFast Powder	—	Protein, carbohydrates, vitamins	190 calories with 8 oz skim milk
SlimFast Breakfast and Lunch bar	—	Protein, carbohydrates, vitamins	150 calories/bar
Super Odrinex	Phenylpropanolamine 25 mg		Immediate release
Thinz Back-to-Nature Timed-Release	Phenylpropanolamine 75 mg PPA		
Thinz-Span Timed Release	Phenylpropanolamine 75 mg		
Ultra SlimFast powder	—	Protein, carbohydrates, vitamins	200 calories with 8 oz skim milk
Ultra SlimFast Nutritional Snack bar	—	Protein, carbohydrates, vitamins	120 calories/bar

Accidental Poisoning

Accidental poisoning is a problem that is common throughout the world. Ingestion is the most common route of poisoning. The most common products ingested are medications, household items (such as cleaners and disinfectants), and oils/perfumes. Children under the age of 6 years are the most common victims of accidental poisonings. When an item is ingested, it is vital that it be identified, if possible, before an OTC antidote is used or the nearest poison control center is called.

Nonprescription drugs used to treat poisonings are syrup of ipecac and activated charcoal.

SYRUP OF IPECAC

Pharmacology

Syrup of ipecac is used to induce vomiting when an overdose or poisoning occurs. Syrup of ipecac causes vomiting by several mechanisms. It has a local irritating effect on the gastrointestinal tract and stimulates the chemoreceptor trigger zone (CTZ) in the brain. Ipecac syrup consists of alkaloids, mainly emetine and cephaline. These two alkaloids are responsible for ipecac's activity on the CTZ. Ipecac's main use is in the treatment of drug overdose/poisonings.

Side Effects

Syrup of ipecac causes minimal systemic toxicity if the recommended doses are not exceeded. If vomiting does not occur after the recommended doses are administered, systemic absorption of emetine may occur, resulting in protracted vomiting, diarrhea, and drowsiness/mild CNS depression.

Drug Interactions

Activated charcoal will adsorb ipecac syrup. However, these two products are commonly used together. If both products are to be used in a case of poisoning, activated charcoal should be used after vomiting has been initiated with the ipecac.

Lifespan Considerations

Geriatric

There are no unique recommendations for the elderly population.

Pediatric

In young children, emetic effects can be induced more quickly by gently bouncing the child. If the child is frightened, giving liquid before the administration of syrup of ipecac may be helpful.

Pregnancy

Syrup of ipecac is an FDA Pregnancy Category C drug. Minimal systemic absorption is expected with its use. In a poisoning situation in which use of ipecac is appropriate, the benefits of reducing absorption of the toxic substance must be weighed against the remote possibility of fetal harm.

Nursing Mothers

It is not known whether syrup of ipecac is excreted in breast milk. Caution should be exercised if ipecac is to be used in a nursing mother.

Patient Education

- Although emesis is usually recommended after suspected drug overdose or ingestion of most chemicals, there are situations in which ipecac should not be used, including the following:
  1. When a corrosive poison has been ingested, such as strong acid or strong alkaline substances (e.g., drain cleaner).
  2. When the patient is comatose or delirious, because vomiting may cause aspiration in these patients.
  3. When the patient has ingested a CNS-stimulant, because vomiting could cause convulsions.
  4. When the patient has ingested a product containing a petroleum-based chemical, such as kerosene, gasoline, or solvents. If these substances are aspirated, severe lung damage can occur.

- If a poisoning or overdose is suspected, call 911 and then promptly obtain a detailed history concerning the poisoning/overdose, including the name of the product ingested, the amount, time since ingestion, symptoms, and any prior treatment attempted. Call the nearest poison control center immediately.
- The recommended doses for each age group should be followed. If vomiting does not occur after 30 to 45 minutes, gastric lavage may be necessary.
- After emesis has occurred, patients should not eat or drink for at least 2 hours. Ipecac will continue to work as long as something is in the stomach.
- Ipecac is sometimes abused by anorexics and bulimics.
- Every home should have a 30-ml bottle of ipecac in case of accidental overdose or poisoning; this product should be kept safely out of children's reach.

ACTIVATED CHARCOAL

Pharmacology

Charcoal acts as an adsorbent by forming a barrier between particulate material (e.g., the drug or poison) and the gastrointestinal mucosa, preventing further absorption of the drug or chemical ingested. To be maximally effective, the charcoal particles must be small, increasing the surface area on which to adsorb the chemical. Commercially available products have 12.5 g to 50 g of activated charcoal in water and/or sorbitol. Sorbitol is added to increase palatability and to decrease gastrointestinal transit time (sorbitol has a laxative effect).

Side Effects

Constipation can occur after taking aqueous solutions; sorbitol-containing products may cause diarrhea, vomiting, and dehydration.

Drug Interactions

Activated charcoal will adsorb ipecac. However, these products are commonly used together. If both products are to be used, activated charcoal should be administered after vomiting has been initiated. *Activated charcoal may reduce absorption of many prescription and nonprescription medications.*

Lifespan Considerations

Geriatric

There are no unique recommendations for the elderly population.

Pediatric

Controversy exists as to whether infants should be given activated charcoal. A local emergency medical facility or poison control center should be consulted for more information.

Pregnancy and Nursing Mothers

Activated charcoal is not absorbed into the bloodstream. It is safe for use in pregnant and nursing women.

Patient Education

- If a poisoning or overdose is suspected, call 911 and then promptly obtain a detailed history concerning the poisoning or overdose, including the name of the product ingested, the amount, time since ingestion, symptoms, and any prior treatment attempted. The nearest poison control center should be called immediately.
- Activated charcoal is ineffective for overdoses or poisonings of mineral acids, alkalies, or cyanide. For a list of agents against which activated charcoal may be useful, contact the local poison control center.
- Activated charcoal should be administered only to conscious individuals.
- Activated charcoal adsorbs gases from the air and should be stored in closed containers.
- When used in combination with gastric lavage, activated charcoal should be used without sorbitol.
- Milk, ice cream, and sherbet decrease the adsorbing capacity of activated charcoal. Do not administer with activated charcoal.
- Activated charcoal is commercially available as ready-to-use suspensions or as a powder that must be mixed with water before administration.

Product Selection

Poisoning is a medical emergency. Every household should have both syrup of ipecac and activated charcoal available. However, medical advice from a poison control center should be sought immediately after the poisoning.

SUGGESTED READING

Larsen LC, Cummings DM: Oral poisonings: guidelines for initial evaluation and treatment, *Am Fam Phys* 57(1):85-92, 1998.

Product Information: Accidental Poisoning

Brand Name	Ingredient	Adult Dose	Pediatric Dose	Comments
Acitdose-Aqua	Activated charcoal (liquid)	25-100 g or 1g/kg or approximately 10 times the amount of poison ingested, as a suspension (4-8 oz of water)		Administer within 30 minutes after ingestion of poison, if possible
Actidose with Sorbitol	Activated charcoal (liquid)	25-100 g or 1 g/kg or approximately 10 times the amount of poison ingested, as a suspension (4-8 oz of water)		Administer within 30 minutes after ingestion of poison, if possible
CharcoAid	Activated charcoal (suspension)	25-100 g or 1g/kg or approximately 10 times the amount of poison ingested, as a suspension (4-8 oz of water)		Administer within 30 minutes after ingestion of poison, if possible

CharcoAid 2000	Activated charcoal (liquid and granules)	25-100 g or 1g/kg or approximately 10 times the amount of poison ingested, as a suspension (4-8 oz of water)	Administer within 30 minutes after ingestion of poison, if possible
Ipecac Syrup	Ipecac (syrup)	15-30 ml followed by 3-4 glasses of water; give an additional 15 ml if vomiting has not occurred after 20 minutes	*Infants <1 year:* **Under medical supervision only.** 5-10 ml, followed by ½ to 1 glass of water *1-12 years:* 15 ml, followed by 1-2 glasses of water; give an additional 15 ml if vomiting has not occurred after 20 minutes (in patients >1 year) / If vomiting does not occur within 30-45 minutes after second dose, gastric lavage may be necessary
Liqui-Char	Activated charcoal (liquid)	25-100 g or 1g/kg or approximately 10 times the amount of poison ingested, as a suspension (4-8 oz of water)	Administer within 30 minutes after ingestion of poison, if possible

External Analgesics

External analgesics should be considered to be adjuncts in the management of pain. None of these agents treat the underlying cause of the pain but rather disguise the pain or block the ability of the body to process the pain sensation. External analgesics (with the exception of capsaicin) are intended for short-term use.

Drugs used for external analgesia are counterirritants and salicylates.

COUNTERIRRITANTS

CAMPHOR
CAPSAICIN
CAPSICUM OLEORESIN
EUCALYPTUS OIL
MENTHOL
METHYL NICOTINATE
METHYL SALICYLATE
MUSTARD OIL
TURPENTINE OIL

Pharmacology

Counterirritants produce superficial irritation or a sensation of warmth or cold in the areas where they are applied. One explanation for the effectiveness of topical analgesics is based on the theory that the intense stimulation of nerve endings in the skin floods the brain with so many impulses that the deeper, visceral pain impulses are crowded out or modified so they are not translated into pain sensations. The exact mechanism of action is unknown.

Capsaicin has a small counterirritant effect but works mainly by depleting substance-P in peripheral nerve fibers. Repeated application of capsaicin causes depletion of substance-P, blocking the ability of the nerve fiber to transmit nerve impulses to the pain center in the brain.

Side Effects

Patients with sensitive skin may experience more local irritation with the application of counterirritant preparations.

Drug Interactions

There is a possible drug interaction between methyl salicylate and warfarin. It is theoretically possible to absorb sufficient salicylate to interact with warfarin, which could cause increased bleeding tendency. However, this has little clinical significance.

Lifespan Considerations

Geriatric

There are no unique recommendations for use in the elderly population.

Pediatric

Use in children under the age of 2 years requires monitoring by a health care professional.

Pregnancy

Camphor is an FDA Pregnancy Category C drug. Animal studies have demonstrated possible effects on the fetus, but there are no adequate studies in humans. There are no data available for the remaining counterirritants. Pregnant women should consult a health care professional before self-administration of counterirritant preparations.

Nursing Mothers

There are no data available in this population.

Patient Education

- Nonpharmacologic methods of producing counterirritation may be used as well. These methods include massage and application of heat. Patients should be advised to avoid using a counterirritant preparation and heat concomitantly because skin necrosis, burning, or blistering may occur.
- These products are for external use only. Patients should be advised not to use these preparations on mucous membranes or around the eyes.
- These products should not be applied to damaged skin or open wounds.
- Hands should be thoroughly washed after application of the products to prevent accidental contact with the eyes.
- Avoid the use of tight, occlusive dressings after application because this may lead to increased redness and irritation.
- Most of these products are toxic if ingested.

- Patients should be advised to use these products no more than 3 or 4 times per day.
- Patients should contact a health care professional for pain persisting more than 7 days or worsening pain.

Product Selection

- The most potent counterirritant preparations include capsaicin, capsicum, mustard oil, and methyl salicylate. These products may cause irritation and redness.
- Menthol and camphor preparations cause a cooling sensation.
- Capsaicin products provide excellent pain relief and are particularly useful for joint pain. However, 2 to 3 weeks of daily use is required to deplete substance-P. The patient must be educated regarding interim pain relief.

Product Information: External Analgesics (Counterirritants)

Brand Name*	Counterirritant
Absorbine Arthritis Strength	4% menthol, capsaicin .025%
Absorbine Jr. Extra Strength	4% menthol
Absorbine Jr. Liniment	1.27% menthol
Analgesic Balm	Methyl salicylate, menthol
Argesic Cream	Methyl salicylate
Arthricare Cream	1.25% menthol, capsaicin 0.25%, methyl nicotinate .25%
ArthriCare Rub Odor Free	0.25% methyl nicotinate, 1.25% menthol, 0.025% capsaicin
Arthricare Triple Medicated Gel	30% methyl salicylate, menthol 1.25%, 0.7% methyl nicotinate
Arthricare Ultra Cream	2% menthol, capsaicin 0.075%
Arthritis Hot Crème	15% methyl salicylate, 10% menthol
Banalg Hospital Strength Lotion	14% methyl salicylate, 3% menthol
Banalg Lotion	14% methyl salicylate, 3% menthol
Ben-Gay Extra Strength Cream	30% methyl salicylate, 8% menthol
Ben-Gay Original Ointment	18.3% methyl salicylate, 16% menthol
Ben-Gay Regular Strength Cream	15% methyl salicylate, 10% menthol
Ben-Gay Ultra Strength Cream	30% methyl salicylate, 10% menthol
Ben-Gay Vanishing Scent Gel	3% menthol, camphor
Betuline Lotion	Methyl salicylate, menthol, camphor
Capzain P Lotion	.025% capsaicin
Capzasin P crème	.025% capsaicin
Deep-Down Rub	15% methyl salicylate, 10% menthol
Dencorub	.025% capsaicin
Dermal-Rub Balm	Methyl salicylate, camphor
Double Ice ArthriCare Gel	4% menthol, 3.1% camphor
Exocaine Medicated Rub	25% methyl salicylate
Exocaine Plus Rub	30% methyl salicylate
Flex-All 454 Gel	Methyl salicylate, menthol, eucalyptus oil
Flex-All 454 Maximum Strength Gel	16% menthol
Flex-All Ultra Plus Gel	16% menthol, 10% methyl salicylate, 3.1% camphor
Gordobalm	Methyl salicylate, menthol, camphor, eucalyptus oil
Gordogesic Crème	10% methyl salicylate
Heet Liniment	15% methyl salicylate, 3.6% camphor, capsicum oleoresin
Icy Hot Balm	29% methyl salicylate, 7.6% menthol

*Refer to individual product labeling for application directions.

Product Information: External
Analgesics (Counterirritants)—cont'd

Brand Name*	Counterirritant
Icy Hot Cream	30% methyl salicylate, 10% menthol
Icy Hot Stick	30% methyl salicylate, 10% menthol
InfraRub Cream	35% methyl salicylate, 10% menthol
MenthoRub Ointment	Eucalyptus oil, turpentine oil, menthol, camphor
Methagual	8% methyl salicylate
Methalgen Cream	Methyl salicylate, menthol, camphor
Minit-Rub	15% methyl salicylate, 3.5% menthol, 2.3% camphor
Muscle Rub Ointment	15% methyl salicylate, 10% menthol
Musterole Deep Strength Rub	30% methyl salicylate, 3% menthol, 0.5% methyl nicotinate
Musterole Extra Strength	Methyl salicylate, 3% menthol, 5% camphor
Panalgesic Gold Liniment	55% methyl salicylate, 1.25% menthol, 3.1% camphor
Sloan's Liniment	0.025% capsaicin, turpentine oil
Soltice Quick-Rub	Methyl salicylate, menthol camphor
Sports Spray	3.5% methyl salicylate, 10% menthol, 5% camphor
Theragesic Cream	15% methyl salicylate, menthol
Therapeutic Mineral Ice Exercise Formula Gel	4% menthol
Vicks VapoRub	2.6% menthol, 4.7% camphor, eucalyptus oil
Wonder Ice Gel	5.25% menthol
Zostrix	0.025% capsaicin
Zostrix-HP	0.075% capsaicin

SALICYLATES

Trolamine salicylate

Pharmacology

The mechanism of action of trolamine salicylate as an external analgesic is not clearly understood. Trolamine salicylate is most likely absorbed into the affected area, where it inhibits synthesis of pain-sensitizing prostaglandins.

Side Effects

Salicylates may be irritating to the skin. External application of salicylates to large areas of skin may lead to significant absorption of salicylate, producing salicylate toxicity.

Drug Interactions

It is theoretically possible to systemically absorb salicylate through the skin to interact with warfarin. Interaction could cause increased bleeding tendency. The clinical significance of this interaction is minor.

Lifespan Considerations

Geriatric

There are no unique recommendations for the elderly population.

Pediatric

Use in children under the age of 2 years requires monitoring by a health care professional.

Pregnancy

There is no information concerning trolamine salicylate risk in pregnancy.

Nursing Mothers

There is no information on salicylate absorption or concentrations in breast milk.

Patient Education

- These products are for external use only. Patients should be advised not to use these preparations on mucous membranes or around the eyes.
- These products should not be applied to damaged skin or open wounds.
- Patients should thoroughly wash their hands after application.
- Patients should be advised to use these products no more than 3 or 4 times per day.
- Patients should contact a health care professional for pain persisting for more than 7 days or worsening pain.

SUGGESTED READING

Kuritzky L: Topical analgesics: are they understood? *Hosp Prac* 15:131-132, 1997.

 Product Information: External Analgesics (Salicylates)

Brand Name*	Active Ingredient
Analgesia Creme	10% trolamine salicylate
Aspercreme	10% trolamine salicylate
Sportscreme	10% trolamine salicylate
Exocaine Odor Free Creme	10% trolamine salicylate
Myoflex	10% trolamine salicylate
Mobisyl	10% trolamine salicylate
Aspercreme Rub	10% trolamine salicylate

*Refer to individual product labeling for application directions.

Fever and Internal Pain

Nonprescription analgesics (pain relievers) have antipyretic (fever reducing) and antiinflammatory properties, with the exception of acetaminophen. The reason for these common effects is that they all block local production of prostaglandins. Prostaglandins are involved in numerous physiologic processes, many of which have not been fully elucidated. Prostaglandins of the E,G, and I series are involved in production of pain, fever, and inflammation. The release of prostaglandin E_2 (PGE_2) in the hypothalamus causes the production of fever. PGEs and PGI_2 sensitize nerve endings to painful stimuli. Prostaglandins E_2 and I_2 are involved in edema formation and the inflammatory response. Levels of prostaglandins are elevated in menstrual fluids. These prostaglandins are thought to contract uterine and gastrointestinal smooth muscle and sensitize nerve fibers to pain, contributing to the symptoms of dysmenorrhea.

In response to local injury, prostaglandins are synthesized. Prostaglandins appear to sensitize pain receptors to pain-eliciting stimuli. Oral analgesics, such as acetaminophen, salicylates, and nonsteroidal antiinflammatory drugs (NSAIDs) reduce prostaglandin formation, thus reducing pain.

Body temperature is maintained by a thermoregulatory center located in the hypothalamus. Fever-producing substances, known as *pyrogens*, appear to increase the thermoregulatory setpoint by enhancing the production of prostaglandins. Antipyretic drugs inhibit prostaglandin biosynthesis, reducing fever. Additionally, acetaminophen, ibuprofen, and aspirin increase the dissipation of heat by causing vasodilation and increased peripheral blood flow.

Inflammation is a normal defense mechanism that occurs in response to insult or injury. Unfortunately, inflammation is often counterproductive. Inflammation occurs in response to chemical mediators such as prostaglandins, histamine, bradykinin, leukotrienes, and other substances. Antiinflammatory drugs reduce inflammation at least in part because they block formation of inflammation-producing prostaglandins.

ACETAMINOPHEN

Pharmacology

Acetaminophen may reduce the formation of pain- and fever-producing prostaglandins in the central nervous system (CNS) and in the periphery. Alternatively, it may cause pain receptors to become less sensitive to pain caused by mechanical or chemical stimulation. Unlike aspirin and NSAIDs, acetaminophen lacks clinically significant antiinflammatory properties.

Side Effects

Side effects are minimal at usual doses. The following side effects have been reported, although they are rare: rash, hypersensitivity, and blood dyscrasias (neutropenia, pancytopenia, leukopenia). Long-term daily use can be associated with renal damage and may contribute to liver damage in patients who consume alcohol on a regular basis.

Overdose

Acetaminophen overdose is a medical emergency. Left untreated, overdose can cause potentially fatal hepatic necrosis and renal tubular necrosis. Overdose is usually accidental in children who mistake the chewable tablets or flavored liquids for candy. Overdose is usually intentional in adults. **If overdose is suspected, the patient should be instructed to seek immediate emergency medical treatment at the closest hospital emergency room.** Early diagnosis is vital in the treatment of overdosage with acetaminophen and begins with a plasma acetaminophen level. However, therapy should not be delayed while awaiting laboratory results if the patient's history suggests a significant overdosage. Aggressive supportive therapy is essential when intoxication is severe. Gastric lavage should be performed in all cases, preferably within 4 hours of the ingestion, followed by a loading dose of N-acetylcysteine (Mucomyst). N-acetylcysteine is the specific antidote for acetaminophen poisoning. An oral loading dose of 140 mg/kg is given, followed by the administration of 70 mg/kg every 4 hours for 17 doses. Treatment is terminated if acetaminophen plasma levels indicate that the risk of hepatotoxicity is low. This is determined by comparison of the acetaminophen plasma level with a published nomogram. Assistance in treatment of patients with acetaminophen overdose can be obtained from the Rocky Mountain Poison Center (800-525-6115). Approximately 10% of poisoned patients who do not receive specific treatment develop severe liver damage; of these, 10% to 20% eventually die of hepatic failure. Acute renal failure may occur in some patients.

Drug Interactions

Acetaminophen has few, if any, *clinically significant* drug–drug interactions. Additive hepatotoxicity is possible when acetaminophen is combined with other hepatotoxic drugs and chemicals, such as alcohol, barbiturates, carbamazepine, and phenytoin. Recently an interaction between acetaminophen and warfarin has been reported to cause increased bleeding tendency. This report notwithstanding, acetaminophen remains the safest analgesic/antipyretic for most patients taking oral anticoagulants.

Lifespan Considerations

Geriatric

Acetaminophen is an excellent pain and fever reducer for geriatric patients because it has no significant side effects or drug interactions, and it is well tolerated. It is highly efficacious in the treatment of osteoarthritis and has a better side effect profile than salicylates and NSAIDs.

Pediatric

Acetaminophen is the preferred pain and fever reducer for children because its use is not associated with Reye's syndrome. Reye's syndrome is a rare but serious condition that has been associated with aspirin and NSAIDs given to children with viral illnesses.

Pregnancy

Acetaminophen is an FDA Pregnancy Category B drug. Large epidemiologic studies have failed to demonstrate an increased rate of congenital anomalies among women who took acetaminophen during pregnancy. Acetaminophen is the preferred analgesic for pregnant women.

Nursing Mothers

Low concentrations of acetaminophen are excreted in breast milk but appear to cause no harmful effects to nursing infants. Both the American Academy of Pediatrics and the WHO Working Group on Drugs and Human Lactation consider acetaminophen use by nursing mothers to be safe.

Patient Education

- Use of acetaminophen suppositories should be avoided when possible because absorption is slow and erratic via the rectal route. If suppositories are the only option, they should be administered at a dosage 25% to 50% higher than the oral dose.
- Alcohol consumption should be determined before acetaminophen is recommended for long-term therapy. Alcohol and other hepatotoxic drugs increase the hepatotoxicity of acetaminophen.
- Acetaminophen has little antiinflammatory activity. It may not be as effective in the treatment of rheumatoid arthritis. It may be used to treat the pain associated with osteoarthritis.
- Acetaminophen should be used cautiously in patients with preexisting hepatic disease, renal disease, or anemia.
- Parents of small children should be educated regarding accidental acetaminophen poisoning. They should be instructed to store acetaminophen (and all other drugs) out of the reach of children.
- Adult patients should not exceed 4 g of acetaminophen daily (8 extra-strength tablets or capsules).

Product Selection

- Adult patients unable to swallow tablets or caplets can take Tylenol Extra Strength Adult Liquid Pain Reliever, which contains 500 mg acetaminophen/15 ml.
- Acetaminophen is available in elixir form (contains alcohol) or in aqueous suspension. The suspension form must be shaken before use to ensure equal distribution of the drug in the suspension.
- Patients should be aware of differences in strengths between formulations. Acetaminophen drops contain 100 mg/ml (80 mg/0.8 ml dropperful). Acetaminophen elixir and suspension contain 160 mg/5 ml. Dosing recommendations should be made in milligrams rather than milliliters. This will decrease the risk of underdosing or overdosing patients if the incorrect liquid preparation is purchased.
- Many of the acetaminophen chewable-tablet formulations contain aspartame and should be avoided in patients with phenylketonuria.

SALICYLATES

Pharmacology

Salicylates (i.e., acetylsalicylic acid [aspirin], choline salicylate, magnesium salicylate, and sodium salicylate) reduce pain, fever, and inflammation by decreasing the formation of pain-sensitizing, fever-producing, and inflammation-producing prostaglandins. Salicylates block prostaglandin production by inhibiting cyclooxygenase, the enzyme required for the conversion of arachidonic acid derivatives to prostaglandins. Salicylates may also decrease cramping associated with menstrual pain by blocking the formation of prostaglandins that cause uterine contraction. The ulcerogenic effects of salicylates are caused in large part by their ability to block the formation of gastroprotective prostaglandins. Salicylates also block the formation of vasodilatory prostaglandins that function to augment renal blood flow. As a result, salicylates can cause constriction of renal vasculature, diminished renal blood flow, and decreased renal function. Aspirin, but not the other salicylates, inhibits platelet aggregation by blocking the formation of thromboxane A_2. Aspirin's antiplatelet activity is utilized for the prevention and treatment of transient ischemia attacks (TIAs) and ischemic strokes and is the basis for its cardioprotective effects against myocardial infarction.

Side Effects

Gastrointestinal disturbances (e.g., heartburn and nausea) are the most common side effects of salicylate use. Frequent or excessive use can cause and/or aggravate gastritis and sometimes gastrointestinal bleeding because of the fact that salicylates block the formation of gastroprotective prostaglandins. Allergic reactions are possible. Aspirin intolerance most commonly occurs in patients with chronic urticaria, asthma, or nasal polyps. Diminished renal function secondary to inhibition of renal prostaglandins is possible.

Overdose

Fatality can occur with doses of 200 mg/kg to 500 mg/kg. Early symptoms are CNS stimulation with vomiting, hyperpnea, hyperactivity, and possibly convulsions. This progresses quickly to depression, coma, respiratory failure, and collapse. These symptoms are accompanied by severe electrolyte disturbances.

Treatment of salicylate overdosage requires a hospital setting. Intensive supportive therapy should be instituted immediately. Plasma salicylate levels should be measured to determine the severity of the poisoning and to provide a guide for therapy. Emptying of the stomach should be accomplished as soon as possible with syrup of ipecac unless the patient is unconscious. In unconscious patients, airway-protected gastric lavage should be done. Absorption can be delayed with activated charcoal. Treatment should proceed according to standard protocol.

Drug Interactions

The following drugs may interact with aspirin.

- **Warfarin.** May cause increased bleeding potential, as evidenced by increased INR. Concomitant use of low-dose aspirin (<325 mg/day) and warfarin is relatively safe. Studies have shown only a minor increase in bleeding potential.
- **Lithium.** May cause increased lithium levels because of competition for renal excretion.
- **Valproic acid.** May cause increased valproic acid levels, causing neurologic toxicity.
- **Sulfonylureas, chlorpropamide, tolazamide, tolbutamide, glyburide, glipizide.** May cause increased hypoglycemic effect with large aspirin doses.
- **Methotrexate.** Causes increased methotrexate activity and toxicity.
- **Probenecid.** May antagonize uricosuric effect of probenecid, aggravating gout.
- **Alcohol.** Increased gastrointestinal irritation and increased risk of gastrointestinal bleeding.

Lifespan Considerations

Geriatric

Geriatric patients are at higher risk for development of ulcers secondary to salicylate use and are more sensitive to the renal effects of salicylates. Salicylates should be used cautiously in this group of patients.

Pediatric

Salicylates should not be given to children 18 years and younger who have influenza or other viral illnesses, such as chicken pox. Reye's syndrome, a rare but potentially serious illness, has been associated with aspirin use in these situations. Because it can be difficult to rule out viral illness, acetaminophen is considered the drug of choice for pain and fever relief in the pediatric patient.

Pregnancy

Aspirin is an FDA Pregnancy Category C drug in the first two trimesters but is a category D drug if used in last trimester. It has been reported that adverse effects were increased in the mother and fetus after chronic ingestion of aspirin. Prolonged pregnancy and labor, with increased bleeding before and after delivery, as well as decreased birth weight and increased rate of stillbirth were correlated with high blood-salicylate levels. Because of possible adverse effects on the neonate and the potential for increased maternal blood loss, aspirin use should be avoided during pregnancy.

Nursing Mothers
Aspirin is excreted in breast milk in low concentrations. Because of potential adverse effects in nursing infants, the American Academy of Pediatrics recommends that aspirin should be taken cautiously by nursing mothers.

Patient Education
- Salicylates should be taken with food to minimize gastrointestinal upset.
- Salicylates are highly effective antiinflammatory agents; however, the large doses required for this indication cannot be tolerated by many patients. High-dose salicylate therapy should be done only under close medical supervision.
- Salicylates should not be used in patients who have previously exhibited hypersensitivity to aspirin and/or NSAIDs. Aspirin should be administered cautiously to patients with asthma, nasal polyps, or nasal allergies.
- Aspirin should not be given to patients with a recent history of gastrointestinal bleeding, patients with bleeding disorders (e.g., hemophilia), or patients taking oral anticoagulants (warfarin) because aspirin inhibits platelet aggregation. Note: Low-dose aspirin (<325 mg/day) can be administered to warfarinized patients with low risk for bleeding. Bleeding risk increases with larger aspirin doses. Salicylates should be used with caution in patients with severe hepatic damage, preexisting hypoprothrombinemia, or vitamin K deficiency, and in those undergoing surgery.
- Salicylates should be used cautiously in patients with decreased renal function, decreased hepatic function, ulcer disease, or bleeding disorders.
- Large doses of salicylates produce a hypoglycemic effect and may enhance the effect of the oral hypoglycemics. If concomitant use is necessary, the dosage of the hypoglycemic agent may need to be reduced while the salicylate is given. This hypoglycemic action may also affect the insulin requirements of diabetics.
- Low-dose aspirin may aggravate gout. Salicylates in large doses are uricosuric agents; smaller amounts may decrease the uricosuric effects of probenecid, sulfinpyrazone, and phenylbutazone.
- Patients receiving large doses of aspirin and/or prolonged therapy may

develop mild salicylate intoxication (salicylism), requiring a dosage reduction. Tinnitus (ringing in the ears) is an early sign of salicylate toxicity.

- Occult gastrointestinal bleeding occurs in some patients. The amount of blood lost is usually clinically insignificant, but with prolonged administration, iron-deficiency anemia may result.

Product Selection

- Enteric-coated formulations cause less gastrointestinal irritation because the aspirin is released in the alkaline environment of the intestine rather than in the stomach. Although fecal blood loss with enteric-coated aspirin is less than that with uncoated aspirin tablets, enteric-coated aspirin tablets should be administered with caution to patients with a history of gastric distress, ulcer, or bleeding problems.
- The buffered product formulations may reduce gastric irritation. These formulations may contain magnesium hydroxide, aluminum hydroxide, calcium carbonate, magnesium oxide, or magnesium carbonate as buffering agents.
- The effervescent product formulations are absorbed more rapidly.
- Choline salicylate, magnesium salicylate, and sodium salicylate are less effective than equivalent doses of aspirin in reducing pain and fever, but might be better tolerated than aspirin in some patients. As a practical matter, patients intolerant of the gastrointestinal effects of aspirin are usually treated with acetaminophen, enteric-coated aspirin, NSAIDs, or prescription products.
- Salicylates may be superior to acetaminophen for treatment of menstrual pain because they block formation of prostaglandins involved in uterine contraction. Thus they may help relieve the "cramping" associated with menstruation.

NSAIDs

Nonsteroidal antiinflammatory drugs (NSAIDs) were developed in an effort to produce products with the potent antiinflammatory actions of high-dose aspirin without the gastrointestinal side effects. NSAIDs have analgesic, antipyretic, and antiinflammatory activity similar to aspirin but cause less gastrointestinal irritation than equivalent antiinflammatory aspirin doses. Like salicylates, NSAIDs inhibit cyclooxygenase and reduce prostaglandin formation, including formation of gastroprotective prostaglandins and those augmenting renal blood flow. Nonprescription NSAIDs include ibuprofen, naproxen, and ketoprofen.

Side Effects

Gastrointestinal side effects (e.g., heartburn and nausea) are the most common side effects. Frequent and/or excessive use can aggravate and/or cause gastritis and sometimes gastrointestinal bleeding because NSAIDs block the formation of gastroprotective prostaglandins. Allergic reactions are possible in patients with aspirin allergy. Diminished renal function secondary to inhibition of renal prostaglandins is possible but more problematic with regular use of prescription-strength doses. NSAIDs also inhibit platelet aggregation, but to a lesser degree than aspirin.

Drug Interactions

There are case reports of drug interactions similar to those reported with aspirin. However, it is obvious given the small number of such reports, that these interactions are insignificant in most cases. The following drugs may interact with NSAIDs:

- **Warfarin.** May cause increased bleeding potential, demonstrated by an increased INR.
- **Lithium.** May increase lithium levels because of competition for renal excretion.
- **Valproic acid.** May increase valproic acid levels, causing neurologic toxicity.
- **Methotrexate.** Increased methotrexate activity and toxicity.
- **Alcohol.** Increased gastrointestinal irritation and risk of gastro-intestinal bleeding.

Lifespan Considerations

Geriatric

NSAIDs should not be recommended for routine use by elderly patients. These patients must be appropriately screened and monitored to avoid adverse effects. Gastritis and NSAID-induced ulcers are particularly common in the older patient. NSAIDs may precipitate renal failure in some patients due to inhibition of renal vasodilatory prostaglandins.

Pediatric

NSAIDs should not be given to children age 18 and younger who have influenza or other viral illnesses, such as chicken pox. Reye's syndrome, a rare but potentially serious illness, been associated with use of aspirin and NSAIDs in these situations. Acetaminophen is considered the drug of choice in the pediatric patient until viral illness is ruled out.

Pregnancy

Ibuprofen, naproxen, and ketoprofen are FDA Pregnancy Category B drugs but are category D drugs if used in the third trimester. Epidemiologic studies have failed to demonstrate an increased risk of congenital anomalies in women taking ibuprofen during the first trimester of pregnancy. There are no epidemiologic studies involving pregnant women taking naproxen or ketoprofen. Animal studies have not demonstrated increased risk during pregnancy.

Prostaglandins are involved in uterine contraction and closure of the ductus arteriosis. NSAIDs may delay labor and/or cause premature closure of the ductus arteriosis if taken late in pregnancy. For this reason, their use should be avoided late in pregnancy.

Nursing Mothers

The American Academy of Pediatrics considers ibuprofen to be safe to use while nursing. The American Academy of Pediatrics and the WHO Working Group on Drugs and Human Lactation consider naproxen to be safe for use while nursing.

Patient Education

- NSAIDs should be taken with food to minimize gastrointestinal side effects.
- Nonprescription NSAID products are sold for relief of occasional pain and/or fever. They are not intended for long-term treatment of chronic pain or inflammation.
- Ibuprofen should be recommended for fevers unresponsive to acetaminophen. It may be more effective in pediatric patients with a temperature above 39° C.
- Antiinflammatory therapy should be conducted only under proper medical supervision because the incidence of adverse effects is significant. From a practical standpoint, the larger antiinflammatory doses of these agents would require multiple tablets of the nonprescription products, making them inconvenient and more costly than higher-strength prescription doses.
- NSAIDS should be used cautiously in patients with decreased renal function, decreased hepatic function, peptic ulcer disease, congestive heart failure, or who are receiving anticoagulants.
- Ibuprofen suspension must be avoided when viral infections or chicken pox cannot be ruled out because of the risk of Reye's syndrome.

General Patient Education

- Adults with fever persisting for more than 5 days should be instructed to contact a health care professional.
- Parents of febrile children should be instructed to contact a health care professional in any of the following situations:
  1. Infants under the age of 6 months with a fever
  2. Children with a temperature greater than 104° F
  3. Children with fever persisting for more than 72 hours
  4. Children with persistent fevers associated with headache, back pain, stiff neck, mental status changes, lethargy, or petechiae
  5. Children with a previous history of febrile seizures
- Fever is a source of discomfort. Removing excess clothing or blankets may help to make patients more comfortable.
- For a body temperature greater than 104° F, external cooling by body sponging with tepid water will increase evaporation and promote heat loss. Alternatively, cool cloths may be placed on the trunk or legs to help lower the body temperature.
- Body temperature should be reassessed approximately 1 hour after the administration of an antipyretic to determine the drug's effectiveness. Reassessment can be made by rechecking the body temperature or by assessing the behavior/discomfort level of the patient.
- Patients should be encouraged to maintain adequate hydration to compensate for the increase in insensible fluid loss.
- There is currently no recommended alternating drug regimen. Health care professionals have different preferences, so patients should consult their health care professional before taking regularly scheduled alternate drugs.

Product Selection

- Ibuprofen suspension has an advantage over acetaminophen in that its duration of action is longer. Ibuprofen suspension is dosed every 6 to 8 hours compared with acetaminophen elixir/suspension, which is dosed every 4 to 6 hours. This avoids the necessity of waking a sleeping child for a dose.
- NSAIDs are probably superior to acetaminophen for treatment of menstrual pain because they block formation of prostaglandins involved in uterine contraction. Thus they may help relieve the "cramping" associated with menstruation.

SUGGESTED READINGS

Amadio Jr. P, Cummings DM, Amadio PB: NSAIDs revisited: selection, monitoring, and safe use, *Postgrad Med* 101(2):257-260, 1997.

Dinarello CA: Thermoregulation and the pathogenesis of fever, *Infect Dis Clin North Am* 10(2):433-449, 1996.

Greenspan JD: Nociceptors and the peripheral nervous system's role in pain, *J Hand Ther* 10(2):257-260.

Ling SM, Bathon JM: Osteoarthritis in older adults, *J Am Geriatr Soc* 46(2):216-225, 1998.

Markenson JA: Mechanisms of chronic pain, *Am J Med* 101(1A):6S-18S, 1996.

Rowsey PJ: Pathophysiology of fever. I. The role of cytokines, *Dimens Crit Care Nurs* 16(4):202-207, 1997.

Rowsey PJ: Pathophysiology of fever. II. Relooking at cooling interventions, *Dimens Crit Care Nurs* 16(5):251-256, 1997.

Product Information: Acetaminophen

Brand Name*	Dose	Other Ingredients	Comments
Anacin Maximum Strength Aspirin Free	500 mg		
Anacin P.M. Aspirin Free	500 mg	Diphenhydramine 25 mg	Diphenhydramine causes drowsiness; marketed for pain relief and sleeplessness
Arthritis Foundation Aspirin Free	500 mg		Enteric coated
Backaid	1000 mg	Pamabrom 50 mg	Efficacy of pamabrom questionable
Bayer Select Maximum Strength Headache Pain Relief Formula	500 mg	Caffeine 65 mg	Caffeine may potentiate the analgesic effect of acetaminophen
Bayer Select Maximum Strength Night Time Pain Relief Formula	500 mg	Diphenhydramine 25 mg	Diphenhydramine causes drowsiness; marketed for pain relief and sleeplessness
Bayer Select Maximum Strength Sinus Pain Relief	500 mg	Pseudoephedrine 30 mg	Nasal decongestant (pseudoephedrine) added to relieve sinus pressure
Bayer Select Menstrual Maximum Strength Multisymptom Formula	500 mg	Pamabrom 25 mg	Pamabrom is a weak diuretic promoted for relief of water retention and bloated feeling; benefit questionable
Bromo-Seltzer	325 mg		Effervescent

*Adult dose: 325 mg to 650 mg every 4-6 hours, or 1000 mg every 6-8 hours. Maximum 4 g/day. Children's dose: 10 mg to 15 mg/kg/dose every 4-6 hrs. Do not exceed 5 doses in 24 hours.

Continued

Product Information: Acetaminophen

Brand Name*	Dose	Other Ingredients	Comments
Congespirin For Children	81 mg	Phenylephrine 1.25 mg	Nasal decongestant (phenylephrine) added to relieve sinus pressure; chewable
Excedrin AF Dual	500 mg	Calcium carbonate 111 mg; magnesium carbonate 64 mg; magnesium oxide 30 mg	Antacids added to formulation; reasoning for this combination not clear
Excedrin Aspirin Free	500 mg	Caffeine 65 mg	Caffeine may potentiate the analgesic effect of acetaminophen
Excedrin Extra Strength	250 mg	Caffeine 65 mg	Caffeine may potentiate the analgesic effect of acetaminophen and aspirin
Excedrin Migraine	250 mg	Caffeine 65 mg	Caffeine may potentiate the analgesic effect of acetaminophen and aspirin
Excedrin PM Aspirin-Free	500 mg	Diphenhydramine 38 mg	Diphenhydramine added to cause drowsiness; marketed for pain relief and sleeplessness
Excedrin Sinus	500 mg	Pseudoephedrine 30 mg	Decongestant (pseudoephedrine) added to relieve sinus pressure
Feverall Junior Strength Suppository	80 g, 120 mg, 325 mg		Because rectal absorption of acetaminophen is erratic, doses 25% to 50% larger than the oral dose should be administered
Liquiprin Infant's Drops	48 mg/ml		Includes calibrated dropper; shake before using
Midol Menstrual Maximum Strength Multisymptom Formula	500 mg	Caffeine 60 mg, pyrilamine 15 mg	Caffeine and pyrilamine may potentiate the analgesic effect of acetaminophen; pyrilamine is a sedating antihistamine

Product	Dose	Ingredients	Notes
Midol Menstrual Regular Strength Multisymptom Formula	325 mg	Pyrilamine 12.5 mg	Pyrilamine may potentiate the analgesic effect of acetaminophen
Midol PM Night Time Formula	500 mg	Diphenhydramine 25 mg	Diphenhydramine causes drowsiness; marketed for relief of pain and sleeplessness
Midol PMS Multisymptom Formula	500 mg	Pamabrom 25 mg; pyrilamine 15 mg	Pamabrom is a weak diuretic purported to relieve water retention and bloated feeling; pyrilamine may potentiate the analgesic effect of acetaminophen
Midol Teen Multisymptom Formula	400 mg	Pamabrom 25 mg	Pamabrom is a weak diuretic purported to relieve water retention and bloated feeling
Mobigesic	400 mg	Magnesium salicylate 325 mg; phenyltoloxamine 30 mg	Phenyltoloxamine is an antihistamine that may potentiate the analgesic effect of acetaminophen
Pamprin Maximum Pain Relief	250 mg	Magnesium salicylate 250 mg; pamabrom 25 mg	Pamabrom is a weak diuretic purported to relieve water retention and bloated feeling
Pamprin Multisymptom Maximum Strength	500 mg	Pamabrom 25 mg; pyrilamine 15 mg	Pyrilamine may potentiate the analgesic effect of acetaminophen; pamabrom is a weak diuretic purported to relieve water retention and bloated feeling
Pamprin PMS	500 mg	Pamabrom 25 mg; pyrilamine 15 mg	Pyrilamine may potentiate the analgesic effect of acetaminophen; pamabrom is a weak diuretic purported to relieve water retention and bloated feeling
Panadol Children's	80 mg		Chewable tablet
Panadol Children's Liquid	32 mg/ml		Includes calibrated dropper
Panadol Junior Strength	160 mg		

Continued

Product Information: Acetaminophen—cont'd

Brand Name*	Dose	Other Ingredients	Comments
Panadol Maximum Strength	500 mg		Includes calibrated dropper
Panadol Infant's drops	80 mg/0.8 ml		
Percogesic	325 mg	Phenyltoloxamine 30 mg	Phenyltoloxamine is an antihistamine that may potentiate the analgesic effect of acetaminophen
Premsyn PMS	500 mg	Pamabrom 25 mg; pyrilamine 15 mg	Pyrilamine may potentiate the analgesic effect of acetaminophen; pamabrom is a weak diuretic purported to relieve water retention and bloated feeling
St. Joseph Aspirin Free for Children	80 mg		
St. Joseph Low Dose Adult Aspirin	81 mg		
Stanback AF Extra Strength	950 mg		
Tempra-1 Drops	80 mg/0.8 ml		Includes calibrated dropper
Tempra-2 Syrup	160 mg/5 ml		
Tempra Quicklets	80 mg		
Tempra-3 Double Strength	160 mg		

Product	Acetaminophen	Other ingredient	Notes
Tylenol Extended Relief	650 mg immediate release; 325 mg continuous release		
Tylenol Extra Strength	500 mg		
Tylenol Extra Strength Adult Pain Reliever Liquid	500 mg/15 ml		
Tylenol Extra Strength Headache Plus	500 mg	Calcium carbonate 250 mg	Calcium carbonate is an antacid; the rationale for the combination is unclear
Tylenol Junior Strength Chewable Tablet	160 mg		Chewable
Tylenol Junior Strength Swallowable	160 mg		
Tylenol Regular Strength	325 mg		
Tylenol Chewable Children's Tablet	80 mg		Cherry or grape flavor
Tylenol Children's Elixir	80 mg/2.5 ml		
Tylenol Children's Suspension	80 mg/2.5 ml		Alcohol free
Tylenol Infant's Drops	80 mg/0.8 ml		
Tylenol Infant's Suspension	80 mg/0.8 ml		Alcohol free

Product Information: Salicylates

Brand Name*	Aspirin	Other Ingredients	Comments
Alka-Seltzer Extra-Strength	500 mg		Effervescent; 588 mg sodium/tablet
Alka-Seltzer Original	325 mg		Effervescent; 567 mg sodium/tablet
Alka-Seltzer PM	325 mg	Diphenhydramine 38 mg	Diphenhydramine may cause drowsiness; marketed for pain relief and sleeplessness
Anacin	400 mg	Caffeine 32 mg	Caffeine may potentiate the analgesic effect of aspirin
Anacin Maximum Strength	500 mg	Caffeine 32 mg	Caffeine may potentiate the analgesic effect of aspirin
Arthritis Foundation Safety Coated Aspirin	500 mg		
Arthritis Pain Formula	500 mg		
Arthropan		Choline salicylate 174 mg/ml	Liquid (equivalent to aspirin 130 mg/ml)
Ascriptin Arthritis Pain	325 mg	Magnesium hydroxide 75 mg; aluminum hydroxide 75 mg	Antacids are added to minimize stomach upset; doubtful that antacid amounts are meaningful
Ascriptin Maximum Strength	500 mg	Magnesium hydroxide 75 mg; aluminum hydroxide 75 mg	Antacids are added to minimize stomach upset; doubtful that antacid amounts are meaningful
Ascriptin Regular Strength	325 mg	Magnesium hydroxide 50 mg; aluminum hydroxide 50 mg	Antacids are added to minimize stomach upset; doubtful that antacid amounts are meaningful
Aspergum	225 mg		Gum
Bayer Aspirin Maximum Strength	500 mg		
Bayer Children's Aspirin	81 mg		Chewable; taken by some adult patients for MI prevention

Product	Aspirin Dose	Other Ingredients	Comments
Bayer Delayed-Release Aspirin Extra Strength	500 mg		Enteric coated
Bayer Delayed-Release Enteric Aspirin Adult Low Strength	81 mg		Enteric coated
Bayer Delayed-Release Enteric Aspirin Regular Strength	325 mg		Enteric coated
Bayer Extended-Release 8 Hr Aspirin	650 mg		Timed release
Bayer Genuine Aspirin	325 mg		
Bayer Plus Buffered Aspirin	325 mg	Calcium carbonate, magnesium carbonate, magnesium hydroxide	Antacids are added to minimize stomach upset; doubtful that antacid amounts are meaningful
Bayer Plus Extra Strength Buffered Aspirin	500 mg	Calcium carbonate, magnesium carbonate, magnesium hydroxide	Antacids are added to minimize stomach upset; doubtful that antacid amounts are meaningful
Bayer Select Maximum Strength Backache Pain Relief Formula		Magnesium salicylate 500 mg	
BC Arthritis Strength	742 mg	Salicylamide 222 mg; caffeine 36 mg	
BC Powder	650 mg	Salicylamide 195 mg; caffeine 32 mg	
BC Tablet	325 mg	Salicylamide 95 mg; caffeine 16 mg	
Bufferin Arthritis Strength Tri-Buffered	500 mg	Calcium carbonate 222 mg, magnesium hydroxide 89 mg, magnesium carbonate 56 mg	Antacids added to minimize stomach upset; efficacy of small amounts of antacids questionable

*Adult dose (aspirin): 325 mg–1000 mg/dose every 4-6 hours. Maximum 4 g/day. *Children's dose (aspirin):* 10-15 mg/kg/dose every 4-6 hours. Maximum 4 g/day.

Continued

Product Information: Salicylates—cont'd

Brand Name	Aspirin	Other Ingredients	Comments
Bufferin Extra Strength Tri-Buffered	500 mg	Calcium carbonate 222 mg, magnesium hydroxide 89 mg, magnesium carbonate 56 mg	Antacids added to minimize stomach upset; efficacy of small amounts of antacids questionable
Bufferin Tri-Buffered	325 mg	Calcium carbonate 158 mg, magnesium hydroxide 63 mg, magnesium carbonate 39 mg	Antacids added to minimize stomach upset; efficacy of small amounts of antacids questionable
Cope	421 mg	Caffeine 32 mg, magnesium hydroxide 50 mg, aluminum hydroxide 25 mg	Caffeine may potentiate the analgesic effect of aspirin; efficacy of small amounts of antacids questionable
Doan's Extra Strength		Magnesium salicylate 580 mg	
Doan's Extra Strength PM		Magnesium salicylate 580 mg; diphenhydramine 25 mg	Diphenhydramine added to cause drowsiness; marketed for pain relieve and sleeplessness
Doan's Regular Strength		Magnesium salicylate 377 mg	
Ecotrin Adult Low Dose	81 mg		Enteric coated
Ecotrin Maximum Strength	500 mg		Enteric coated
Ecotrin Regular Strength	325 mg		Enteric coated
Empirin	325 mg		
Halfprin Low Strength Enteric Coated	162 mg		Enteric coated
Stanback Original Formula	650 mg	Caffeine 32 mg; salicylamide 200 mg	

Product Information: NSAIDs

Brand Name*	NSAID	Other	Comments
Actron	Ketoprofen 12.5 mg		
Advil	Ibuprofen 200 mg		
Advil Children's Strength tablets	Ibuprofen 100 mg		
Advil Suspension	Ibuprofen 100 mg/5 ml		Must be shaken before use
Aleve	Naproxen sodium 220 mg		
Arthritis Foundation Ibuprofen	Ibuprofen 200 mg		
Bayer Select Ibuprofen Pain Reliever/Fever Reducer	Ibuprofen 200 mg		
Excedrin IB	Ibuprofen 200 mg		
Midol Cramp Formula	Ibuprofen 200 mg		
Motrin IB	Ibuprofen 200 mg		
Motrin IB Sinus	Ibuprofen 200 mg	Pseudoephedrine 30 mg	Decongestant (pseudoephedrine) added to relieve sinus pressure

*Adult dose: Ibuprofen, 200 mg to 400 mg every 4-6 hours. Maximum 1.2 g/day. Naproxen, 220 mg every 8-12 hours. Maximum 660 mg/24 hours. Ketoprofen, 12.5 mg every 4-6 hours. No more than 25 mg in any 6-hour period, and no more than 75 mg in any 24-hour period. Children's dose: Ibuprofen, 5 mg/kg/dose to 10 mg/kg/dose every 6-8 hours. Maximum 40 mg/kg/day. There are no recommended children's doses for naproxen and ketoprofen.

Continued

Product Information: NSAIDs—cont'd

Brand Name*	NSAID	Other	Comments
Motrin Chewable tablets	Ibuprofen 50 mg		
Motrin Children's Drops	Ibuprofen 50 mg/1.25 ml		Much more concentrated than suspension; dose accordingly
Motrin Junior Strength	Ibuprofen 100 mg		
Motrin Pediatric Suspension	Ibuprofen 100 mg/5 ml		Shake well before administering dose
Nuprin	Ibuprofen 200 mg		
Orudis-KT	Ketoprofen 12.5 mg		
PediaCare Fever Drops	Ibuprofen 50 mg/1.25 ml		Much more concentrated than suspension; dose accordingly

Insomnia

Insomnia is a common complaint. It is not a disease; it is a symptom or complaint that is usually caused by other factors. Some of the causes of insomnia include:

- Stress
- Anxiety or tension
- Pain
- Breathing problems
- Medications
- Depression

Everyone suffers from an occasional inability to sleep. This is usually related to stress or anxiety about something that has happened or is about to happen. This is normal and usually corrects itself within a couple of days. Sleep aids may be appropriate for this type of insomnia. If the stress or anxiety is severe, the inability to sleep may continue causing short-term insomnia.

Certain antihistamines are used to treat occasional insomnia.

ANTIHISTAMINES

Antihistamines are used primarily for the treatment of allergies. Certain antihistamines are also used as sleep aids because they cause significant drowsiness. The antihistamines used as sleep aids are diphenhydramine and doxylamine.

Pharmacology

All antihistamines are capable of causing drowsiness; however, the degree of lipid solubility determines the ability of a given antihistamine to penetrate the blood-brain barrier and gain access to the central nervous system (CNS). Diphenhydramine and doxylamine are highly lipid soluble and cause the most significant drowsiness. Antihistamines are not ideal sleep aids because they cause other side effects that can be bothersome.

Side Effects

Diphenhydramine and doxylamine can cause drowsiness, dry mouth, constipation, blurred vision, and urinary retention. Additionally, because they readily cross the blood-brain barrier, diphenhydramine and doxylamine can also antagonize the actions of acetylcholine within the CNS, leading to acute confusional states and delirium, especially in the elderly.

Precautions/Interactions

Diphenhydramine and doxylamine can interact with many prescription drugs. When taken with analgesics, anxiolytics, sleeping pills, or alcohol, excessive drowsiness may occur. When taken with tricyclic antidepressants or antispasmodics, both excessive drowsiness and excessive dry mouth may occur. Caution must be exercised in persons being treated for glaucoma, urinary retention or incontinence, or colon spasms.

Lifespan Considerations

Geriatric

Diphenhydramine is often recommended as a sleep aid for older patients, based on the theory that it is not habit forming and that it is "gentle." However, diphenhydramine and doxylamine should be used cautiously in geriatric patients because these medications can cause acute delirium. The cause of the delirium can be direct antagonization of central cholinergic function or urinary retention secondary to diphenhydramine.

Pediatric

Diphenhydramine and doxylamine are not recommended for use in children for the treatment of insomnia. The reasons for insomnia should be explored.

Pregnancy

Studies of women who took diphenhydramine during pregnancy did not demonstrate a higher than expected frequency of fetal anomalies. Therapeutic doses of diphenhydramine are unlikely to pose a substantial teratogenic risk, but the data are insufficient to state that there is no risk. Benefit versus risk must be weighed.

Nursing Mothers

The American Academy of Pediatrics considers antihistamines to be safe for use while nursing.

Patient Education

Before taking sleep aids, the following principles of good sleep hygiene should be practiced by patients:

- Go to bed and get up about the same time each day.
- Engage in relaxing activities before going to bed.
- Exercise regularly, but not late in the evening.
- Avoid eating meals or large snacks immediately before going to bed.
- Eliminate daytime naps.
- Avoid caffeine after noon.
- Avoid alcohol or nicotine late in the evening.
- Minimize excessive light and noise.
- If unable to fall asleep, get out of bed and engage in a relaxing activity (e.g., watching television, reading a book) until tired.

Product Selection

Because diphenhydramine is available generically, there is no reason to recommend a more expensive product marketed as a sleep aid.

SUGGESTED READING

Hartman PM: Drug treatment of insomnia: indications and newer agents, Am Fam Phys 51(1):191-194, 197-198, 1995.

Product Information: Insomnia	
Brand Name	**Ingredient**
Compoz	Diphenhydramine
Nervine Nighttime Sleep Aid	Diphenhydramine
NiteLite	Diphenhydramine
Nytol	Diphenhydramine
Nytol Maximum Strength	Doxylamine
Sleepinal	Diphenhydramine
Sominex	Diphenhydramine
Tranquil Plus	Diphenhydramine
Unisom Nighttime Sleep Aid	Doxylamine
Unisom Sleepgels	Diphenhydramine

Smoking Cessation

Nicotine is the addictive ingredient in tobacco products. It binds to acetylcholine receptors in the brain, causing stimulation and psychologically rewarding effects. Receptor stimulation results in increased alertness, better cognitive functioning, and relaxation in many individuals. Nicotine addiction is complex and often difficult to overcome. Selected programs including nicotine-replacement products can improve the individual's chance of quitting smoking and minimize the negative effects of withdrawal.

Drugs used in smoking cessation are the nicotine transdermal system (patch) and nicotine chewing gum.

Pharmacology

Nicotine products (patches and chewing gum) replace the nicotine that would have been received from smoking or chewing tobacco, relieving withdrawal symptoms such as restlessness, irritability, sleep disturbances, and weight gain. Although smoking cessation products do replace nicotine, the amount of nicotine received can be controlled and titrated downward as part of a smoking cessation program. Immediate benefit is realized from avoiding the carcinogens in tobacco products and increasing oxygen-carrying capacity of hemoglobin because carbon monoxide contained in cigarette smoke competes with oxygen for hemoglobin binding.

Side Effects

Side effects caused by nicotine replacement products are usually insignificant because the amount of nicotine received in smoking cessation products is usually less than the patient received from tobacco products. The side effects and adverse effects caused by use of tobacco products (including, but not limited to, effects on the cardiovascular and respiratory systems) may be more significant than side effects caused by nicotine replacement products.

In general, nicotine may cause heart palpitations and irritate stomach ulcers. These products should be used with caution in patients with heart disease, irregular heartbeats, uncontrolled high blood pressure, and stomach ulcers.

Nicotine Patches

Skin irritation (pruritus, redness, burning, edema) is the most common side effect of nicotine patches, and may be due to the patch and/or adhesive. Redness generally resolves within 24 hours. Insomnia, vivid/abnormal dreaming, and headache may occur in some individuals. Insomnia may be caused by the transdermal nicotine or unrelieved symptoms of nicotine withdrawal. In addition, transdermal nicotine patches that are applied for 24 hours (e.g., Nicoderm CQ) may cause a higher incidence of insomnia.

Nicotine Chewing Gum

Mouth and throat soreness occur in approximately one third to one half of the individuals who use nicotine gum. Jaw-muscle ache may also occur secondary to the actions of chewing. Nausea, vomiting, and hiccups can occur in some individuals, and are usually caused by chewing too quickly.

Drug Interactions

Use of nicotine and CNS stimulants such as caffeine and theophylline may result in additive CNS stimulation (e.g., fine tremor, tachycardia, insomnia, anxiety, nervousness). The practice of cigarette smoking stimulates the metabolism of a number of drugs, decreasing their effectiveness. When smoking ceases, metabolism will eventually return to normal. Blood levels of the following medications may increase as the result of smoking cessation:

Acetaminophen	Oxazepam
Caffeine	Pentazocine
Furosemide	Propranolol
Imipramine	Theophylline
Insulin	

Lifespan Considerations

Geriatric

Geriatric patients suffer from insomnia more often than younger patients. Geriatric patients should be educated regarding the possibility of insomnia related to nicotine.

Pediatric

Nicotine products are not recommended for persons under the age of 18 unless monitored by a health care professional. There are limited data on the risks and benefits of nicotine therapy in young patients.

Pregnancy/Nursing Mothers

The nicotine transdermal system is an FDA Pregnancy Category D drug. Nicotine chewing gum is a category C* drug. Nicotine may harm unborn babies and newborns, thus tobacco products and nicotine replacement products should be avoided during pregnancy and while nursing. However, if the patient is continuing to smoke more than 10 to 15 cigarettes per day and has failed efforts to quit without medication, nicotine replacement may be a viable option.

Patient Education

- Nicotine replacement products aid individuals who wish to overcome their addiction to nicotine. These products will help control the symptoms of nicotine withdrawal but they do not magically cause patients to stop smoking. They should be utilized as a part of a smoking cessation program.
- Patients should be advised to avoid smoking and chewing tobacco while using nicotine products because of the increased risk of side effects.
- Nicotine patches should be applied to a nonhairy, clean, dry area of the skin. The patch should not be continually applied to the same spot, but rotated to a different site with each application.
- Patients should immediately wash their hands after application of a nicotine patch. Nicotine on the hands could get into the eyes, nose, or other mucosal membranes and cause irritation.
- Patients should dispose of nicotine patches by sticking the edges of the patch together and placing it in the child-resistant disposal tray provided. This procedure avoids accidental nicotine exposure to children and pets.
- When using nicotine gum, patients should avoid eating or drinking for 15 minutes before and while chewing the gum. Absorption of the nicotine gum is reduced when acidic beverages such as coffee, juice, or soft drinks are consumed while the gum is being used.
- Nicotine gum should be chewed slowly over 30 minutes. If the gum is chewed too rapidly, the nicotine may be released too quickly, causing unpleasant side effects.
- For overdosages of the nicotine transdermal system, patients should remove the patch, wash the skin with water, and dry. Soap should be

---

*Nicotine chewing gum was initially labeled a category X drug on FDA approval; however, it has since been upgraded to a category C drug.

avoided because it may increase absorption of the nicotine. Nicotine will still have systemic effects for several hours because of absorption into the bloodstream. Individuals may need to be referred to an acute care setting if symptoms such as tremor or tachycardia are severe. If a patch has been ingested, the patient should be referred to a local acute care facility.
- For overdosages of nicotine chewing gum, vomiting can be induced with syrup of ipecac if the patient is conscious and emesis has not occurred.

Product Selection

- Although it may appear that the transdermal nicotine patch is more effective than the gum, there have been limited, direct-comparable trials between the two medications (Henningfield, 1995). Both agents are more effective when combined with nonpharmacologic therapy (e.g., behavioral therapy).
- Dosing guidelines (listed in the Product Information table) are manufacturer recommendations. However, studies have demonstrated the following suggestions (Henningfield, 1995):
  Nicotine chewing gum: For initial dosing, patients should be given one dose of 2-mg gum in place of every two cigarettes. For patients who smoke more than 20 cigarettes per day, one dose of 4-mg gum should be used in place of every three to four cigarettes. Titrate the quantity of gum according to relief of nicotine withdrawal symptoms and side effects.
  Nicotine transdermal system: Patients who smoke more than 10 cigarettes per day should be treated with the highest dose available (21-mg patch). Patients who smoke fewer than 10 cigarettes per day should begin with the midrange transdermal dose (15-mg or 14-mg patch).
- Nicotine replacement products work better in individuals who have a high "physical" type of nicotine dependence. "Physical" dependence can be correlated with the smoking habits of patients who do the following:
  Smoke more than 15 cigarettes daily
  Prefer brands of cigarettes with nicotine levels more than 0.9 mg
  Usually inhale the smoke frequently and deeply
  Smoke the first daily cigarette within 30 minutes of awakening
  Find it difficult to refrain from smoking in nonsmoking areas
- If vivid nightmares or sleep disturbances develop, consider removing the nicotine patch at bedtime. However, doing so may result in

nicotine craving and reduction in the overall effectiveness of the product.

• After the maximum recommended duration is exceeded, therapy should be reevaluated. (The maximum duration recommendation is included in the Product Information table for each individual product.)

SUGGESTED READINGS

Gora ML: Nicotine transdermal systems, *Ann Pharmacother* 27:742-750, 1993.
Haxby DG: Treatment of nicotine dependence, *Am J Health-Sys Pharm* 52:265-281, 1995.
Henningfield JE: Nicotine medications for smoking cessation, *N Engl J Med* 333:1196-1203, 1995.

 Product Information: Smoking Cessation

Brand Name	Dosing	Comments
Nicoderm CQ Patches (21 mg/14 mg/7 mg)	Apply daily at the same time each day; remove the old patch when the new patch is applied	Recommended to be used for 10 weeks maximum in the following step-wise manner: 21-mg patch daily for the first 6 weeks; 14-mg patch daily for the next 2 weeks; 7-mg patch daily for the last 2 weeks
Nicorette gum (2 mg and 4 mg)	*Weeks 1-6:* 1 piece every 1-2 hours *Weeks 7-9:* 1 piece every 2-4 hours *Weeks 10-12:* 1 piece every 4-8 hours Do not exceed 24 pieces per day	Recommended to be used for 12 weeks maximum
Nicotrol Patches (15 mg)	Apply daily in the morning on waking and remove at bedtime	Recommended to be used for 6 weeks maximum

FDA Pregnancy Categories

A No risk demonstrated to the fetus in any trimester.
B No adverse effects in animals, no human studies available.
C Only given after risks to the fetus are considered; animal studies have shown adverse reactions, no human studies available.
D Definite fetal risks, may be given in spite of risks if needed in life-threatening conditions.
X Absolute fetal abnormalities; not to be used any time during pregnancy.

Alcohol-Free Products

ANALGESICS

Advil (Children's)
Liquiprin
Motrin (Children's)
Panadol Children's Chewable Tablets
Panadol Children's Drops
Panadol Children's Liquid
PediaCare Fever
PediaCare Fever Drops
Tempra 1 Drops
Tempra 2 Syrup
Tempra 3 Chewable Tablets
Tylenol Children's Elixir
Tylenol Children's Suspension
Tylenol Infants Concentrated Drops
Tylenol Infants Suspension Drops

ANTIFLATULENTS

Mylicon Children's Drops

ANTIDIARRHEALS

Kaopectate Advanced Formula
Kaopectate Children's Liquid
Pepto-Bismol Suspension

ANTIEMETICS

Emetrol Solution

COLD/COUGH/ALLERGY

Chlor-Trimeton Allergy Syrup
Creomulsion
Diabetic Tussin
Dimetapp Children's Allergy Syrup
Dimetapp Decongestant Pediatric Drops
Motrin Children's Suspension
PediaCare Cough-Cold Drops
PediaCare Decongestant Infant's Drops
PediaCare Nightrest Liquid
Robitussin CF Syrup
Robitussin Cough & Congestion Liquid
Robitussin DM
Robitussin Pediatric Cough Syrup
Robitussin Pediatric Drops
Robitussin Pediatric Night Relief Liquid
Robitussin PE Syrup
Safe Tussin 30
Scot-Tussin DM Liquid
Scot-Tussin Expectorant
Scot-Tussin Original Liquid
Scot-Tussin Senior Liquid
Triaminic DM
Triaminic Expectorant
Triaminic Infant Decongestant Drops
Triaminic Night Time
Triaminicol Cold & Cough Liquid
Tylenol Children's Allergy-D Liquid
Tylenol Children's Sinus Liquid
Tylenol Children's Suspension
Tylenol Cold Children's Drops
Tylenol Flu Children's Suspension
Vicks 44E Pediatric Liquid
Vicks DayQuil Liquid
Vicks NyQuil Children's

MOUTH/THROAT PRODUCTS

Orajel Baby
Orajel Baby Nighttime
Gly-Oxide Liquid

LAXATIVES

Agoral Emulsion
Colace Liquid
Kondremul Plain Liquid
Phillips Milk of Magnesia Liquid
Senokot Children's Syrup

VITAMINS/MINERALS

Poly-Vi-Sol Drops
Poly-Vi-Sol with Iron Drops
Theragran Liquid
Tri-Vi-Sol Drops
Tri-Vi-Sol with Iron Drops

Sugar-Free Products

ANALGESICS

Panadol Children's Chewable Tablets
Panadol Children's Drops
Panadol Children's Liquid
Tempra 1 Drops
Tempra 2 Syrup
Tempra 3 Chewable Tablets
Tylenol Children's Suspension Liquid
Tylenol Infant's Drops
Tylenol Infant's Suspension Drops

ANTACIDS/ANTIFLATULENTS

Alka-Mints
Amphojel Suspension
Amphojel Tablets
Di-Gel Liquid
Gaviscon Liquid
Pepto-Bismol Liquid
Pepto-Bismol Tablets
Riopan Plus Suspension
Riopan Suspension
Tagamet HB Tablets
Titralac Plus Liquid
Titralac Plus Tablets
Tums E-X Chewable Tablets
Zantac 75 Tablets

ANTIDIARRHEALS

Diasorb Suspension
Donnagel Chewable Tablets
Donnagel Liquid
Pepto-Bismol Liquid
Pepto-Bismol Tablets

COUGH/COLD/ALLERGY

Cerose-DM Liquid
Codimal-DM Syrup
Diabetic Tussin DM
Dimetane-DX Cough Syrup
Dimetapp Allergy Children's
Novahistine Elixir
Robitussin CF Syrup
Safe Tussin 30
Scot-Tussin DM
Scot-Tussin Expectorant
Scot-Tussin Original

LAXATIVES

Citrucel Sugar Free Powder
Doxidan Capsules
Fiberall Powder
Haley's MO
Hydrocil Instant Powder
Kondremul Emulsion
Konsyl Effervescent Powder
Konsyl Powder
Maalox Daily Fiber Therapy
Metamucil Smooth Texture
Surfak Capsule

MOUTH/THROAT PRODUCTS

Orajel Baby
Tanac Liquid

VITAMINS/MINERALS

Bugs Bunny Complete
Bugs Bunny with Extra C
Bugs Bunny with Iron
Caltrate 600 Tablets
Geritol Complete Tablets
Iberet Liquid
One-A-Day Essential Tablets
One-A-Day Maximum Formula Tablets
One-A-Day Women's Formula Tablets
Posture Tablets
Tri-Vi-Sol Drops
Vi-Daylin ADC Drops
Vi-Daylin Drops
Vi-Daylin Plus Iron ADC Drops
Vi-Daylin Plus Iron Drops

GENERAL INDEX

Glycerine in artificial tears, 167
Glycopyrrolate in interactions
  with antihistamines, 218
  with diphenhydramine, 224
Goiter in iodine deficiency, 317
Gold salts as photosensitizer, 148
Gotu kola in weight reduction,
  343, 345
Green soap as photosensitizer, 148
Grepafloxacin as photosensi-
  tizer, 148
Griseofulvin as photosensitizer, 148
Growth
  fetal impairment of, in iodine
    deficiency, 317
  retardation of, in calcium
    deficiency, 312
Guaifenesin
  in allergy, 204
  in common cold and flu, 226-227,
    233, 234, 236, 238, 243,
    245-247, 251-254, 256, 260,
    269-271
Guarana in weight reduction,
  343, 345
Guidelines for weight loss, 336, 338

H

H₂ antagonists
  and calcium needs, 313
  in indigestion, 47-49
  in vitamin B₁₂ deficiency, 306
H₂ receptors interacting with ketoconazole, 48
Haemophilus influenzae and neomycin, 85
Hair care in dandruff, 114
Haloperidol as photosensitizer, 148
Hamamelis water in hemorrhoids,
  41, 45
Health information dissemination
  and self-care, 1
Heart
  arrhythmias of
    with epinephrine, 214
    in magnesium deficiency, 319
    with vasoconstrictors, 42
  disturbances of, in potassium de-
    ficiency, 319
  stimulation of, with deconges-
    tants, 191

Heart disease and vitamin E, 301
Heart failure and vitamin B₁
  deficiency, 302
Hemochromatosis in iron toxic-
  ity, 315
Hemolysis
  in vitamin C toxicity, 307
  in vitamin E deficiency, 300
Hemorrhage
  capillary, in vitamin C defi-
    ciency, 307
  intracranial, with phenylpropanol-
    amine, 339
Hemorrhoids, 41-46
Hepatic damage with acetaminophen, 364
Hepatic nutritional formula, choosing, 285
Hepatotoxicity and vitamin B₃ toxicity, 304
Herbal products, 321, 322
Hexachlorophene as photosensi-
  tizer, 148
Histamine; *see* H₂ antagonists
Homosalate in sunscreens, 147
Hydralazine as photosensitizer, 148
Hydrochlorothiazide as photosensitizer, 148
Hydrocortisone
  in hemorrhoids, 41, 45
  in poison ivy, 103
  in psoriasis, 135-137
  topical, in sunburn, 150, 152
  for vaginal irritation, 279
Hydroflumethiazide as photosensitizer, 148
Hydrogen peroxide in canker and
  cold sores, 173-174
Hydroxychloroquine as photosensitizer, 148
Hydroxycholecalciferol, 299, 300
Hydroxyethylcellulose
  in artificial tears, 166
  in dry mouth, 175-177
Hydroxypropyl methylcellulose
  in artificial tears, 166, 167
Hyoscyamine in interactions
  with antihistamines, 188, 218
  with diphenhydramine, 224
Hypercalcemia in calcium toxicity, 312

PRODUCT INDEX